W9-DDO-732

Nutritional Management of Digestive Disorders

Nutritional Management of Digestive Disorders

Edited by
Bhaskar Banerjee

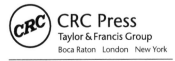

CRC Press
Taylor & Francis Group
Boca Raton   London   New York

CRC Press is an imprint of the
Taylor & Francis Group, an **informa** business

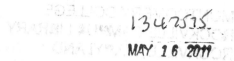
CRC Press
Taylor & Francis Group
6000 Broken Sound Parkway NW, Suite 300
Boca Raton, FL 33487-2742

© 2011 by Taylor and Francis Group, LLC
CRC Press is an imprint of Taylor & Francis Group, an Informa business

No claim to original U.S. Government works

Printed in the United States of America on acid-free paper
10 9 8 7 6 5 4 3 2 1

International Standard Book Number: 978-1-4200-8654-6 (Hardback)

Library of Congress Cataloging-in-Publication Data

Nutritional management of digestive disorders / editor, Bhaskar Banerjee.
    p. ; cm.
  Includes bibliographical references and index.
  ISBN 978-1-4200-8654-6 (hardcover : alk. paper)
  1. Gastrointestinal system--Diseases--Diet therapy. I. Banerjee, Bhaskar.
  [DNLM: 1. Digestive System Diseases--diet therapy. 2. Nutrition Therapy--methods. WI 140 N9765 2011]

RC816.N88 2011
616.3'0654--dc22
                                          2010004493

Visit the Taylor & Francis Web site at
http://www.taylorandfrancis.com

and the CRC Press Web site at
http://www.crcpress.com

To my family for their enduring support

throughout my career

Contents

Preface

Nutrition is inseparably intertwined with disorders of digestion, and this compact book, written by many prominent authors, covers not only the traditional areas of nutrition, but embraces new disorders, novel therapies, and important recent developments to present a text with a distinctive collection of important, practical topics.

Chapters are dedicated to nutritional assessment, parenteral nutrition in hospitalized patients, and home nutritional support, which is needed for an increasing number of patients. The scientific basis and management of celiac disease and eosinophilic esophagitis are thoroughly discussed. Management of conditions that can impact nutritional status, such as disorders of swallowing and chronic nausea and vomiting, are described with practical steps in their management.

New and exciting developments, such as the use of probiotics in irritable bowel syndrome and antibiotic-associated diarrhea, are included, and the role of nutrition in acute pancreatitis and liver disease extensively discussed.

In addition to presenting the reader with descriptions of established endoscopic techniques of enteral access and enteral nutrition, a separate chapter is dedicated to expanding metal stents that are now increasingly used to overcome malignant obstructions of the upper gastrointestinal (GI) tract.

The epidemic of obesity is introduced by a chapter devoted to weight management by diet, exercise, and drugs, followed by a comprehensive account of bariatric surgery. The often overlooked, but vital topic of nonalcoholic fatty liver disease is portrayed, along with the relationship between obesity and gastrointestinal cancer as well as the role of macro- and micronutrients in preventing colon cancer. To contrast this, the role of nutrition and dietary supplements in inflammatory bowel disease is described, followed by a chapter on the short bowel syndrome, adverse effects of parenteral nutrition on the liver, and small intestine transplantation. To put these recent developments into perspective, the book begins with a chapter that recounts the history of nutritional therapy in gastrointestinal disorders.

Nutritional Management of Digestive Disorders not only covers the traditional areas of nutrition, but includes new and emerging fields to produce a unique blend of topics in a compact text. I am extremely grateful to all the outstanding authors who have made this work possible.

Bhaskar Banerjee

Editor

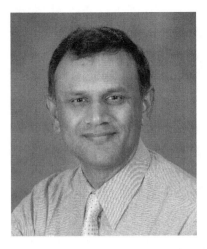

Bhaskar Banerjee, MD, AGAF, received his medical degree from the University of London, England, in 1983. He is the chief of gastroenterology at the University of Arizona College of Medicine in Tucson. Dr. Banerjee is a professor of medicine, optical sciences, and biomedical engineering at the University of Arizona and is the director of the Gastroenterology Fellowship program. Prior to his current position, he was a professor of medicine in the division of gastroenterology, Washington University School of Medicine in St. Louis. Throughout his career, Dr. Banerjee has been involved in the education of medical students, residents, and gastroenterology fellows. He has lectured and published widely and serves on the editorial boards of scientific journals. His clinical interests are in the luminal gastrointestinal diseases, particularly the detection and management of gastrointestinal cancer and its relationship to obesity. Dr. Banerjee's research interests are in the use of biomarkers in gastrointestinal cancer and in developing novel optical techniques of early cancer detection. He has discovered a unique method of detecting cancer cells using the optical properties of an intracellular molecule and is working on other techniques of cellular imaging in gastrointestinal disease. Dr. Banerjee is a fellow of the American Gastroenterological Association and a member of the Educational Affairs Committee of the American College of Gastroenterology.

Contributors

Bhaskar Banerjee, MD
Section of Gastroenterology
University of Arizona
Tucson, Arizona

Francis W. Chan, MD
Section of Digestive Diseases
Yale University School of Medicine
New Haven, Connecticut

Ashwini Davison, MD
The Johns Hopkins Hospital
Baltimore, Maryland

Alessandrina Freitas, MD
Department of Surgery
Emory University School of Medicine
Atlanta, Georgia

Mario Guslandi, MD, FACG
Gastroenterology Unit
San Raffaele University Hospital
Milan, Italy

C. Prakash Gyawali, MD, MRCP
Division of Gastroenterology
Washington University School of
 Medicine
St. Louis, Missouri

Laura S. Harkness, PhD, RD
Nutrition Sciences
Pepsico Nutrition
Pepsico R&D
Valhalla, New York

Peter David Howdle, BSc, MD, FRCP
Leeds Institute of Molecular Medicine
St. James's University Hospital
Leeds, United Kingdom

Carol Ireton-Jones, PhD, RD, LD, CNSD
Professional Nutrition Therapists
Dallas, Texas

Priya A. Jamidar, MD
Section of Digestive Diseases
Yale University School of Medicine
New Haven, Connecticut

Manreet Kaur, MD
Washington University School of
 Medicine
St. Louis, Missouri

Khalid Khan, MD
Department of Surgery
University of Arizona College of
 Medicine
Tucson, Arizona

Kevin M. Korenblat, MD
Division of Gastroenterology
Washington University School of
 Medicine
St. Louis, Missouri

Robert Martindale, MD, PhD
Division of General Surgery
Oregon Health Sciences University
Portland, Oregon

Laura E. Matarese, PhD, RD, LDN, FADA, CNSD
Thomas Starzl Transplantation
 Institute
University of Pittsburgh Medical Center
Pittsburgh, Pennsylvania

Rémy F. Meier, MD
Gastroenterology, Hepatology, and
    Nutrition Department
Medical University Clinic
Liestal, Switzerland

Gerard E. Mullin, MD
Integrative GI Nutrition Services
The Johns Hopkins Hospital
Baltimore, Maryland

Melissa Munsell, MD
The Johns Hopkins Hospital
Baltimore, Maryland

Yume Nguyen, MD
Division of Gastroenterology
Washington University School of
    Medicine
St. Louis, Missouri

Mathias Plauth
Klinik für Innere Medizin
Dessau, Germany

Ryan F. Porter, MD
Washington University School of
    Medicine
St. Louis, Missouri

Petr Protiva, MD
Division of Gastroenterology
Yale University School of Medicine
New Haven, Connecticut
and
Breslow Lab
Rockefeller University
New York, New York

**Eamonn M. M. Quigley, MD, FRCP,
FACG, FACG, FRCPI**
Alimentary Pharmabiotic Centre
Department of Medicine
University College Cork
Cork, Ireland

Waqar A. Qureshi, MD
Baylor College of Medicine
Houston, Texas

Carol Redel, MNS, MD
Pediatric Gastroenterology, Hepatology,
    and Nutrition
GROW and Feeding Disorders Clinic
Baylor College of Medicine
Houston, Texas

Dominic Reeds, MD
Division of Geriatrics and Nutritional
    Science
Washington University School of
    Medicine
St. Louis, Missouri

Gregory S. Sayuk, MD, MPH
Division of Gastroenterology
Washington University School of
    Medicine
St. Louis, Missouri

Alain M. Schoepfer, MD
Department of Gastroenterology
Inselspital/Bern University Hospital
Bern, Switzerland

Tatjana Schütz
Gastroenterologie/Hepatologie/
    Endokrinologie
Charité Universitätsmedizin
Berlin, Germany

David S. Seres, MD, PNS
Medical Nutrition and Nutrition
    Support Service
Division of Preventative Medicine and
    Nutrition
Department of Medicine
Columbia University Medical Center
New York, New York

Fergus Shanahan, MD, BSc, FRCP (UK); FRCPI, FRCP, FRCP (C), FACG
Alimentary Pharmabiotic Centre
Department of Medicine
University College Cork
Cork, Ireland

Alex Straumann, MD
Department of Gastroenterology
Kantonsspital Olten
Olten, Switzerland

Shelby Sullivan, MD
Washington University School of
    Medicine
St. Louis, Missouri

John F. Sweeny, MD, FACS
Division of General and
    Gastrointestinal Surgery
Emory University School of Medicine
Atlanta, Georgia

Piyush Tiwari, MD
Department of Medicine
University of Arizona
Tucson, Arizona

1 The History of Medical Nutrition Therapy in the Treatment of Gastrointestinal Disorders

Laura S. Harkness

CONTENTS

1.1 INTRODUCTION

Medical nutrition therapy has changed substantially since Hippocrates first empha-sized the importance of diet to human health in the fifth century BCE. In particular, there have been significant advances in the nutrition management of gastrointes-tinal diseases and surgical interventions that have enabled patients to return to health. Yet, despite Hippocrates' recognition of the importance of diet to help

1

recovery from illness, the history of dietary treatment from Galen (fourth century CE) until the mid-1800s has predominantly been treatments of starvation and purging. Robert Graves, in 1849, decided that rather than starve his patients, to give them food and beverages during treatments for typhus resulting in an improved mortality rate.[1]

The advent of modern medical nutrition therapy has its roots in the work of nutrition pioneers of the nineteenth and twentieth century. In the United States, the names of scientists Lusk, Chittenden, Mendel, McCollum, Atwater, Rose, Goldberger, Sherman, and Leverton stand out for their tremendous contributions to the basic science of nutrition. Key discoveries in the evolution of medical nutrition therapy include the determination of essential nutrients, advances in body composition analysis and anthropometry, work on metabolism and energy expenditure during illness and injury, and refinement of the objective process of nutrition assessment. It was from this work, as well as others, that the first Recommended Dietary Allowances was published by the National Research Council to provide a guide for planning normal and therapeutic diets with a goal toward good nutrition, and the era of modern medical nutrition therapy was fully here.[2]

1.2 DIETARY TREATMENT OF GASTROINTESTINAL DISEASES

1.2.1 Peptic Ulcer Disease

The dietary treatment of peptic ulcer disease has changed substantially over the past century. Prior to the discovery of *Helicobacter pylori* and the use of antibiotic regimens, it was thought that excess gastric acid production was the primary cause of peptic ulcer disease. Dietary treatment was centered on reducing gastric acid production and providing symptomatic relief of pain. Perhaps the most widely used dietary treatment for peptic ulcers was the Sippy Diet, which was prescribed as recently as the 1970s.[3] The Sippy Diet consisted of frequent small feedings of milk or milk and cream given every hour. As the patient reported less pain, soft cooked eggs, cooked cereals, custards, cream soups, cottage cheese or cream cheese, and milk toast were added. It was thought that giving frequent, small feedings to ensure continuous food in the stomach would neutralize acid. Foods that stimulated gastric acid production including meat extracts, tea, coffee, cola-based beverages, spices (pepper, mustard), sugar, and acids (vinegar, pickles, fruit, and fruit juice) were also eliminated.[4] In addition, low residue diets were used to reduce risk of mechanical irritation. In patients with a hemorrhaging peptic ulcer, there were diets specifically prescribed for bleeding ulcers that consisted of mixing gelatin, glucose, cream, and milk,[5] and in the case of a Danish physician, Meulengracht, a pureed diet of meat, liver, poultry, fish, eggs, mashed potatoes, vegetables, fruit, custard, ice cream, and puddings.[4]

As early as the 1950s, there was debate about the usefulness of these diets including the Sippy Diet. Schneider, in 1956, published research demonstrating that spices, such as cloves, cinnamon, paprika, and sage, did not increase gastric acid production in patients.[6] But, as recent as the 1990s, elimination diets were still being used to reduce gastric acid production. Diets that eliminated caffeine and theobromine-containing foods, such as coffee, tea, and chocolate, were prescribed. Today, there is no evidence to suggest that specific foods affect the etiology of peptic ulcer disease, even for foods that are potent inducers of gastric acid.[7] The only notable exception may be for fiber. A high fiber diet is associated with reduced risk of ulcers.[7,8]

1.2.2 Gastrointestinal Disorders and Diet Therapy

The bland diet was often prescribed for a variety of gastrointestinal disorders and consisted of low fiber, reduction of foods that stimulate gastric acid secretion, and neutralization or dilution of gastric contents.[9] Foods, including high fiber foods that were thought to induce mechanical irritation to mucous membranes, were restricted. Permitted foods included low fiber foods, young vegetables rather than overripe vegetables, refined cereals, and cooked or pureed fruits and vegetables, since it was thought that cooking softened and disintegrated the fiber. Strong flavored or sulfur-containing vegetables, such as onions, broccoli, cabbage, cucumber, green pepper, dried beans and peas, corn, Brussels sprouts, and turnips were eliminated. In addition, since it was not known what foods stimulated gastric acid, many foods were limited or eliminated from the diet, including meat soups and gravies, smoked meats, prepared meats (frankfurters, deli meats, sausage), fatty meat, relishes, ketchup, mustard, pepper, horseradish, meat sauces, vinegar, candy, and pickles. For treatment as a method to reduce gastric acid or to neutralize gastric acid, foods that contained "highly emulsified" fats were used. These foods included whole milk, cream, butter, and egg yolk.[4,9] Based on the Sippy Diet theory, it was thought that milk had high buffering properties and became a primary constituent of the bland diet. Patients were advised to consume one quart of milk per day, including milk or cream at each meal and in-between meals.

Frequently high protein, low fat, bland, low residue, or high fiber diets are prescribed to treat gastrointestinal diseases. The origins of these diets can be traced to the 1940s and 1950s. For example, in 1953, a number of case reports of patients receiving high protein, low fat diets with supplemental vitamins, and minerals for Crohn's disease and ulcerative colitis were published.[10]

More recently the use of these diets, including low fat, low residue, and bland diets has declined as scientific studies have demonstrated no clinical benefit in treating gastrointestinal disease.[11–14] Low fat diets were frequently prescribed for patients with conditions including inflammatory bowel disease, gallbladder disease, ulcerative colitis, and Crohn's disease. A number of studies have demonstrated no association between dietary fat intake and symptoms of gallbladder disease.[15] In addition, research during the past 40 years demonstrated that significant fat malabsorption only occurs when there is massive inflammation or immediate postmassive small bowel resection.[16,17] Of interest, Jeejeeboy and colleagues demonstrated that patients recovered optimally when given a high kilocalorie (kcalorie), high protein diet with both fat and carbohydrate as the source of kcalories.[18] This was shown in patients with an intact colon. Previously, it was thought that fat restriction was needed when the colon was intact due to long chain fatty acid binding with divalent cations.

The most important component of dietary management for gastrointestinal disease is to provide adequate nutrition to maintain or restore weight. Liberal provision of kcalories and protein as well as treating any underlying nutritional deficiencies should be the hallmark of current dietary therapy. The major problem with highly restrictive diets is that they frequently are inadequate in one or more nutrients including kcalories. In addition, they tend to be less appetizing than regular diets and result in inadequate intake. Specialized diets that restrict fat, fiber, or specific foods should be reserved for individual cases and liberalized as quickly as possible.

1.3 POSTSURGICAL DIETS

1.3.1 DUMPING SYNDROME DIET

Surgical procedures can often result in impaired digestion and absorption. Truncal vagotomy with pyloroplasty, truncal vagotomy with antrectomy, gastroduodenostomy, and gastrojejunostomy often lead to dumping syndrome, a condition in which foods and liquids enter the intestines too rapidly. This leads to severe pain, diarrhea, and malabsorption as the digestive and absorptive capacity of the intestine is overwhelmed. The change in the medical treatment for peptic ulcer disease has resulted in a striking decrease in surgical intervention, especially truncal vagotomy with pyloroplasty and truncal vagotomy with antrectomy. Current dietary treatment for dumping syndrome is aimed at symptomatic control and prevention of malnutrition. The primary focus of nutrition management is to eliminate large volumes of food and liquids from entering the intestinal tract. Small frequent meals, separating liquids from solids, and reduced intake of simple sugars to decrease hyperosmolar load are commonly prescribed. Other interventions include the addition of soluble fibers, higher protein if needed, and treatment of any underlying nutrient deficiencies. This dietary treatment has not changed substantially since the early 1950s when patients were given high protein and low carbohydrate regimens in six to eight small meals with liquids 30 minutes after meal consumption.

One notable exception in the dietary treatment history for postsurgical intervention was prescribed for a brief period in the 1950s. Developed by Pittman and Robinson, the process consisted of a three-stage approach called "Routines."[19] Routine I, prescribed for one month, consisted of eggs, bacon, lean meat, butter, and margarine. Routine II followed for one month, allowed the addition of cream, cream cheese, nuts and limited quantities of bread, cereals, and vegetables. Routine III consisted of separating liquids from solids with fluids consumed 30 minutes after a meal. In addition, patients were told to eat regularly and frequently, to relax before and after a meal, to eliminate all forms of sugar, and to omit milk and milk products until tolerated. Most of these treatment regimens are no longer used to manage dumping syndrome. However, patients are still advised to follow parts of Routine III, separating liquids from solids, limiting simple sugars, and watching for intolerance to milk and fat.

1.4 ENTERAL NUTRITION

The development of enteral nutrition therapy is a notable medical achievement because it enables provision of nutrients directly into the gastrointestinal tract for patients who cannot meet their nutrition needs orally. Enteral nutrition therapy has a long history starting with rectal feedings in ancient Egypt and Greece to modern day specialty formulas and techniques. It is particularly interesting that the enteral nutrition solutions used today can be traced to developments from the 1930s and to delivery techniques that were first introduced in 1910.

1.4.1　Rectal Feedings

Rectal feedings were the preferred route for enteral nutrition until the early part of the 1900s when gastric and small bowel feedings became the chosen method. The history of rectal feedings dates to ancient Egypt and Greece, where rectal feeding consisting of enemas of wine, milk, whey, wheat, and barley broths were used to promote good health and treat diarrhea.[20] There was a belief that reverse peristalsis could lead to colonic absorption of nutrients and would provide adequate nutrition to meet the patient's needs. Rectal feeding devices included a piece of pipe with a bladder tied to one end, long pieces of rubber tubing attached to funnels or wooden syringes, and wooden syringes that were used to push solutions into the rectum.[21]

Rectally fed mixtures included ingredients, such as raw beef, eggs, milk, liquor, tobacco, wax, red wine, blood, and beef broths.[21] Many proponents of rectal feedings advocated using pancreatic glands from a recently slaughtered animal. In fact, case reports of patients fed rectally include a patient with esophageal stenosis, who was given enemas of a raw beef mixed with hog's pancreas.[22] This mixture was pushed into the patient's rectum twice per day. The physician, in this case, noted that "the patient was so well fed by that means that he had not visibly lost fluid when he died, after apoplectic symptoms eight days after the time these enemas had been first used." The most famous case of rectal feedings was that of President Garfield after he was shot during an assassination attempt.[23] President Garfield was rectally infused with peptonized beef broth, beef peptonoid, and whiskey every four hours during the 79 days that he survived after being shot. President Garfield is reported to have died from infection and internal bleeding since the surgeons could not locate and remove the bullet.

1.4.2　Nasal and Gastric Feedings

Historical accounts report that development of gastric feeding devices and solutions started during the sixteenth century. The first report of enteral feeding was in 1598, when Capivacceus, a Venetian physician, used a hollow tube to put liquid down a patient's esophagus. Other reports include that of Aquapendente, in 1617, who passed a small silver nasopharyneal tube to feed a patient with tetanus. Von Helmont, in 1646, fashioned a flexible tube using leather for esophageal feeding. And, Boerhave, in 1710, used Von Helmont's leather tube to feed into the stomach. In 1790, Hunter became the first physician to use a nasogastric tube made of a whale bone probe covered with eel skin and attached to a bladder pump.[24]

During the eighteenth and nineteenth centuries, one method to provide enteral feedings was via nasal and oral routes. Feedings were delivered using a rubber tube or oral feedings using a rigid spout. Feeding solutions, during this time, consisted of ingredients, such as warm milk, eggs, wine, whiskey, sugar, custard, mashed mutton, and broth.[25-27] For the treatment of children with diphtheria, Morrison in 1895, used a mixture of cream, brandy, tincture of nux vomica (the seed of an Asian tree that contains the alkaloids strychnine and brucine), and a digestive ferment that consisted of liquor of pancreaticus and essence of pepsin.[28] The use of nasogastric tubes continued to increase and became the preferred method by the early part of the twentieth century, although saline solutions were still infused rectally until 1940. During this time, Einhorn, developed a nasogastric tube that was weighted on one end to allow it to pass into the duodenum.[29]

1.4.3 SMALL BOWEL FEEDING

The development of the nasogastric weighted tube was the turning point in the development and refinement of enteral nutrition. Several physicians made improvements to Einhorn's techniques to help with intolerance to the feeding solution, since patients were given milk, raw eggs, salt, butter, lactose, and sugar. Morgan and Jones proposed a method to administer the feeding solution drop-by-drop instead of bolus,[30,31] and Gross and Held designed a larger tube with a heavier weight that passed to the duodenum faster than the Einhorn tube.[32] In 1918, Andresen introduced jejunal feeding by passing a tube into the jejunum during surgery and feeding a solution of 200 ml peptonized milk, 15 g glucose, and 8 ml whiskey every two hours postsurgery to reach 2500 kcalories in 24 hours.[33]

Refinement of the nasojejunal tube and enteral feeding solution can be credited to two groups: Abbott and Rawson and Stengel and Ravdin. Abbott and Rawson developed a double lumen tube with one opening in the stomach for suction and one in the jejunum for feeding.[34] Stengel and Ravdin used the Abbott tube to feed patients with a partially digested solution.[35]

1.4.4 DEVELOPMENT OF ENTERAL FORMULAS

Refinement to the feeding solutions occurred during the same time as technical changes were made to the feeding systems and tubes. In the early part of the 1900s, Morgan heated and strained the food mixtures and, in 1939, Stengel and Ravdin developed a feeding solution that contained a sterile mix of acidified skim milk, commercial pepsin, sodium bicarbonate, sodium chloride, dextrose, fish liver oil, thiamin chloride, nicotinic acid, and vitamin C. In addition, Stengel and Ravdin designed the first casein hydrolysate. Commercial companies had started to develop enteral products that could be used to supplement kitchen-prepared mixtures by the later part of 1930. Companies including Mead Johnson and Wyeth-Ayerst were producing mixtures of homogenized solid food substances, combinations of supplemented dairy products, and elemental food products.[21] In 1954, Pareira et al.[36] collaborated with Mead Johnson to produce a tube feeding solution made of powdered whole milk, nonfat milk solids, dextrose, eight vitamins, and eight minerals.

It was during this time in the 1950s that Barron and colleagues at Henry Ford Hospital in Detroit, Michigan, argued that enteral solutions made from food in hospital kitchens were nutritionally superior to commercially prepared formulas.[37,38] Hospitals produced tube feeding solutions in their kitchens using standard food ingredients.[39] The Henry Ford Hospital method was much more sophisticated than the standard hospital-produced solution because it used a food mill that had been adapted to produce large quantities of liquefied baby food and blenderized hospital diets. An interesting part of the history of hospital feedings was concern for the patient being able to feel as if he/she is eating. Patients were initially given alternating boluses of milk and water and then progressed to tube feeding solutions. The tube feeding solution was warmed to room temperature and served in a teapot on a tray, so that the feeding looked like the patient was receiving a standard tray.[4]

The development of chemically defined enteral solutions parallels the development of parenteral nutrition solutions in the 1950s and 1960s. Hospitals were increasingly becoming concerned about two significant issues: malnutrition and infections. These concerns led to a large-scale study of chemically defined formulas by the National Institutes of Health and the Vivonex Corporation.[40-42] Both animal and human studies were conducted using purified L-amino acids with procedures to ensure optical purity, highly purified grades of crystalline glucose monohydrate and sucrose, 16 vitamins analyzed for purity and potency, 15 minerals, and purified ethyl linoleate. During the 1960s and 1970s, proponents for chemically defined enteral products continued to promote the benefits of these solutions, but it was during this time that the first successful animal and human cases of total parenteral nutrition (TPN) were published.[43,44] This resulted in a shift to the use of TPN as the nutrition therapy of choice for patients who could not ingest food orally.

Advocates for enteral nutrition continued to promote the use of the gastrointestinal tract as the primary way to provide nutrition to patients, even in patients with minimal intestinal tract. The Codelid Elemental diet (also referred to as the Space diet, since it was modeled after the U.S. Space Program diet) consisting of 18 purified amino acids, sucrose, 11 minerals, 12 water soluble vitamins, 3 fat soluble vitamins, and ethyl linoleate was given to patients with short bowel syndrome secondary to massive resection, fistulas, pancreatitis, ulcerative colitis, and Crohn's disease.[45,46] In most cases, the patients recovered. Other studies followed and proved that elemental diets could be successfully provided to patients with fistulas and short bowel due to surgical resections via jejunostomy feedings.

1.4.5 MODERN ENTERAL NUTRITION THERAPY

Enteral nutrition has evolved significantly from the original delivery and feeding solutions of the 1800s and 1900s. Commercial refinement of enteral formulas, tubing, and pumps continues today with more than 100 commercial products available and a variety of tubes and pumps for optimizing delivery. However, one of the most notable achievements that contributed to today's formulas occurred in 1970. The Wisconsin formula, which was developed by Gormican and Catli in collaboration with Gerber Products Company, was designed to provide the energy-yielding nutrients in the ratio found in a regular diet; 30% of the energy as fat, 20% as protein, 50% as carbohydrate.[47] This was a marked departure from elemental diets, which contained minimal fat. The enteral products used today rely on the idea of feeding the carbohydrate, protein, and fat ratio found in a regular diet. As demonstrated by Stengel and Ravdin in 1939, the use of protein hydrolysates and lactose-free carbohydrates is still successful today.

The composition of enteral products varies substantially, from intact nutrients for general use to specialized products for treating clinical conditions. Formulas include polymeric solutions that provide more intact ingredients, such as whole proteins, monomeric formulas that require less digestion with proteins in the form of peptides and carbohydrates as partially hydrolyzed starch, modular solutions to provide separate macro- or micronutrients, and specialized formulas to treat metabolic or clinical conditions. Enteral nutrition support is focused on supporting nutritional needs, weight gain or maintenance, preventing complications associated with malnutrition, infection, malabsorption, and intolerance as well as modulating the immune system and the body's response to injury and illness.

1.5 PARENTERAL NUTRITION

Parenteral nutrition (PN) is a lifesaving therapy for patients who cannot be adequately nourished by oral or enteral feeding. As a modern therapy, PN has been available clinically for approximately 50 years, but the history of PN dates back to the early 1600s.[44,48] In 1656, Christopher Wren gave intravenous injections (IVs) and infusions of wine and ale to dogs using a goose quill attached to a pig's bladder. Wren was able to demonstrate that the IV solutions caused the same effect as alcohol provided orally.[1,49] During the same time, Lower and King[51,52] reported IV feeding and blood infusions with dogs and, in one case, a young man. The dogs and the young man reportedly survived. Other early researchers included William Courten who, in 1678, gave IV olive oil to dogs that did not survive, thus depicting the need for specialized IV lipid solutions.[53] The first successful IV infusion of saline solutions was achieved by the Scottish physician, Thomas Latta, when he infused salt and water into a cholera patient who recovered and survived.[54] Hodder, in 1873, reportedly infused milk into three cholera patients, two who recovered.[55] The first total parenteral nutrition use in humans occurred in 1904 when Friedrich infused subcutaneously peptone, fat, glucose, and salt.[1] Unfortunately for the patients, this method proved to be too painful and Friedrich abandoned subcutaneous infusion of PN.

1.5.1 GLUCOSE IN PARENTERAL NUTRITION

In 1859, Claude Bernard made a key discovery that resulted in numerous experiments with IV glucose administration. He discovered the importance of glucose and liver glycogen in metabolism, by demonstrating that intravenous glucose was not immediately excreted in the urine.[49] Subsequently, the first infusion of glucose in humans was reported in 1896 by Beidl and Krauts and was soon followed by a series of studies by Woodyatt (in 1915).[48,56] Woodyatt and colleagues conducted a series of timed infusions using a pump to ensure constant delivery of solutions. In the experiments, they varied the infusion rate to establish a dose-response relationship. By this method, Woodyatt determined that an infusion of 0.85 g of glucose/kg/h did not cause glucosuria. Soon after, Mattas[57] used a continuous drip infusion of glucose, which led to subsequent work by Zimmerman, who gave IV solutions through a catheter in the superior vena cava.[58]

Carbohydrates were recognized as a principal component of metabolism, an inexpensive energy source, and easy to manufacture for PN solutions. This recognition led to many trials testing differing forms of carbohydrate in PN, which were largely unsuccessful. Substitutes for glucose were extensively researched including fructose and invert sugar; however, infusion caused higher levels of lactate and pyruvate than did infusion of glucose.[59] In addition, fructose infusion resulted in higher urinary electrolyte losses, including phosphate, sodium, and potassium.[60,61] Glycerol was also used as a source of energy and was well tolerated in animals and humans in small doses, but large doses caused hemolysis, hypotension, and convulsions.[59]

During the 1960s and 70s, glucose was used as the primary source of energy for PN in the United States, since lipid emulsions had not yet been accepted for use in humans. It was during this time that high doses of glucose were given via central venous access because it was thought that trauma increased energy needs significantly. A number of clinical problems resulted from use of high doses of IV glucose as the primary energy source, including liver steatosis, fever, essential fatty acid deficiency, hyperglycemia, and insulin resistance.

1.5.2 PROTEIN

Elman, in 1937, gave the first successful IV infusions of amino acids, as a protein hydrolysate, in man.[62,63] Elman was a student of William Rose, the discoverer of essential amino acids. Prior to Rose and Elman's work, Danish physicians Henriques and Anderson (in 1913) showed that nitrogen equilibrium could be maintained in a goat with an IV solution of beef protein hydrolysate, glucose, and electrolytes.[64] These studies by Elman, Rose, and Henriques formed the basis for many investigations into using amino acids in PN solutions. Protein hydrolysates, crystalline amino acids, and racemic forms of amino acids were all researched following Elman's work.[59] Many of these solutions resulted in side effects, including vomiting, nausea, and increased ammonia and urea. The initial protein hydrolysates were produced using an acid treatment, which destroyed tryptophan. This problem was solved in 1944 by Wretlind when he produced an enzymatic hydrolysate of casein called Aminosol.[65] It is particularly interesting that Aminosol contained impurities, which caused trace element contamination of the solution. This resulted in patients receiving trace elements as a beneficial effect and leading to fewer deficiencies of trace elements.[49]

Crystalline amino acid solutions were introduced by Bansi and colleagues in 1964.[50] Soon after, Wretlind developed Vamin, a more complete crystalline amino acid solution that was effective at maintaining postoperative nitrogen balance. In these solutions, it was technically challenging to include tyrosine, cysteine, cystine, and glutamine. This problem was solved with the advent of dipeptides in the 1980s, which improved solubility and stability.[66]

1.5.3 LIPID

A major effect was undertaken to find methods to prepare fat emulsions since it was recognized that fat is an excellent kcalorie source. Unfortunately most experiments with fat emulsions caused severe adverse reactions in animals and humans. Following the studies of Courten in the late 1600s, researchers continued to search for methods to successfully infuse fat via IV. From 1920 to 1960, researchers in the United States and Japan worked diligently to develop lipid infusions that could be tolerated by humans. In Japan, a number of researchers, including Yamaka, Sato, and Nomura, tested hundreds of differing lipid solutions and emulsifiers, particularly using lecithin with good tolerance in animals.[49,59] In the United States, Geyer, Stare, and Meng were working on lipid research during the same period of time.[59,67-69] Meng gave a complete parenteral solution to dogs using an olive oil emulsion for four weeks with no adverse reactions; nevertheless, this solution was not tolerated by humans.

It was not until 1960 that the first IV lipid emulsion, called Lipomul, was produced by the Upjohn Company.[70] Lipomul was the result of research conducted by Meng and Canham (from the U.S. Army Research and Development Command).[71] Cottonseed oil was used in Lipomul, which cause significant adverse effects in humans including chills, fever, vomiting, hypoxia, and hypotension. In 1965, the entire issue of the *American Journal of Clinical Nutrition* was devoted to articles from a symposium on intravenous fat emulsions.[71] The high level of toxicity of the lipid emulsions led to a distrust of lipid infusions in the United States and continued use of providing kcalories from glucose alone. This reliance of glucose for kcalories continued until the mid-1970s. Intralipid was the first nontoxic lipid emulsion to be designed that was made from soybean oil and egg yolk phospholipids, as the emulsifier. It was introduced in 1961 by Wretlind and Schuberth,[72] but not available for use in the United States until 1975. Intralipid, consisting of long-chain fatty acids, made it possible to use fat-soluble vitamins in TPN solutions.

1.5.4 First Successful Total Parenteral Nutrition

Research conducted during the 1960s by Dudrick, Wilmore, Vars, Rhodes, and Rhoades at the University of Pennsylvania Harrison Department of Surgery Research Laboratories on adult dogs and, later beagle puppies, led to a landmark paper on the first human infant fed with PN.[43,73,74] Relying on previous work from Elman, Geyer, and Zimmerman, among others cited in this chapter, Rhoades and Dudrick, with colleagues, initiated a series of experiments to successfully develop and refine PN.[75] During the experiments on beagle puppies, the researchers solved a number of key problems associated with PN; namely, provision of all required substrates to support normal growth and development, sterilization of the solution, maintenance of sterility, safe and nonreactive long-term central venous catheters, and dependable infusion pumps to standup to the activity of a puppy.[75] In addition to solve the problem with the lack of commercially available IV fat soluble vitamins, the researchers asked the U.S. Vitamin Corporation to develop a water-soluble form of fat-soluble vitamins.

The first clinical application of the PN in humans was conducted on six malnourished adult surgical patients.[75] It was during the care of these patients that several clinical issues were discovered and remedied. Key observations included noting that severe hypophosphatemia (a symptom of refeeding syndrome) occurred in a severely malnourished patient and that gravity-drip infusion was inaccurate and resulted in hypovolemia, hyperglycemia, and glycosuria. This discovery caused the researchers to use infusion pumps from the laboratory to deliver continuous steady doses to the patients and, as a result, led to the use of pumps to infuse IV liquids in critically ill patients. After successfully treating the six adult patients, the next patient put on PN was a one-month-old infant.[44]

In 1968, Wilmore and Dudrick reported on the case of an infant, who had undergone surgery for atresia, sustained for five months on PN as her sole source of nutrition.[44] This was the first case report of long-term PN being able to support life. A number of key nutrition insights were gained during this case, including the need for adequate vitamin D to prevent rickets and the need to provide essential fatty acids. Fat was provided by feeding the infant's parents high fat meals, drawing blood from the parents, and infusing the fatty plasma into the infant. Over the course of the next years, many patients were successfully treated with PN. This led to parenteral nutrition becoming the primary nutrition therapy during the 1970s and 1980s for postsurgical patients who could not eat for more than a few days and who suffered from acute illnesses.[76–81] It was during this time that Dr. Rhoades introduced the term hyperalimination.

1.5.5 Modern Parenteral Nutrition

Parenteral nutrition today is for patients who cannot be fed orally or via enteral nutrition and require nutrition support during a critical time period. Specific guidelines are in place, which help clinicians determine appropriate use of PN. These criteria are detailed in the *American Society for Parenteral and Enteral Nutrition Guidelines for the Use of Parenteral and Enteral Nutrition in Adult and Pediatric Patients*.[81] Parenteral nutrition is no longer a substitute or preferential modality for enteral nutrition, as enteral nutrition is the appropriate method of nutrition support in patients with a working gastrointestinal tract. As early as 1980 and continuing to the present day, clinicians and researchers have recognized that PN frequently resulted in higher rates of complications in patients.[83–90] In fact, a meta-analysis conducted by Klein et al.[91] demonstrated that both preoperative and postoperative enteral nutrition support results in lower incidence of postoperative complications. Moreover, while preoperative PN reduced overall risk of complications by 10%, postoperative PN increases overall risk by 10%.

Current parenteral nutrition solutions and delivery system have been refined to include all-in-one mixtures infused using electronic pumps. Special care is taken to prevent infections and bacterial contamination. Solutions include water, glucose monohydrate, lipid emulsions of soybean oil, triglycerides, and egg yolk phospholipids, and amino acids with vitamins and minerals. Clinical research with PN is focused on reducing complications, such as hepatic dysfunction, gallstones, metabolic bone disease, bowel function as well as improving patient outcome. Newer innovations include use of medium chain triglycerides, omega 3 fatty acids, and short chain fatty acids as well as addition nonessential and conditionally essential amino acids (taurine, arginine, glutamine) that may be beneficial for patients on PN or with special clinical needs.

1.6 CONCLUSION

The nutritional management of gastrointestinal disease has changed markedly in the past 100 years. Advances in formulations and delivery systems continue as greater scientific understanding of immune function and disease pathologies is advanced. Medical nutrition therapy continues to be refined, although it is clear that restrictive diets, whether as food, beverages, enteral feeding solutions, or parenteral nutrition solutions, are not useful for most patients and can result in potential deficiencies of essential nutrients and calories as well as increased complications. Restrictive diets and feeding prescriptions should be limited to individual cases when it is clear that there is a therapeutic role. Use of liberal diets and nutritional solutions that provide adequate calories and nutrients to patients, in combination with medical management, result in the best patient outcomes.

REFERENCES

1. Allison SP. History of nutrition support in Europe pre-ESPEN. *Clin Nutr* 2003;S2;S2–3.
2. Food and Nutrition Board, National Research Council: Recommended Dietary Allowances 1942, Washington, D.C.
3. Sippy B. Gastric and duodenal ulcer. Medical cure by an efficient removal of gastric juice corrosion. *JAMA* 1915;64:1625–1630.
4. Cooper LF, Barber EM, Mitchell HS, Rynbergen HJ. *Nutrition in Health and Disease. 14th Edition.* Philadelphia: JB Lippincott Company;1963.
5. Andresen AF. The peptic ulcer problem. *NY State J Med* 1949;49:2811–2919.
6. Deluca V, Gray SJ, Schneider MA. The effect of spice ingestion upon the stomach. *Am J Gastroenterol* 1956;26:722–732.
7. Ryan-Harshman M, Aldoori W. How diet and lifestyle affect duodenal ulcers: Review of the evidence. *Can Fam Physician* 2004;50:727–732.
8. Rydning A, Berstad A. Dietary fiber and peptic ulcer. *Scan J Gastroenterol* 1986;21:1–5.
9. Robinson CH. Dietotherapy: The bland diet. *J Clin Nutr* 1954;2:206–210.
10. Burke J. The treatment of steatorrhea in Crohn's Disease. *Brit Med J* 1953;1:239–242.
11. Serrena A, Hedemann MS, Bach Knudsen KE. Influence of dietary fiber on luminal environment and morphology in the small and large intestine of sows. *J Anim Sci* 2008;86:2217–2227.
12. Korzenik JR, Case Closed? Diverticulitis: Epidemiology and fiber. *J Clin Gastroenterol* 2006;40:S112–116.
13. Levenstein S, Prantera C, Luzi C, D'Ubaldi A. Low residue or normal diet in Crohn's disease: A prospective controlled study in Italian patients. *Gut* 1985;26:989–993.
14. Ritchie JK, Wadsworth J, Lennard-Jones JE, Rogers E. Controlled multicentre therapeutic trial of an unrefined carbohydratae, fiber rich diet in Crohn's disease. *Br Med J* 1987;29:517–520.
15. Madden AM. Changing perspectives in the nutritional management of disease. *Proc Nutr Soc* 2003;62:765–772.
16. Filipsson S, Hulten L, Lindstedt G. Malabsorption of fat and vitamin B12 before and after intestinal resection for Crohn's disease. *Scand J Gastroenterol* 1978;13:529–536.
17. Dyer NH, Dawson AM. Malnutrition and malabsorption in Crohn's disease with reference to the effect of surgery. *Br J Surg* 1973;60(2):134–140.

18. Woolf GM, Miller C, Kurian R, Jeejeebhoy KN. Nutritional absorption in short bowel syndrome: Evaluation of fluid, calorie, and divalent cation requirements. *Dig Dis Sci* 1987;32:8–15.
19. Pittman AC, Robinson FW. Dumping syndrome; control by diet. *J Am Diet Assoc* 1958;34:596–602.
20. Randall HT. The History of Enteral Nutrition. In: Rombeau JL, Caldwell MD, ed. *Enteral and Parenteral Nutrition.* Philadelphia: WB Sanders;1984:1–10.
21. Harkness L. The history of enteral nutrition therapy: From raw eggs and nasal tubes to purified amino acids and early postoperative jejunal delivery. *J Am Diet Assoc* 2002;102:399–404.
22. Brown-Sequard CE. Feeding per rectum in nervous afflictions. *Lancet* 1878;1:144.
23. Bliss DW. Feeding per rectum: As illustrated in the case of the late President Garfield. *Med Rec* 1882;22:64–69.
24. Pareira MD, Conrad EJ, Hicks W, Elman R. Therapeutic nutrition with tube feeding. *JAMA* 1954;156:810–816.
25. Dukes CA. A simple mode of feeding some patients by nose. *Lancet* 1876;2:394–395.
26. Coulston TS. Forcible feeding. *Lancet* 1872;2:797–798.
27. Hott E. Gavage (forced feeding) in the treatment of acute diseases in infancy and childhood. *Med Rec* 1894;45:524–525.
28. Morrison WA. The value of the stomach tube in feeding after intubation, based on twenty-eight cases: Also its use in post-diptheric paralysis. *Boston Med Surg J* 1895;132:127–130.
29. Einhorn M. Duodenal alimentation. *Med Rec* 1910;78:92–94.
30. Morgan WG. Duodenal aliminentation. *Am J Sci* 1914;148:360–368.
31. Jones CR. Duodenal feedings. *Surg Gynecol Obstet* 1916;22:236-240.
32. Gross MH, Held IW. Duodenal alimentation. *JAMA* 1915;65:520–523.
33. Andresen AFR. Immediate jejunal feeding after gastro-enterostomy. *Ann Surg* 1918;67:565–566.
34. Abbott WO. Fluid and nutritional maintenance by the use of the intestinal tract. *Ann Surg* 1940;1:32–36.
35. Stengel A, Ravdin IS. The maintenance of nutrition in surgical patients with a description of the orojejunal method of feeding. *Surgery* 1939;6:511–523.
36. Pareira MD. *Therapeutic Nutrition with Tube Feeding.* Springfield, Ill: Charles C. Thomas;1959.
37. Barron J, Falls LS. Tube feeding with liquefied whole food. *Surg Forum* 1953;iv:519–522.
38. Barron J. Preparation of natural food for tube feeding. *Henry Ford Hosp Bull* 1953;1:13–17.
39.. Robinson CH. Dietotherapy: Liquid diets. *J Clin Nutr* 1953;1;476–477.
40. Greenstein JP, Birnbaum SM, Winitz M, Otey MC. Quantitative nutritional studies with water-soluble chemical defined diets. *Arch Biochem Biophys* 1957;72:396–416.
41. Winitz M, Seedman DA, Graft. Studies in metabolic nutrition employing chemically defined diets. *Am J Clin Nutr* 1970;23:525–545.
42. Couch RB, Watkins DM, Smith RR, Rosenberg LE, Winitz M, Birnbaum SM, Otey MC, Greenstein JP. Clinical trials of water-soluble chemically defined diets. *Fed Proc* 1960;19:13–21.
43. Dudrick SJ, Wilmore DW, Vars HM. Long-term total parenteral nutrition with growth in puppies and positive nutrition balance in patients. *Surg Form* 1967;18:356–357.
44. Wilmore DW, Dudrick SJ. Growth and development of an infant receiving all nutrients exclusively by vein. *JAMA* 203;1968,140–144.
45. Thompson WR, Stephens RV, Randall HT, Bowen JR. Use of the "Space Diet" in management of a patient with extreme short bowel syndrome. *Am J Surg* 1969;117:449–456.

46. Stephens RV, Randall HT. Use of a concentrated, balanced, liquid elemental diet for nutritional management of catabolic states. *Ann Surg* 1969;170;642–667.
47. Gormican A, Catli E. Nutritional and clinical responses of immobilized patients to sterile milk-based feedings. *J Chron Dis* 1972;25:291–303.
48. Vinnars E, Wilmore D. Jonathan Rhoads Symposium Papers. History of parenteral nutrition. *JPEN* 2003;27:225–232.
49. Vinnars E, Hammarqvist F. 25th Arvid Wretlind's Lecture, 25 years of ESPEN, the history of nutrition. *Clin Nutr* 2004;23:955–962.
50. Bansi HW, Juergens P, Mueller G, Rostin M. Metabolism in intravenous administration of nutritional solutions, with special reference to synthetically composed amino acids solutions. *Klin Wocheschr* 1964;42:332–52.
51. Lower T. The method observed in transfusing blood out of one live animal into another. *Philos Trans R Soc Lond* 1667;1:353–358.
52. Lower R, King E. An account of the experiment of transfusion practiced upon a man in London. *Philos Trans R Soc Lond* 1667;2:557–564.
53. Courten W. Experiments and observations of the effects of several sorts of poisons upon animal made at Montpelier in the years 1678 and 1679 by the late William Courten. *Philos Trans R Soc Lond* 1712;27:485.
54. Latta T. Relative to the treatment of cholera by copious injection of aqueous and saline fluids into the veins. *Lancet* 1831:274.
55. Hodder EM. Transfusion of milk in cholera. *Practitioner* 1873;19:517.
56. Woodyatt PD, Sansum WD, Wilder RM. Prolonged and accurately times IV injections of sugar: A preliminary report. *J Am Med Assoc* 1915;65:2067–2070.
57. Mattas R. The continued intravenous drip. *Ann surg* 1924;5:643–661.
58. Zimmerman T. Intravenous tubing for parenteral therapy. *Science* 1945;101:567–568.
59. Geyer RP. Parenteral Nutrition. *Physiol Rev* 1960;40:150–168.
60. Beal JM, Smith JL, Frost PM. Studies in the utilization of fructose administered intravenously in man. *Surgery* 1953;33:721.
61. Hoenig V, Schuck O, Fischer O, Hoenigova J, Patova V. Hypophosphaturia after intravenous administration of glucose and fructose. *Act Med Scand* 1958;161:79–84.
62. Elman R, Weiner DO. Intravenous alimentation with special reference to protein (amino acid) metabolism. *J Am Med Assoc* 1939;112:796–802.
63. Elman R. Amino acid content of the blood following intravenous injection of hydrolyzed protein. *Proc Soc Exp Bio Med* 1937;37:437–440.
64. Cuthbertson DP. Symposium on surgery and nutrition. *Proc Nutr Soc* 1980;39:101–104.
65. Wretlind A. The amino acid content of the blood following intravenous injection of hydrolyzed casein. *Acta Phys Scand* 1952;27:189–203.
66. Vinnars E, Bergstrom J, Furst P. Comparative nitrogen balance studies with an amino-acid solutions based on nutritional studies against two protein-based solutions. *Acta Anaesthesiol Scan Suppl* 1973;53:76–80.
67. Stare FJ. Recollections of pioneers of nutrition: Establishment of the first department of nutrition in a medical center. *J Am Coll Nutr* 1989;8:248–252.
68. Meng HC, Early F. Study of complete parenteral alimentation in dogs. *J Lab Clin Med* 1949;34:1121–1132.
69. Waddell WR, Van Itallie TB, Geyer RP, Stare FJ. Liver function during intravenous infusion of emulsified fat to humans. *Ann Surg* 1953;138:734–740.
70. Wretlind A, Szczygiel B. Total parenteral nutrition. History. Present time. Future. *Pol Merkur Lekarski* 1998;4:181–185.
71. Mueller JF, Canham JE. Symposium on intravenous fat emulsions. *Am J Clin Nutr* 1965;16:1–3.

72. Schuberth O, Wretlind A. Fat emulsions for intravenous nutrition. Pharmacological and clinical experiences: Intravenous infusion of fat emulsions, phosphatides, and emulsifying agents. *Nord Med* 1963;69:13–17.
73. Rhode Cm, Parkins W, Tourtellotte D, Vars H. Method of continuous intravenous administration of nutritive solutions suitable for prolonged studies in dogs. *Am J Physiol* 1949;59:409–411.
74. Dudrick SJ, Wilmore DW, Vars HM. Long-term total parenteral nutrition with growth, development, and positive nitrogen balance. *Surgery* 1968;64:134–162.
75. Dudrick SJ. A 45-year obsession and passionate pursuit of optimal nutrition support: Puppies, pediatrics, surgery, geriatrics, home TPN, ASPEN, et cetera. *JPEN* 2005;29:272–287.
76. Shaw SN, Elwyn DH, Askanazi J, Iles M, Schwarz Y, Kinney JM. Effects of increasing nitrogen intake on nitrogen balance and energy expenditure in nutritionally depleted adult patients receiving parenteral nutrition. *Am J Clin Nutr* 1983;37:930–940.
77. Mullen JL, Hargrove WC, Dudrick SJ, Fitts WT, Rosato EF. Ten years experience with intravenous hyperalimentation and inflammatory bowel disease. *Ann Surg* 1978;187:523–529.
78. Sitzmann JV, Steinborn PA, Zinner MJ, Cameron JL. Total parenteral nutrition and alternative energy substrates in treatment of severe acute pancreatitis. *Surg Gynecol Obstet* 1989;168:311–317.
79. Silberman H, Dixon NP, Eisenberg D. The safety and efficacy of a lipid-based system of parenteral nutrition in acute pancreatitis. *Am J Gastroenterol* 1982;77:494–497.
80. Dudrick SJ, Wilmore DW, Steiger E. Spontaneous closure of traumatic pancreatoduodenal fistulas with total intravenous nutrition. *J Trauma* 1970;10:542–553.
81. Silberman H. Freehauf M, Fong G. Parenteral nutrition with lipids. *J Am Med Assoc* 1977;238:1380–1382.
82. ASPEN 2009 http://www.nutritioncare.org/Library.aspx.
83. Latham PS, Menkes E, Phillips MJ, Jeejeebhoy KN. Hyperalimentation-associated jaundice: An example of a serum factor inducing cholestasis in rats. *Am J Clin Nutr* 1985;41:61–65.
84. Gramlich L, Kichian K, Pinilla J, Rodych NJ, Dhaliwal R, Heyland DK. Does enteral nutrition compared to parenteral nutrition result in better outcomes in critically ill adult patients? A systematic review of the literature. *Nutrition* 2004;20:843–848.
85. Kalfarentzos F, Kehagias J, Mead N, Kokkinis K, Gogos CA. Enteral nutrition is superior to parenteral nutrition in severe acute pancreatitis: Results of a randomized prospective trial. *Br J Surgery* 1997;84:1665–1669.
86. Chen SS, Donmoyer C, Zhang Y, Hande SA, Lacy DB, McGuinness OP. Impact of enteral and parenteral nutrition on hepatic and muscle glucose metabolism. *JPEN* 2000;24:255–260.
87. Koffler M, Imamura T, Inman L. Deleterious effects of chronic intravenous glucose overload and their possible prevention by glucagon. *Horm Metabol Res* 1987;19:672.
88. McClave SA, Greene LM, Snider HL, Makk LJK, Cheadle WG, Owens NA, Dukes LG, Goldsmith LJ. Comparison of the safety of early enteral vs parenteral nutrition in mild pancreatitis. *JPEN* 1997;21:14–20.
89. de Vree JML, Romijn JA, Mok KS, Mathus-Vliegen LMH, Stoutenbeek CP, Ostrow JD, Tytgat GNJ, Sauerwein HP, Olferink RP, Groen AK. Lack of enteral nutrition during critical illness is associated with profound decrements in biliary lipid concentrations. *Am J Clin Nutr* 1999;70:70–77.

90. Grau T, Bonet A, Rubio M, Mateo D. Liver dysfunction associated with artificial nutrition in critically ill patients. Critical Care 2007;11 epub http://ccforum.com/content/11/1/R10.
91. Klein S, Kinney J, Jeejeebhoy K, Alpers D, Hellerstein M, Murray M, Twomey P. Nutrition support in clinical practice: Review of published data and recommendations for future research directions. *JPEN* 1997;21:133–156.

2 Assessment of Nutritional Status

Laura E. Matarese

CONTENTS

2.1 INTRODUCTION

Good nutrition is essential for the well-being and health of the patient with gastrointestinal (GI) disease. Nutrition deals with the very crux of existence. Historically, malnutrition has been associated with poverty, poor sanitation, and lack of resources often occurring in underdeveloped countries. However, with the abundance of food, lack of exercise, and overall higher standard of living, obesity and chronic disease linked to diet has become epidemic and is also considered to be a form of malnutrition. Nutritional health results from an intricate balance between nutrient intake and requirements. When requirements exceed intake, malnutrition ensues and encompasses a wide spectrum of physiological alterations including undernutrition and specific micronutrient deficiencies. When intake exceeds requirements, malnutrition in the form of obesity and its co-morbidities result. Malnutrition leads to a sequence of metabolic and pathological events with physiological alterations, reduced organ and tissue function, loss of body mass, and eventually death (Figure 2.1). In the setting

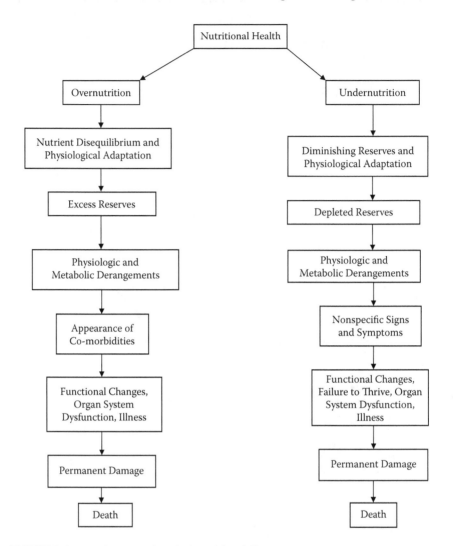

FIGURE 2.1   Development of clinical nutritional disease.

of gastrointestinal disease, nutrient intake may be adequate, but malabsorption and biochemical alterations can lead to significant nutrient deficiency with biochemical and physiological changes over a relatively short period of time. Additionally, nutrient requirements are elevated during periods of active disease states, infection, postsurgical stress, or general need for repletion; or, oral intake may be reduced in the face of illness.

Nutritional assessment is an evaluation of the nutritional status of individuals or populations through measurements of food and nutrient intake and evaluation of nutrition-related health indicators. The goal is to identify those individuals who will require nutrition intervention. Since most nutrition interventions carry some risk, the degree of malnutrition and the potential benefit must be considered when deliberating the decision to provide these therapies. Nutrition intervention should be provided to those patients who are most likely to progress to critical malnutrition. The ability to identify individuals at nutritional risk and to effectively augment their health status through improved nutrition has made nutritional assessment an important skill for health professions concerned about making healthcare more cost effective. Despite the abundance of clinical data surrounding the use of subjective and objective assessment tools to identify malnutrition, no single measure has been proved to be comprehensive, accurate, and cost-efficient in all patients. This is due in part to the fact that clinically available measures, such as anthropometrics and serum proteins, are frequently distorted by the parallel influences of malnutrition and disease on body composition and function.[1] The predictive ability of nutritional assessment techniques are also affected by the reproducibility and error in the measurements themselves as well as narrowly defined standards for comparison. Ultimately, there is no substitute for good clinical judgment. Nonetheless, nutritional assessment is an important component in the care of the patient with GI disease. Nutritional assessment and the provision of nutrition support should be part of the total integration of care.

2.2   NUTRITIONAL ASSESSMENT METHODS

A comprehensive nutritional assessment encompasses data collection and evaluation from several different categories: history, physical examination, anthropometry and body composition analysis, and biochemical evaluation. Within each category are numerous subcategories of both subjective and objective components. The advantages and limitations of each are presented with a special emphasis on the potential applications of each method in the assessment of the patient with GI disease. However, the strength and value of the nutritional assessment lies in the integration of these components into the overall clinical picture, which is used to identify malnutrition and formulate a treatment plan.

2.2.1   PATIENT HISTORY

The history elicits subjective information from the patient, family, or caregivers and is the first step in the clinical assessment of nutritional status. Information obtained from a detailed history contributes to a more accurate assessment of nutritional status. Results from the history may prompt the clinician to investigate areas of possible deficiency and forms the basis for a more focused physical examination and judicious use of laboratory studies. Even after nutrition intervention has been initiated, ongoing patient histories may provide information as to why the patient's nutritional state is not responding to therapy. The historical portion of the nutritional assessment is divided into medical, medication usage, nutrition, and psychosocial (Table 2.1).

2.2.1.1   Medical History

The medical history is critical in determining the adequacy of nutritional status. Inadequacies and the potential causes of these deficits are often obtained from a thorough review of the patient's medical record and a focused interview with the

TABLE 2.1
Components of Nutrition-Oriented History

Medical History

- Present and previous illnesses or trauma interfering with nutritional status
- Presence of fever, chills, or myalgias
- Usual level of activity with any remarkable changes
- Diagnostic tests evaluating organ function
- Chronic diseases and/or surgical procedures affecting the GI tract
- Length of the remnant small and large intestine and presence of the ileocecal valve
- Presence and location of GI tubes, surgical drains, stomas, or fistulae
- Hydration status
- Changes in urinary or bowel habits (diarrhea, constipation, steatorrhea)

Medication Usage

- Current prescriptions
- Over-the-counter medications
- Vitamin, mineral or herbal supplements, meal replacements
- Appetite stimulants or suppressants
- Allergies to medications, enteral or parenteral nutrition components, or medical supplies

Nutrition History

- Food habits, eating patterns, diet restrictions, factors influencing nutrient intake, aversions, or allergies
- Recent weight loss or gain, time frame (≤ six months), stated versus documented, intentional versus unintentional, has weight stabilized or has patient continued to lose/gain?
- Usual body weight 20% more or less than ideal
- Dysphagia, dysgeusia, anorexia, early satiety, nausea, vomiting, diarrhea, constipation steatorrhea, gastroesophageal reflux, abdominal pain
- Intake of commercial and/or nonconventional nutritional supplements
- Enteral, parenteral, oral rehydration, or intravenous fluid and electrolyte regimens

Psychosocial Information

- Altered mental states including depression, anxiety, and confusion
- Low education and/or income levels
- Drug or alcohol addiction
- Tobacco use
- Absence of social support
- Housing, finances, ability to purchase and prepare food
- Activity level

patient, family, or caregiver. Understanding the pathophysiology of various disease states, illness, surgical procedures, and medication interactions is necessary to identify interactions that may put a patient at nutritional risk. The onset and duration of the patient's current health problems provide insight into the changes in GI function that may possibly alter nutritional status. The configuration of the GI tract for those patients who have had previous surgeries is important in determining the extent of

TABLE 2.2

Nutritional Consequences of GI Surgery

Type of Surgery	Potential Nutritional Consequences
Esophagus	
Resection/replacement	• Early satiety
Gastric pull-up	• Weight loss due to inadequate intake
	• Increased protein loss secondary to catabolism
	• Rapid gastric emptying of hypertonic fluids
Colonic interposition	• Early satiety
	• May need short-term enteral or parenteral nutrition
	• May require antidumping diet
Stomach	
Partial gastrectomy/vagotomy	• Early satiety
	• Delayed gastric emptying of solids
	• Rapid emptying of hypertonic fluids
	• Malabsorption of vitamins and minerals due to achlorhydria
Total gastrectomy	• Dumping syndrome
	• Malabsorption of vitamins and minerals due to achlorhydria
	• Bezoar formation
Bariatric surgery	• Malabsorption of vitamins and minerals due to achlorhydria, nonavailability of bile acids and pancreatic enzymes
Intestine	
Ileal resection	• Malabsorption of bile salts and vitamin B12
	• Poor jejunal adaptation
	• Rapid intestinal transit
Extensive bowel resection	• Large fluid and electrolyte losses
	• Nutrient malabsorption
	• Gastic acid hypersecretion
	• Rapid gastric emptying
	• Rapid intestinal transit

GI dysfunction. Review of operative reports and directed questions to the surgeon can help to construct an accurate diagram. Although any surgical procedure could potentially impact nutritional status, operations on the GI tract can have significant nutritional consequences (Table 2.2).[2–10]

2.2.1.2 Medications

Prescription and over-the-counter medications as well as vitamin, mineral, and nontraditional medications, such as herbal and alternative remedies, should be reviewed for polypharmacy, nutrient drug interactions, and potential influence on nutritional status. Many drugs commonly used in the treatment of GI disorders, such as corticosteroids, narcotics, immunosuppressants, chemotherapy, antidiarrheals, laxatives, somatostatin analogues, diuretics, and antibiotics can impact bowel function, appetite, fluid and electrolyte balance, and overall nutritional status. Unfortunately, there are many GI patients with chronic disorders who eventually develop narcotic dependence.

2.2.1.3 Nutrition

The nutrition history provides data concerning the patient's eating habits and patterns, dietary restrictions, food intolerance, and factors influencing nutrient intake. A thorough nutrition history can provide valuable insight into past dietary interventions and potential nutrient deficiencies or excesses. Nutrient deficiencies are identified with relative certainty when a detailed, accurate dietary intake record is compared with carefully estimated daily requirements. However, the assessment of dietary patterns may be skewed by high intraindividual variability in food intake, frequent withholding of intake for diagnostic testing or surgical procedures, or inaccurate reporting of intake on behalf of the patient, family, or caregiver. An evaluation of GI symptoms that may be trigged by oral intake can provide an indication of disease conditions that affect nutritional status. Key questions, such as the incidence of nausea, vomiting, anorexia, or early satiety, can clue in the clinician to possible deficiencies. Many patients with GI disorders will voluntarily restrict oral intake in order to minimize GI output. Oral intake should be evaluated with reference to GI losses so that adjustments in fluid provisions, antidiarrheal medications, or dietary composition can be implemented.

There are different methods available to perform a dietary assessment. No single best method exists for measuring dietary intake. There are two techniques that are generally used in the clinical setting. The first is a dietary history or 24-hour recall in which the patient is asked to verbally report all foods and beverages consumed on a typical day. The clinician then asks probing questions to ascertain the frequency and amounts of consumption of specific foods or food groups in order to evaluate the reliability of the interview. This is quick to perform, has a low respondent burden, but does not give data representative of an individual's usual intake. The second method is a 24- to 72-hour nutrient intake record or food diary. With this technique the patient or caregiver is asked to record all foods and beverages consumed during the specific time frame. The method does not rely on memory, can provide detailed intake data, but requires a high degree of respondent cooperation. An experienced registered dietitian can assess the adequacy of overall energy, protein, fluid, and micronutrient intake based on information obtained from a thorough diet history by translating foods consumed into nutrient intake. For larger epidemiological studies, a survey tool is generally employed.

2.2.1.4 Psychosocial

The maintenance of adequate nutrient intake and compliance with nutrition therapy is often altered in the patient with social, economic, or psychological challenges. These situations can significantly impact an individual's ability to comply with medical and nutritional therapy. Information regarding the patient's living arrangements, social support systems, access to medical care, activity level, food purchasing and preparation capabilities, and religious practices allows the clinician to tailor the nutrition care plan for optimal success. The use of alcohol, tobacco, and illicit drugs should also be investigated. For those receiving specialized nutrition therapies, such as home parenteral or enteral nutrition, it is important to ensure the patient's ability to obtain and safely administer the therapy as directed. Both nutritional and medical therapies will be enhanced when the patient is evaluated and treated as a whole, including the psychological, emotional, and cognitive needs using the skills of a multidisciplinary team.

2.2.2 NUTRITION-FOCUSED PHYSICAL EXAM

The physical examination corroborates and adds to the findings obtained by history. The addition of the nutrition-focused aspects is valuable in detecting nutritional deficiencies or excesses. These include both macro- and micronutrient deficiencies (Table 2.3). The most obvious physical markers of chronic protein-energy malnutrition are temporal or skeletal muscle wasting and loss of subcutaneous fat in the face, triceps, waist, and thighs. Rapidly proliferating bodily tissues (i.e., hair, skin, nails, oral cavity, and eyes) tend to respond more promptly to nutrient deficiencies than other tissues. Thin, dry, easily pluckable hair can signify protein or protein-calorie deficiency, whereas dryness, scaling, or roughened bumps of the skin may indicate essential fatty acid deficiency. Protein deficiency is also observed with excessive bruising, edema, or delayed wound healing. Common manifestations of micronutrient deficiencies in GI patients include zinc, magnesium, and B vitamins. This is often due to impaired ability to digest and absorb as well as the large GI losses from excessive diarrhea or ostomy effluent.

An evaluation of fluid balance is also an important component of the nutritional assessment. Malabsorption, chronic illness, and surgery can lead to severe hypoalbuminemia and fluid retention presenting as edema, ascites, or anasarca. Dehydration due to substantial fluid loss from gastric suctioning, vomiting, diarrhea, excessive ostomy output, and fistula or wound drainage is also possible. This can be physically detected by assessing skin turgor and examining mucous membranes. Physical findings should be integrated with daily weight changes, laboratory values, intake and output records, and appearance of urine and stool to ascertain overall fluid balance.

The patient's subcutaneous adipose stores should be evaluated as these represent energy reserves and are depleted in chronic malnutrition. This is common in patients with GI disorders. For those patients who are obese, the location and deposition of the adipose tissue can signal the potential for other risk factors. Body fat distribution can be classified into two types: (1) upper body, android, or male type; and (2) lower body, gynoid, or female type.[11] Patients with android obesity or central adiposity seem to be at greater risk for other diseases. Android obesity has been associated with co-morbidities, such as cardiovascular disease, insulin resistance, hyperinsulinemia, noninsulin-dependent diabetes mellitus, hypertension, hyperlipidemia, stroke, and even increased mortality.[12-15]

An evaluation of the functional capacity of the GI tract is especially important for any patient with a history of GI disease. This can be accomplished using techniques of inspection, auscultation, percussion, and palpation. Bowel sounds, level of abdominal distention, and presence of tenderness is assessed to rule out ileus or bowel obstruction. Data from the physical assessment of bowel function should be combined with radiologic and laboratory tests along with a history of early satiety, postprandial pain, nausea, vomiting, flatus, diarrhea, or constipation to provide a comprehensive evaluation along with a treatment plan.

TABLE 2.3
Physical Signs of Macronutrient and Micronutrient Deficiency

Protein

- Mental confusion, hyperirritability, apathy
- Thinning, dull, easily pluckable hair; traverse depigmentation of hair
- Edema, anasarca
- Delayed wound healing, decubitus ulcers
- Traverse ridging of nails
- Hepatomegaly
- Decreased baseline temperature
- Cellophane appearance of skin

Protein-energy

- Dry, dull hair
- Hollowed cheeks
- Mottled teeth with cavities
- Loss of balance
- Muscle weakness and overall wasting

Essential fatty acids

- Xerosis (scaly, flaky dermatitis of the extremities)
- Thrombocytopenia
- Follicular hyperkeratosis
- Dry, dull hair
- Nasolabial seborrhea

Thiamine (Vitamin B1)

- Wernicke's-Korsakoff encephalopathy
- Peripheral neuropathy
- Ophthalmoplegia
- Heart failure
- Edema
- Pour wound healing, pressure ulcers

Riboflavin (Vitamin B2)

- Angular stomatitis
- Cheilosis
- Atrophic lingual papillae
- Glossitis

Pyridoxine (Vitamin B6)

- Angular stomatitis
- Cheilosis
- Glossitis
- Peripheral neuropathy

Ascorbic acid (Vitamin C)

- Perifollicular hyperkeratosis
- Hemorrhage
- Corkscrew hair
- Swollen, retracted, bleeding gums
- Poor wound healing

Vitamin A

- Night blindness
- Bitot's spots
- Xerosis
- Hyperkeratosis of skin

Vitamin D

- Osteomalacia
- Rickets
- Tetany

Vitamin E

- Hemolytic anemia
- Neuropathy

Vitamin K

- Bleeding
- Increased prothrombin time (PT)

Iron

- Hypochromic microcytic anemia
- Weakness
- Cheilosis
- Pale conjunctiva

Zinc

- Apathy
- Alopecia
- Poor wound healing
- Dysgeusia
- Skin rash
- Nasolabial seborrea

Copper

- Microcytic hypochromic anemia, leukopenia, neutropenia
- Menke's syndrome

Chromium

- Glucose intolerance
- Peripheral neuropathy
- Metabolic encephalopathy

TABLE 2.3 (CONTINUED)
Physical Signs of Macronutrient and Micronutrient Deficiency

Cobalamin (Vitamin B12)
- Megaloblastic anemia
- Pernicious anemia
- Angular lingual papillae
- Dementia
- Ataxia

Folate
- Pancytopenia
- Glossitis
- Stomatitis
- Atrophic lingual papillae

Selenium
- Dilated cardiomyopathy
- Keshan's disease
- White nails

2.2.3 ANTHROPOMETRY AND BODY COMPOSITION ANALYSIS

Anthropometry is the measurement of physical parameters that deal with the physical dimensions, proportions, and composition of the human body as well as the study of related variables that affect them. Body weight is one of the most important measurements in nutritional assessment. Weight, which is relative to height and frame size, is often used as a tool to determine nutritional status and risk. Changes in usual body weight should be ascertained. It is important to note the percent of weight loss as well as the rate of weight loss. Unintentional weight loss greater than 10% is associated with a poor clinical outcome.[16,17] However, it is often difficult to assess true tissue loss. Weight fluctuations are common in GI disease due to malabsorption and side effects of corticosteroid therapy and dehydration. It is especially important to note any significant increase or decrease in GI losses via stomas, drains, tubes, or fistulae.

The body mass index (BMI) is calculated as weight in kilograms divided by height in meters squared. A BMI of 14 to 15 is associated with significant mortality. However, measurements of body weight in patients in hospitals and intensive care units and those with liver disease, cancer, and renal failure are confounded by changes in body water due to dehydration, edema, and ascites. Additionally, healthy BMI indices will vary for individuals of different populations and cultures.

There are other more sophisticated measures available including isotope dilution, bioelectrical impedance analysis (BIA), bioelectrical impedance spectroscopy (BIS), dual-energy x-ray absorptiometry (DXA) neutron-activation analysis, computerized axial tomography, and magnetic resonance imaging. Although these methods are accurate, they are not practical in the clinical setting. The only methods that are available for wide clinical application in nutritional assessment are BIA and BIS. Both of these techniques have shown that reduced fat-free mass increases length of stay in hospitalized patients. However, limitations exist in the generalization of these equations to the patient with GI disorders, particularly if they have large fluid losses from high output ostomies. Water and electrolyte disturbances, which are common in intestinal failure, may skew impedance measurements leading to over- or underestimation of malnutrition in this population.[18,19] Pichard et al. studied the use of BIA in chronically ill patients and confirmed the need for disease-specific BIA equations.[19]

2.2.4 Muscle Function Assessment

In addition to measuring the amount of lean muscle, there is interest in measuring the functional capacity of the muscle mass. This may provide a more meaningful evaluation than a static measurement of absolute muscle mass. Deficits in muscle function have been linked to nutritional depletion and higher incidences of postoperative complications among hospitalized patients.[20–22]

Several methods exist for the assessment of muscle function in the hospital and ambulatory clinics. One of the simplest functional tests for alert and cooperative patients is grip strength, measured with a small, portable handgrip dynometer. In a study of 120 patients undergoing elective major abdominal surgery, the most useful index to determine postoperative complications was hand-grip dynamometry, which predicted 90% of those who developed complications.[23] A grip strength below 85% of standard for age and sex was found by Webb et al. to be the most specific predictor of postoperative risk; however, research has yet to show the benefits of preoperative nutrition support in the at-risk population.[24]

Handgrip strength was also found to be significantly less in chronically energy-deficient and underweight young males as compared to those who were well-nourished but underweight or of normal weight status.[25] This implies a potential use of grip strength in the differentiation of patients with similar weights, but conflicting nutritional status.

2.2.5 Laboratory

Historically, hepatic transport proteins have been used to assess nutritional status. These proteins can be categorized into negative and positive acute-phase proteins (Table 2.4). It is the negative acute phase proteins that are often used as a tool for nutritional assessment. Serum levels of these proteins are largely affected by variations in synthesis, degradation, and distribution seen with chronic malnutrition or acute stress. Despite these confounding factors, they have long been used to evaluate nutritional status and guide nutrition intervention strategies. There were 12 early studies published that correlated serum protein concentrations with duration of nutrition support, anthropometric measurements, morbidity, and mortality, and concluded or assumed that nutrition was the primary causative variable.[26] However, these studies overlooked the influence of inflammatory metabolism as well as the mediators of inflammatory metabolism.[27] Later studies, however, suggested that the changes in these markers were actually caused by inflammation. There were 11 studies that correlated serum proteins concentrations with morbidity and mortality, some inflammatory makers, and concluded that inflammation is the primary causative variable.[26]

During acute stress and inflammation there are significant changes in protein metabolism. Albumin levels often fall dramatically in response to increased degradation, decreased synthesis with preferential use of amino acids for production

TABLE 2.4
Acute Phase Proteins

Negative	Positive
Albumin (Alb)	Fibrinogen
Transferrin (TFN)	Prothrombin
Thyroxine-Binding Prealbumin (TBPA)	Antihemophiliac
Rentinol Binding Protein (RBP)	Plasminogen
Fibronectin	Complement proteins
Insulin-like Growth Factor (IGF)	Alpha 1 antitrypsin
	Alpha 1 antichymotrypsin
	Pancreatic secretory trypsin inhibitor
	Haptoglobin
	Ceruloplasmin
	C-reactive Protein (CRP)

of acute phase proteins, and increased vascular permeability with redistribution of albumin to extravascular spaces.[28] During obligatory muscle and connective tissue proteolysis, stress depresses albumin levels.[29] This proteolysis is mediated by leukocyte pyrogen (IL-1) in sepsis and trauma.[30] Nitrogen balance studies have been used to evaluate protein status. But these equations measure net balance (intake and output) and do not measure synthesis and breakdown for which an isotopic tracer is required.[31] The issue becomes more complicated when considering total body protein versus hepatic protein metabolism. In a study of protein metabolism during sepsis and multiple injury, hepatic proteins were measured 5, 10, 15, and 21 days after injury in 24 critically ill patients who were hemodynamically stable and compared to total body protein metabolism.[32] Hepatic proteins returned to normal levels, total body proteolysis continued, and energy expenditure increased. The authors concluded that normalization of hepatic protein metabolism was independent of total body protein metabolism.

The degree of inflammation must be considered in assessing nutritional status and nutrition intervention. Nutrition support alone is inadequate to prevent loss of lean body mass during inflammation. Many medical conditions are also inflammatory states. Many conditions that afflict GI patients, such as trauma, infection, pancreatitis, cachexia, rheumatoid arthritis, advanced age, obesity, and periodontal disease, are also considered inflammatory states. Nutrition support during inflammatory metabolism probably supports acute phase metabolism, although this has not been proven. In the absence of successful interruption of inflammatory metabolism, the anabolic phase of recovery is the time for nutritional repletion.

The metabolism of these protein markers is different in uncomplicated conditions of nutrient intake deficit and may be more clinically useful. In chronic uncomplicated starvation, serum albumin concentrations are maintained near normal due to decreased catabolism and shifts in distribution from extra- to intravascular spaces.[33,34] In a study of very low calorie diets with different compositions, obese adults were given 1,200 and 180 to 500 calorie weight loss diets for 20 days.[35] In the 1,200 calorie group, serum albumin, thyroxine binding prealbumin (TBPA), and retinol binding protein (RBP) remained the same. However, in the very low calorie group, PAB and RBP decreased at day 5 and remained constant. Changes in plasma proteins during acute nutritional deprivation in healthy human subjects were evaluated. Albumin, transferrin (TFN), and fibronectin concentrations during acute nutrient deprivation and refeeding in healthy adults were monitored over a 15-day trial, which included 5 days of normal diet, 4 days of nothing but water followed by 10 days of a normal diet.[36] Fibronectin decreased by day 2 of starvation. Albumin and TFN remained the constant. During refeeding fibronectin normalized, TFN decreased, and albumin increased. The authors concluded that the changes in albumin and TFN reflect changes in intravascular fluid volume. However, fibronectin responded immediately to both stimuli: starvation and refeeding. In other uncomplicated examples of starvation, such as anorexia nervosa, serum transport protein concentrations remain relatively stable.[37, 38]

Overall, serum transport protein concentrations do not change in uncomplicated states of undernutrition. The fast turnover proteins change quickly with deprivation and feeding, but are obscured by infection. These changes reflect the state of normal undernutrition versus inflammatory metabolism with or without undernutrition. During uncomplicated undernutrition (adaptive starvation), lean body mass and protein loss is minimized, substrate metabolism adapts to increased fat and ketone oxidation. This is reversed by provision of exogenous substrate in the form of nutrition. During inflammatory metabolism, nitrogen loss is accelerated by muscle catabolism and hepatic protein metabolism is radically altered. This state cannot be reversed by exogenous substrate provision (nutrition). During acute phase metabolism, there is a heightened immune response, tissue repair, and substrate mobilization. Hepatic protein metabolism is changed to facilitate this process.[39] During this period, negative acute phase proteins decrease synthesis by at least 25%, while positive acute phase proteins increase synthesis by 25%.

It is enticing to use these proteins as determinates of nutritional status as they are readily available for general use. They are still important tools to be used clinically. Serum proteins are strong prognostic indicators of morbidity,[40] mortality,[41] length of hospital stay,[42] and surgical risk[43] among hospitalized patients. However, they have little to do with nutritional status. The question becomes what is the best use of hepatic positive and negative acute phase proteins in nutrition assessment and monitoring? They do indicate metabolic state. They also indicate the severity of illness and inflammation. They predict the potential need for nutrition interventions; not to normalize serum assays, but because acute and chronic illness and trauma cause anorexia.

2.2.6 MICRONUTRIENT STATUS

Vitamins and trace elements are substances that function as co-enzymes in metabolism and are essential in small quantities. Laboratory assessment of vitamins and trace elements can be useful in detecting subclinical nutrient deficiencies or excess before physical signs manifest. For many of these nutrients, tissue or hair analysis represents the most accurate method of assessment. However, these are not practical in a clinical setting. For the patient with GI disorders, it may be prudent to measure serum levels of these micronutrients particularly if the GI disorder results in decreased intake, malabsorption, or increased GI losses. This is especially important for those individuals on long-term parenteral nutrition. In these instances, the micronutrient composition of the parenteral nutrition formula can be customized. Even for those patients not on specialized nutrition support, the abnormal vitamin and trace levels should be repleted with oral supplementation.

2.2.7 Subjective Global Assessment

Assessment of nutritional status is complex. Unfortunately, no single parameter is able to consistently determine the degree and type of malnutrition in all types of patients. Baker et al.[44] and Detsky et al.[45] developed the technique of subjective global assessment (SGA) based on the principle that findings from a routine clinical examination can correlate with objective measurements and predict clinical outcomes with greater accuracy than objective measurements in a wide range of patient populations.[46,47] The SGA classification is described as follows:

1. History
   - Weight change
   - Change in dietary intake patterns over time
   - Presence of gastrointestinal symptoms persisting for more than two weeks
   - Change in functional capacity over time
   - Primary diagnosis and level of metabolic demand
2. Physical
   - Degree of loss of subcutaneous fat
   - Degree of muscle wasting
   - Degree of edema
   - Degree of ascites
   - Presence of mucosal, cutaneous, or hair abnormalities
3. Subjective Global Assessment Rating
   - A = well nourished
   - B = moderately (or suspected of being) malnourished
   - C = severely malnourished

This subjective approach defines malnourished patients as those who are at increased risk for medical complications and who will most likely benefit from nutritional intervention. The basis of this assessment is to determine whether nutrient metabolism has been altered because of reduced food intake, maldigestion, or malabsorption; whether any effects of malnutrition on organ function and body composition have occurred; and whether the patient's disease process influences nutrient requirements. Unlike traditional methods that rely on objective anthropometric and biochemical data, SGA is based on four elements of the patient's history (recent weight loss, changes in usual diet, presence of significant gastrointestinal symptoms, and the patient's functional capacity) and three elements of the physical examination (loss of subcutaneous fat, muscle wasting, and presence of edema or ascites).

SGA is relatively simple to use. Additionally, despite the subjective nature, the results are reproducible when used by trained clinicians. The interrater reproducibility among nurses and medical residents using SGA was 91% agreement,[46] and among medical residents and specialists in clinical nutrition with 79% agreement.[48]

The ability of SGA to predict outcome and adequately assess nutritional status has been compared to other traditional methods. In a prospective analysis of 59 surgical patients, the predictive value of SGA was compared to different standard techniques.[45] Preoperative SGA was a better predictor of postoperative infectious complications than serum albumin, TFN, delayed cutaneous hypersensitivity, anthropometry, creatinine height index, and the prognostic nutritional index. Combining SGA with some of the traditional markers of nutritional status increased the ability to identify patients who developed complications from 82 to 90% and also increased the percentage of patients who were identified as malnourished but who did not develop postoperative complications from 25 to 30%. Thus, by increasing sensitivity, the number of patients who might receive unnecessary nutrition intervention is reduced.

The ability of SGA to predict body composition was evaluated in a study, which compared SGA to bioelectrical impedance (BIA) measurements of fat-free mass (FFM). FFM was significantly lower in patients classified as severely malnourished by SGA than in those classified as well nourished by SGA.[49] However, SGA classification did not correlate with BIA measurements of FFM in a study of 47 intestinal failure patients receiving home parenteral nutrition.[50] The authors concluded that SGA in combination with a weight history would be sufficient for the assessment of malnutrition in this population.

SGA also has been shown to be a powerful predictor of postoperative complications. Several studies have reported successful use of the SGA to predict complications in general surgical patients,[48] patients on dialysis,[51–53] and liver transplant patients.[54] In each of these studies, significantly more complications were observed in the severely malnourished versus moderate and mildly malnourished patients.

2.3   PREDICTION OF COMPLICATIONS AND DECISION TO INTERVENE

Can nutritional assessment predict which patients will have complications and which patients will benefit from nutrition intervention? There is a clear distinction between prediction of complications and prediction of those who will benefit from nutrition intervention. While many of the tools for nutritional assessment predict potential complications, they may not be able to adequately identify patients who would benefit from nutrition support. Since nutritional support therapies do carry some risk, the potential benefit-to-risk ratio must be considered before instituting. Some of the assessment tools identify patients who have had reduced intake, other tools demonstrate the degree of illness. The exact impact of nutrition on disease outcome has not been clearly demarcated in all disease states. Yet, there is no clinical condition that benefits from malnutrition. It seems intuitive that the provision of nutrition to malnourished patients would produce positive outcomes. However, to date, there have not been any prospective controlled clinical trials demonstrating that providing nutrition support to malnourished patients influences outcome. A retrospective subgroup analysis of a large multicenter trial found that parenteral nutrition given preoperatively to severely malnourished patients or those at nutritional risk decreased postoperative complications.[55]

2.4   IMPACT OF NUTRITION ON DISEASE

There is an intimate relationship between nutrition and GI disease. GI disease may result in undernutrition or frank malnutrition as a consequence of loss of appetite, maldigestion, malabsorption, or increased metabolic demand. It is clear that an inadequate intake of food over time will result in the physiological, body composition, functional, cognitive, and psychological changes that together constitute a state of malnutrition. Malnutrition can result in an increase in the risk of disease. Conversely, malnutrition can be a consequence of GI disease either by increased metabolic demand or reduced nutrient intake.

When intake is poor or absent for a prolonged period, weight loss is associated with organ failure and death (see Figure 2.1). Life-threatening undernutrition is classified as a loss of about one-third of body weight or a BMI $\leq$ 15 kg/m^2. Death will ensue when 40% of lean tissue is lost during acute starvation and 50% is lost during chronic starvation.[56] During the Irish Republican Army (IRA) hunger strikes, previously healthy lean individuals survived between 57 and 73 days without food.[57] The mean weight loss of the group was 38% and one-third of them died. Thus, in the absence of disease, one can anticipate that previously normally nourished adults may die of starvation in approximately 60 days. Superimpose illness and injury onto this, and one can anticipate death much sooner in the hospitalized patient. Studley showed that if patients lost more than 20% of their body weight prior to surgery for peptic ulcer disease, they had a 33% mortality compared with 4% if less than 20% body weight had been lost.[58] Keys and colleagues conducted a number of studies on conscientious objectors to World War II to evaluate the physiological effects of starvation and refeeding.[59] Thirty-two male volunteers were semistarved during a six-month period with an average consumption of 1,570 kcal, 50 gm of protein, and 30 gm of fat. The resulting decline in organ system functions was systematically recorded. Nutritional deprivation had a negative impact on every organ system studied including the GI tract. The subjects developed diarrhea, peptic ulcers, changes in gastric motility, and even changes in the position of the stomach.

The effects of undernutrition on the GI tract are particularly important. Apart from its role in digestion and absorption, the GI tract constitutes a major immune organ, acting as a barrier to prevent the translocation of bacteria into the body. Adequate nutrition is important to preserve gut barrier function. The intestine is unique in that it is nourished by two mechanisms, from the circulation and from nutrients passing directly through the lumen.[60] The epithelial cells of the gut have extraordinary turnover and are renewed every two to three days. Luminal nutrients are the most potent stimulus for mucosal cell proliferation and intestinal adaptation. Interestingly, luminal and systemic starvation can occur separately as when a patient is supported with parenteral nutrition, but receives no nutrition via the enteral route. Alternatively, a patient may be chronically depleted, but may be able to maintain a minimal enteral intake in the form of diet or tube feeding. The diet may or may not contain all the necessary nutrients or the patient may not receive adequate amounts of tube feeding to maintain the health of the GI tract.

The effects of acute and chronic undernutrition in the presence of disease relate to the end result of altered immune function, impaired wound healing, and overall decrease in functional status. This ultimately translates into increased length of stay (LOS), increased hospital costs as well as greater morbidity and mortality. The associations between malnutrition and poor outcome are not confined to the general surgical population. Similar findings have been demonstrated in GI and liver disease. Alberino and colleagues studied 212 hospitalized patients with liver cirrhosis clinically for two years or until death.[61] Severe depletion of muscle mass and body fat were found to be independent predictors of survival. The inclusion of anthropometric measurements in the Child–Pugh score, the prognostic score used most with liver disease, improved its prognostic accuracy. These data demonstrate that malnutrition is an independent predictor of survival in patients with liver cirrhosis.

In a prospective study of 1,053 cirrhotic patients, Child–Pugh classification as well as clinical and biochemical variables were used to assess the severity of cirrhosis and to determine whether malnutrition was a risk factor for mortality in cirrhotic patients.[62] Nutritional status was evaluated both by anthropometric and clinical measurements. In the univariate analysis, the presence of muscle depletion and/or reduction in fat deposits was associated with a higher risk of mortality.

There are data to suggest that a significant proportion of patients undergoing liver transplantation are nutritionally compromised and that this affects patient infection, susceptibility, graft function, and mortality, which may possibly be improved by nutritional intervention. In a prospective study, the effect of nutritional status on outcome in 102 consecutive adult patients undergoing elective orthotopic liver transplantation was examined. Midarm muscle circumference was calculated.[63] Patient outcome variables included time spent in the intensive care unit, total time in hospital, infectious complications, and mortality. Graft outcome variables included early graft function, peak aspartate transaminase, alkaline phosphatase, bilirubin, and prothrombin time. There were significantly more bacterial infections in the malnourished group and a difference in mortality up to six months postoperatively. Additionally, there were significant differences between the malnourished and the well-nourished patients for peak alkaline phosphatase and peak prothrombin. In a retrospective analysis of 99 orthotopic liver transplants, severely malnourished patients require more blood products during surgery and have prolonged postoperative length of stay in hospital.[64]

Severe preoperative malnutrition has a positive predictive value for mortality in patients with gastric cancer. In a prospective study of 40 patients with gastric adenocarcinoma treated surgically, patients who died presented with a significantly greater preoperative cellular immunosuppression than those who survived.[65]

Postoperative mortality correlated significantly with hypoalbuminemia and weight loss. Clearly there is evidence that nutrition impacts the clinical course of the patient with GI disease.

2.5 CONCLUSION

Malnutrition produces a wide range of physiological effects ranging from biochemical alterations, clinical manifestations, and, ultimately, death. Although, the full extent of the relationship between nutrition and disease has not been fully elucidated, there is no clinical condition that benefits from a state of malnutrition. Malnutrition also increases the need for healthcare and healthcare resources. The more severe the malnutrition, the more costly the intervention required and the greater the risk in providing the intervention. The goal of nutritional assessment is to identify those patients who are or may become malnourished. Assessment of nutritional status at first glance appears intuitive. But it is a complex process and encompasses all body systems. Once malnutrition has been identified, a plan for safe and effective intervention must follow. The nutritional assessment must continue during the nutrition therapy in order to ensure safe and effective therapy.

REFERENCES

1. Klein S, Kinney J, Jeejeebhoy K, et al. Nutrition support in clinical practice: review of published data and recommendations for future research directions. National Institutes of Health, American Society for Parenteral and Enteral Nutrition, and American Society for Clinical Nutrition. *Jpen: Journal of Parenteral & Enteral Nutrition.* May–Jun 1997;21(3):133–156.
2. Brolin RE, Gorman JH, Gorman RC, et al. Are vitamin B12 and folate deficiency clinically important after Roux-en-Y gastric bypass? *Journal of Gastrointestinal Surgery.* Sep–Oct 1998;2(5):436–442.
3. Escalona A, Perez G, Leon F, et al. Wernicke's encephalopathy after Roux-en-Y gastric bypass. *Obesity Surgery.* Sep 2004;14(8):1135–1137.
4. Halverson JD. Vitamin and mineral deficiencies following obesity surgery. *Gastroenterology Clinics of North America.* Jun 1987;16(2):307–315.
5. Koffman BM, Greenfield LJ, Ali, II, Pirzada NA. Neurologic complications after surgery for obesity. *Muscle & Nerve.* Feb 2006;33(2):166–176.
6. Love AL, Billett HH. Obesity, bariatric surgery, and iron deficiency: true, true, true and related. *American Journal of Hematology.* May 2008;83(5):403–409.
7. Madan AK, Orth WS, Tichansky DS, Ternovits CA. Vitamin and trace mineral levels after laparoscopic gastric bypass. *Obesity Surgery.* May 2006;16(5):603–606.
8. Malinowski SS. Nutritional and metabolic complications of bariatric surgery. *American Journal of the Medical Sciences.* Apr 2006;331(4):219–225.
9. Skroubis G, Sakellaropoulos G, Pouggouras K, Mead N, Nikiforidis G, Kalfarentzos F. Comparison of nutritional deficiencies after Roux-en-Y gastric bypass and after biliopancreatic diversion with Roux-en-Y gastric bypass. *Obesity Surgery.* Aug 2002;12(4):551–558.
10. Tan JC, Burns DL, Jones HR. Severe ataxia, myelopathy, and peripheral neuropathy due to acquired copper deficiency in a patient with history of gastrectomy. *Jpen: Journal of Parenteral & Enteral Nutrition.* Sep–Oct 2006;30(5):446–450.

11. National Task Force on the Prevention and Treatment of Obesity: overweight, obesity, and health risk. *Archives of Internal Medicine.* Apr 10 2000;160(7):898–904.
12. Despres JP, Moorjani S, Lupien PJ, Tremblay A, Nadeau A, Bouchard C. Regional distribution of body fat, plasma lipoproteins, and cardiovascular disease. *Arteriosclerosis.* Jul–Aug 1990;10(4):497–511.
13. Lemieux S, Prud'homme D, Bouchard C, Tremblay A, Despres JP. A single threshold value of waist girth identifies normal-weight and overweight subjects with excess visceral adipose tissue. *American Journal of Clinical Nutrition.* Nov 1996;64(5):685–693.
14. Wang Y, Rimm EB, Stampfer MJ, Willett WC, Hu FB. Comparison of abdominal adiposity and overall obesity in predicting risk of type 2 diabetes among men[see comment]. *American Journal of Clinical Nutrition.* Mar 2005;81(3):555–563.
15. Bray GA, Champagne CM. Obesity and the metabolic syndrome: implications for dietetics practitioners. *Journal of the American Dietetic Association.* Jan 2004;104(1):86–89.
16. Stanley KE. Prognostic factors for survival in patients with inoperable lung cancer. *Journal of the National Cancer Institute.* Jul 1980;65(1):25–32.
17. Dewys WD, Begg C, Lavin PT, et al. Prognostic effect of weight loss prior to chemotherapy in cancer patients. Eastern Cooperative Oncology Group. *American Journal of Medicine.* Oct 1980;69(4):491–497.
18. Royall D, Greenberg GR, Allard JP, Baker JP, Harrison JE, Jeejeebhoy KN. Critical assessment of body-composition measurements in malnourished subjects with Crohn's disease: the role of bioelectric impedance analysis. *American Journal of Clinical Nutrition.* Feb 1994;59(2):325–330.
19. Pichard C, Kyle UG, Slosman DO. Fat-free mass in chronic illness: comparison of bioelectrical impedance and dual-energy x-ray absorptiometry in 480 chronically ill and healthy subjects. *Nutrition.* Sep 1999;15(9):668–676.
20. Russell DM, Leiter LA, Whitwell J, Marliss EB, Jeejeebhoy KN. Skeletal muscle function during hypocaloric diets and fasting: a comparison with standard nutritional assessment parameters. *American Journal of Clinical Nutrition.* Jan 1983;37(1):133–138.
21. Klidjian AM, Foster KJ, Kammerling RM, Cooper A, Karran SJ. Relation of anthropometric and dynamometric variables to serious postoperative complications. *British Medical Journal.* Oct 4 1980;281(6245):899–901.
22. Hunt DR, Rowlands BJ, Johnston D. Hand grip strength—a simple prognostic indicator in surgical patients. *Jpen: Journal of Parenteral & Enteral Nutrition.* Nov–Dec 1985;9(6):701–704.
23. Klidjian AM, Archer TJ, Foster KJ, Karran SJ. Detection of dangerous malnutrition. *Jpen: Journal of Parenteral & Enteral Nutrition.* Mar–Apr 1982;6(2):119–121.
24. Webb AR, Newman LA, Taylor M, Keogh JB. Hand grip dynamometry as a predictor of postoperative complications reappraisal using age standardized grip strengths. *Jpen: Journal of Parenteral & Enteral Nutrition.* Jan–Feb 1989;13(1):30–33.
25. Vaz M, Thangam S, Prabhu A, Shetty PS. Maximal voluntary contraction as a functional indicator of adult chronic undernutrition. *British Journal of Nutrition.* Jul 1996;76(1):9–15.
26. Fuhrman MP, Charney P, Mueller CM. Hepatic proteins and nutrition assessment. *Journal of the American Dietetic Association.* Aug 2004;104(8):1258–1264.
27. Jensen GL. Inflammation as the key interface of the medical and nutrition universes: a provocative examination of the future of clinical nutrition and medicine. *Jpen: Journal of Parenteral & Enteral Nutrition.* Sep–Oct 2006;30(5):453–463.
28. Vanek VW. The use of serum albumin as a prognostic or nutritional marker and the pros and cons of IV albumin therapy. *Nutrition in Clinical Practice* 1998 Jun;13(3): 110–122 (88 ref).

29. Lakshman K, Blackburn GL. Monitoring nutritional status in the critically ill adult. *Journal of Clinical Monitoring.* Apr 1986;2(2):114–120.
30. Moldawer LL, Bistrian BR, Sobrado J, Blackburn GL. Muscle proteolysis in sepsis or trauma. *New England Journal of Medicine.* Aug 25 1983;309(8):494–495.
31. O'Keefe SJ, Moldawer LL, Young VR, Blackburn GL. The influence of intravenous nutrition on protein dynamics following surgery. *Metabolism: Clinical & Experimental.* Dec 1981;30(12):1150–1158.
32. Clark MA, Hentzen BT, Plank LD, Hill GI. Sequential changes in insulin-like growth factor 1, plasma proteins, and total body protein in severe sepsis and multiple injury. *Jpen: Journal of Parenteral & Enteral Nutrition.* Sep–Oct 1996;20(5):363–370.
33. Hoffenberg R, Black E, Brock JF. Albumin and gamma-globulin tracer studies in protein depletion states. *Journal of Clinical Investigation.* Jan 1966;45(1):143–152.
34. James WP, Hay AM. Albumin metabolism: effect of the nutritional state and the dietary protein intake. *Journal of Clinical Investigation.* Sep 1968;47(9):1958–1972.
35. Scalfi L, Laviano A, Reed LA, Borrelli R, Contaldo F. Albumin and labile-protein serum concentrations during very-low-calorie diets with different compositions. *American Journal of Clinical Nutrition.* Mar 1990;51(3):338–342.
36. Chadwick SJ, Sim AJ, Dudley HA. Changes in plasma fibronectin during acute nutritional deprivation in healthy human subjects. *British Journal of Nutrition.* Jan 1986;55(1):7–12.
37. Van Binsbergen CJ, Odink J, Van den Berg H, Koppeschaar H, Coelingh Bennink HJ. Nutritional status in anorexia nervosa: clinical chemistry, vitamins, iron and zinc. *European Journal of Clinical Nutrition.* Nov 1988;42(11):929–937.
38. Barbe P, Bennet A, Stebenet M, Perret B, Louvet JP. Sex-hormone-binding globulin and protein-energy malnutrition indexes as indicators of nutritional status in women with anorexia nervosa. *American Journal of Clinical Nutrition.* Mar 1993;57(3):319–322.
39. Gabay C, Kushner I. Acute-phase proteins and other systemic responses to inflammation.[erratum appears in *N Engl J Med* 1999 Apr 29;340(17):1376]. *New England Journal of Medicine.* Feb 11 1999;340(6):448–454.
40. Anderson CF, Wochos DN. The utility of serum albumin values in the nutritional assessment of hospitalized patients. *Mayo Clinic Proceedings.* Mar 1982;57(3):181–184.
41. Apelgren KN, Rombeau JL, Twomey PL, Miller RA. Comparison of nutritional indices and outcome in critically ill patients. *Critical Care Medicine.* May 1982;10(5):305–307.
42. dos Santos Junqueira JC, Cotrim Soares E, Rodrigues Correa Filho H, Fenalti Hoehr N, Oliveira Magro D, Ueno M. Nutritional risk factors for postoperative complications in Brazilian elderly patients undergoing major elective surgery. *Nutrition.* Apr 2003;19(4):321–326.
43. Mears E. Outcomes of continuous process improvement of a nutritional care program incorporating serum prealbumin measurements[see comment]. *Nutrition.* Jul–Aug 1996;12(7–8):479–484.
44. Baker JP, Detsky AS, Wesson DE, et al. Nutritional assessment: a comparison of clinical judgement and objective measurements. *New England Journal of Medicine.* Apr 22 1982;306(16):969–972.
45. Detsky AS, Baker JP, Mendelson RA, Wolman SL, Wesson DE, Jeejeebhoy KN. Evaluating the accuracy of nutritional assessment techniques applied to hospitalized patients: methodology and comparisons. *Jpen: Journal of Parenteral & Enteral Nutrition.* Mar–Apr 1984;8(2):153–159.
46. Detsky AS, McLaughlin JR, Baker JP, et al. What is subjective global assessment of nutritional status? *Jpen: Journal of Parenteral & Enteral Nutrition.* Jan–Feb 1987;11(1):8–13.

47. Jeejeebhoy KN, Baker JP, Wolman SL, et al. Critical evaluation of the role of clinical assessment and body composition studies in patients with malnutrition and after total parenteral nutrition. *American Journal of Clinical Nutrition.* May 1982;35(5 Suppl):1117–1127.

48. Hirsch S, de Obaldia N, Petermann M, et al. Subjective global assessment of nutritional status: further validation. *Nutrition.* Jan–Feb 1991;7(1):35–37; discussion 37–38.

49. Kyle UG, Unger P, Mensi N, Genton L, Pichard C. Nutrition status in patients younger and older than 60 y at hospital admission: a controlled population study in 995 subjects. *Nutrition.* Jun 2002;18(6):463–469.

50. Egger NG, Carlson GL, Shaffer JL. Nutritional status and assessment of patients on home parenteral nutrition: anthropometry, bioelectrical impedance, or clinical judgment?[see comment]. *Nutrition.* Jan 1999;15(1):1–6.

51. Fenton SS, Johnston N, Delmore T, et al. Nutritional assessment of continuous ambulatory peritoneal dialysis patients. *ASAIO Transactions.* Jul–Sep 1987;33(3):650–653.

52. Young GA, Kopple JD, Lindholm B, et al. Nutritional assessment of continuous ambulatory peritoneal dialysis patients: an international study. *American Journal of Kidney Diseases.* Apr 1991;17(4):462–471.

53. Enia G, Sicuso C, Alati G, Zoccali C. Subjective global assessment of nutrition in dialysis patients. *Nephrology Dialysis Transplantation.* 1993;8(10):1094–1098.

54. Hasse J, Strong S, Gorman MA, Liepa G. Subjective global assessment: alternative nutrition-assessment technique for liver-transplant candidates. *Nutrition.* Jul–Aug 1993;9(4):339–343.

55. The Veterans Affairs Total Parenteral Nutrition Cooperative Study Group. Perioperative total parenteral nutrition in surgical patients. *New England Journal of Medicine.* Aug 22 1991;325(8):525–532.

56. Massry SG, Smogorzewski M. The hunger disease of the Warsaw Ghetto. *American Journal of Nephrology.* Jul 2002;22(2–3):197–201.

57. Elia M. Metabolic response to starvation, injury and sepsis. In: Payne-James J, Grimble, G, Silk, D, ed. *Artificial Nutrition Support in Clinical Practice.* London: Greenwich Medical Media; 2001:1–24.

58. Studley HO. Percentage of weight loss as a basic indicator of surgical risk in patients with chronic peptic ulcer disease. *Journal of the American Medical Association* 1936;106:458–460.

59. Keys A, Brozek, J., Henschel, A., Michelsen, O., Taylor, H.L. *The Biology of Human Starvation.* Minneapolis: University of Minnesota Press; 1950.

60. Roediger WE. Famine, fiber, fatty acids, and failed colonic absorption: does fiber fermentation ameliorate diarrhea? *Jpen: Journal of Parenteral & Enteral Nutrition.* Jan–Feb 1994;18(1):4–8.

61. Alberino F, Gatta A, Amodio P, et al. Nutrition and survival in patients with liver cirrhosis. *Nutrition.* Jun 2001;17(6):445–450.

62. Merli M, Riggio O, Dally L. Does malnutrition affect survival in cirrhosis? PINC (Policentrica Italiana Nutrizione Cirrosi). *Hepatology.* May 1996;23(5):1041–1046.

63. Harrison J, McKiernan J, Neuberger JM. A prospective study on the effect of recipient nutritional status on outcome in liver transplantation. *Transplant International.* 1997;10(5):369–374.

64. Stephenson GR, Moretti EW, El-Moalem H, Clavien PA, Tuttle-Newhall JE. Malnutrition in liver transplant patients: preoperative subjective global assessment is predictive of outcome after liver transplantation. *Transplantation.* Aug 27 2001;72(4):666–670.

65. Rey-Ferro M, Castano R, Orozco O, Serna A, Moreno A. Nutritional and immunologic evaluation of patients with gastric cancer before and after surgery. *Nutrition.* Oct 1997;13(10):878–881.

3 Management of Disorders of Deglutition

Ryan F. Porter and C. Prakash Gyawali

CONTENTS

3.1 DEFINITIONS

Dysphagia is the sensation arising from impediment or obstruction to the passage of food from the mouth to the stomach.[1,2] Dysphagia is typically described as food "hanging up" or "sticking" on attempted swallowing. A careful history can lead to the cause of dysphagia in greater than 80% of patients with up to 80% accuracy.[3,4] *Odynophagia* refers to pain during the act of swallowing.[1] *Globus* is distinct from dysphagia and describes a sensation of fullness, discomfort, or a lump in the throat that is constant and does not interfere with swallowing.[1] In fact, globus may actually improve during swallowing. Most patients with globus do not have evidence of organic oropharyngeal or esophageal disease despite exhaustive investigation.[1]

There are two categories of dysphagia: oropharyngeal dysphagia and esophageal dysphagia.[1] Oropharyngeal or transfer dysphagia results from impairment of the transfer of food from the mouth into the proximal esophagus.[1,5] This can result from poor oral preparation of the bolus, weak pharyngeal contraction, inadequate opening of the upper esophageal sphincter (UES), and/or lack of coordination between pharyngeal contraction and UES relaxation. Skeletal muscles involved in these events are innervated by the lower cranial nerves. Consequently, neuromuscular dysfunction related to cerebrovascular accidents or Parkinson's disease is the most frequent mechanism of oropharyngeal dysphagia. Structural obstructive processes, such as webs, luminal narrowings, extrinsic compression, and tumors are much less frequent.[1,6] Common causes of dysphagia and odynophagia are:

Oropharyngeal or Transfer Dysphagia
    Neuromuscular Diseases
        Central Nervous System Diseases
            Cerebrovascular accident
            Parkinson's disease
            Amyotrophic lateral sclerosis
            Central nervous system tumor
            Dementia
            Spinocerebellar degeneration
        Cranial Nerve Diseases
            Diabetes Mellitus
            Paraneoplastic syndromes
            Toxins, e.g., lead poisoning and other neurotoxins
        Myopathic Disorders
            Inflammatory myopathies (e.g., polymyositis, dermatomyositis, collagen vascular disorders)
            Muscular dystrophies
            Thyroid dysfunction (hyperthyroidism, myxedema)
            Myasthenia gravis
            Amyloidosis
            Primary cricopharyngeal dysfunction
        Structural Lesions
            Mucosal and luminal lesions

        Oropharyngeal and proximal esophageal carcinoma
        Benign esophageal tumor
        Esophageal web and stricture
        Corrosive damage
        Head and neck surgery
        Foreign body ingestion
        Radiation related changes
      Extrinsic Lesions
        Thyroid enlargement
        Cervical vertebral osteophytes
        Lymph node enlargement
        Vascular anomalies
    Esophageal Dysphagia
      Structural Lesions
        Mucosal and Luminal Lesions
          Gastroesophageal reflux disease
          Peptic stricture
          Eosinophilic esophagitis
          Esophageal tumors (benign and malignant)
          Congenital esophageal webs and strictures (e.g., Schatzki ring)
          Radiation related stricture
          Corrosive and pill related esophagitis
          Postsurgical change (postfundoplication, anastomotic stricture)
          Foreign body
          Radiation changes
        Extrinsic Lesions
          Vascular anomalies (dysphagia lusoria, dysphagia aortica)
          Thoracic vertebral osteophytes
          Mediastinal tumors (lymph node enlargement, benign and malignant tumors)
          Obstructing lesions of the gastric cardia
      Neuromuscular Diseases
        Spastic and Hypermotility Disorders
          Achalasia
          Diffuse esophageal spasm
          Nonspecific spastic disorders
          Isolated incomplete LES relaxation
        Hypomotility Disorders
          Idiopathic hypomotility
          Hypomotility associated with systemic disorders (e.g., connective tissue disease, scleroderma, diabetes mellitus, hypothyroidism)
  Odynophagia
      Infectious esophagitis
        Candida albicans
        Herpes simplex

> Cytomegalovirus
> Varicella
> Foreign body ingestion
> Corrosive ingestion
> Pill esophagitis
> Reflux esophagitis

Neoplasms

Esophageal dysphagia refers to dysphagia arising from disorders in the tubular esophagus, particularly the distal two-thirds, which consists of smooth muscle innervated by intramural neural plexuses with central control.[1,2] Preprogrammed neural mechanisms of esophageal peristalsis are usually robust and are infrequently affected by systemic or central nervous system disorders. Therefore, structural etiologies are more common causes of esophageal dysphagia than neuromuscular disorders (see list above). Mucosal or intrinsic esophageal lesions that narrow the lumen of the esophagus, and conditions in the mediastinum that compress or encase the esophagus can result in esophageal dysphagia. Disorders that disrupt peristalsis in the smooth muscle esophagus or impair lower esophageal sphincter (LES) relaxation are encountered less frequently.[1,7] Organic dysphagia refers to dysphagia from a demonstrable structural abnormality, in contrast to functional dysphagia where symptoms exist, but no organic etiology is identified even after extensive investigation.

Impaired swallowing can lead to malnutrition, weight loss, and dehydration.[8] Older patients are particularly prone to these complications. Although benign causes of dysphagia can also result in malnutrition and weight loss, these symptoms are more marked and progress more rapidly with malignant dysphagia. Body weight and nutritional status of the patient are indirect indicators of disease duration and severity and need to be assessed during physical examination.

3.2 EVALUATION

3.2.1 OROPHARYNGEAL DYSPHAGIA

At the outset, it is important to accurately assess structural and physiologic mechanisms responsible for oropharyngeal dysphagia, and when possible, determine the underlying cause. Additionally, the safety and practicality of oral feeding needs to be addressed.[1]

A careful history and physical examination complemented with videofluoroscopic swallowing evaluation are essential initial steps. Associated symptoms originating in the oral cavity or oropharynx are common, consisting of drooling, spillage of food or saliva from the mouth because of poor muscular tone, inability to chew, and difficulty in propelling the food bolus into the pharynx. Symptoms of pharyngeal dysfunction include nasal regurgitation of food, tracheal aspiration with coughing, choking episodes or aspiration pneumonia, the need to swallow repeatedly to clear food from the pharynx, dysarthria, and dysphonia. Dysphagia occurring within a second of attempted swallowing is usually oropharyngeal in origin. Symptoms related to xerostomia, or dry mouth, can be mistaken for oropharyngeal dysphagia if a careful history is not obtained.[1] The physical examination should assess for evidence of lower cranial nerves palsies, stroke,

Parkinson's disease, and muscular dystrophies. Patients with myasthenia gravis may complain of fatigability, with worsening symptoms as the day progresses.[1,8]

Assessments for oral and neck masses, lymph nodes, goiters, evidence of previous tracheostomy, head and neck surgery, and radiotherapy are also important. Specific treatments are available for toxic and metabolic myopathies, myasthenia gravis, inflammatory polymyopathies, and certain neoplasms.[8] These conditions should be identified and treated appropriately.

3.2.1.1   Clinical Bedside Evaluation

The first step in the evaluation of oropharyngeal dysphagia is a clinical bedside swallowing evaluation, which consists of clinical assessment of the structural and functional integrity of the oropharyngeal swallowing mechanism, and cranial nerve function.[6] The oral mucosa is inspected to determine salivation and state of dentition. Integrity of cranial nerves is assessed with a careful neurologic examination. Bedside clinical assessment can detect aspiration during the swallowing of liquids with a sensitivity of 97% and a specificity of 69%.[9] In stroke patients, the following six clinical features have been associated with a risk for aspiration when compared to documented aspiration on videofluoroscopy: (1) dysphonia, (2) dysarthria, (3) abnormal volitional cough, (4) abnormal gag reflex, (5) cough on trial swallow, and (6) voice change on trial swallow.[6,10] The presence of two of these six features has an accuracy of 92% in identifying aspiration risk, while the presence of four features increases specificity.[10–12] The occurrence of dysphagia within the first 24 hours after a stroke increases the risk for aspiration pneumonia.[13] In patients with amyotrophic lateral sclerosis and other degenerative disorders, the presence of dysarthria may correlate with oropharyngeal dysphagia.[14] Formal testing of swallowing and intervention to prevent aspiration pneumonia is indicated in these instances.

3.2.1.2   Videofluoroscopic Examination

A modification of the barium swallow is the standard in the evaluation of oropharyngeal dysphagia. This consists of a dynamic videofluoroscopic examination of the swallowing mechanism, using boluses of varying consistencies.[8,15] Aspiration of the administered bolus into the airway can be easily identified (Figure 3.1). This

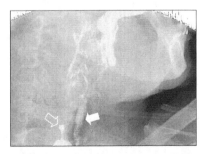

FIGURE 3.1   Aspiration of barium on modified barium swallow: A modified barium swallow in a stroke victim showing a trickle of barium in the larynx and trachea (solid arrow), anterior to the barium column in the esophagus (open arrow). On testing with multiple food consistencies, aspiration occurred with liquids but not with thickened and viscous foods.

examination may be combined with nasal endoscopy for real-time visualization of the pharynx during the act of swallowing and involves the use of special techniques, such as swallowing maneuvers and postures to correct dysfunction. Detailed analysis of physiologic events associated with normal swallowing is performed, along with measurement of bolus transit times.[15] Identification of postdeglutitive pharyngeal residue during videofluoroscopy correlates with an increased aspiration risk.[16] In one series, 90% of 608 dysphagic patients had evidence of aspiration or other swallowing abnormalities resulting in a change in management in 83%.[17]

3.2.1.3   Nasal Endoscopy

Endoscopic assessment is of immense value in assessing the structural integrity of the oropharynx, and addressing aspiration risk with better accuracy compared to clinical examination. A small videoendoscope is introduced through the nostril to assess the pharynx, larynx, and nasopharynx in patients presenting with symptoms suggestive of oropharyngeal dysphagia.[18,19] Flexible endoscopic evaluation of swallowing with sensory testing (FEESST) consists of transnasal fiberoptic endoscopy of the naso- and oropharynx with assessment of laryngopharyngeal sensory discrimination thresholds, using an endoscopically delivered pulse of air to stimulate the mucosa innervated by the superior laryngeal nerve. The technique is safe and well tolerated.[18,19]

3.2.1.4   Imaging Studies

When structural lesions are suspected, computerized tomography (CT) and magnetic resonance imaging (MRI) scans are useful, particularly in the evaluation for central nervous system (CNS) tumors, head and neck tumors, but also CNS lesions, such as stroke, that may be responsible for oropharyngeal neuromuscular dysfunction.[1] Invasion of nerves and musculature responsible for the initiation of swallowing can also be ascertained.

3.2.1.5   Electrodiagnostic Techniques

Distinction between neurogenic and myogenic causes of muscle weakness is sometimes required, and can be achieved with electromyography of the submental muscle, and sometimes the cricopharyngeus.[20] Piezoelectric sensors can be used to study movements of the larynx during swallowing.

3.2.1.6   Laboratory Tests

Blood tests are useful in the diagnosis and follow-up of toxic and metabolic myopathies.[1] The diagnosis of myasthenia gravis can be confirmed by detection of serum acetylcholine receptor antibodies. Serum creatinine phosphokinase is elevated in inflammatory disorders of muscle; erythrocyte sedimentation rate, C-reactive protein, and antinuclear antibody may also be abnormally elevated. Elevated thyroid hormone levels in association with low thyroid-stimulating hormone levels suggest hyperthyroidism or thyrotoxicosis.

3.2.2 Esophageal Dysphagia

As with oropharyngeal dysphagia, careful clinical assessment should precede investigative procedures in the evaluation of esophageal dysphagia. Structural disorders, which predominate as causes of esophageal dysphagia, impair passage of a food bolus, and therefore the initial symptom is usually dysphagia to solids (see above list in Section 3.1). Fixed narrowings from intrinsic esophageal or extrinsic lesions may leave enough patency in the esophageal lumen to allow unimpaired passage of liquids.[1,21] Mild dysphagia to solids can be overcome by chewing food well and drinking liquids to push down the solid bolus. Heartburn is reported by up to 75% of patients with a peptic esophageal stricture; patients with adenocarcinoma associated with Barrett's esophagus also report long-standing heartburn.[22,23] Although, the absence of heartburn does not exclude these conditions, as 25 to 30% of patients with dysphagia from peptic strictures or esophageal adenocarcinoma may have no heartburn at presentation.[24,25] Immunosuppressed patients are prone to esophagitis from opportunistic infections, and may present with dysphagia and odynophagia.[26] Common infections include candida, herpes simplex, and cytomegalovirus, but reflux esophagitis remains in the differential diagnosis. Pill esophagitis can present with dysphagia and odynophagia,[21] and the usual culprits are doxycycline, potassium chloride, alendronate, nonsteroidal antiinflammatory agents, and quinidine.

Disorders that affect esophageal peristalsis can result in dysphagia to both solids and liquids. A long history of dysphagia and regurgitation is seen with achalasia, the prototypical neuromuscular disorder of the tubular esophagus. Chest pain and aspiration pneumonia can occur, and weight loss is common in later stages of the disease.[7] Collagen vascular diseases (typically scleroderma and CREST syndrome, but also rheumatoid arthritis and systemic lupus erythematosus) can be associated with esophageal hypomotility resulting in dysphagia. Severe hypomotility of the esophageal body and hypotonicity of the lower esophageal sphincter can predispose to significant gastroesophageal reflux disease (GERD), sometimes complicated by esophageal strictures, Barrett's esophagus, or even adenocarcinoma.[21,27] Physical examination is usually not particularly revealing, but may demonstrate evidence of collagen vascular disease, or scleroderma (e.g., arthritis, calcinosis, telangiectasia, sclerodactyly, rashes). Lymph nodes, especially in the supraclavicular area, may be seen in neoplastic disorders and oral thrush can be a marker of esophageal candidiasis.[21]

Dysphagia from a benign etiology is generally static or only slowly progressive without significant nutritional impairment or weight loss. Benign esophageal webs or strictures may result in intermittent, short-lived, discrete, symptomatic episodes separated by symptom-free intervals lasting varying periods. In contrast, significant weight loss may occur from dysphagia due to neoplasms.[21,28] The acute onset of esophageal-type dysphagia during a meal suggests food impaction.[1] However, acute onset with symptoms and signs of neurologic impairment may be seen with acute stroke. Both of these situations may result in aphagia or inability to swallow. Dysphagia from obstructive processes in the tubular esophagus may be localized to a point in the chest either above or at the level of the lesion causing the obstruction. Pharyngeal lesions causing dysphagia are typically localized to the front of the neck. Localization of symptoms correspond to the actual site of the lesion in as many as

74% in one series,[29] but localization to the suprasternal notch has limited value in predicting the site of the obstructing lesion. While localization to the cervical region does not necessarily indicate an oropharyngeal process, oropharyngeal dysphagia is never localized to the retrosternal region.[8,21]

3.2.2.1 Upper Endoscopy

Upper endoscopy is preferred as the initial investigative study, and is the test of choice when biopsies or therapeutic dilations are contemplated.[30,31] Since GERD and benign obstructions are the most common diagnoses in dysphagic patients, endoscopy is a reasonable initial test of choice in the primary care setting.[32] In addition to establishing the diagnosis of dysphagia in most instances, endoscopy allows detailed visual inspection of mucosal lesions, enables collection of tissue samples for histopathologic analysis, and offers therapeutic potential.[30] Endoscopy is more sensitive than barium studies in the evaluation of esophageal mucosal lesions and esophagitis. In cost comparisons, initial endoscopy with therapeutic intent is more cost effective than barium swallows if benign obstructive processes are suspected.[32]

3.2.2.2 Barium Studies

Barium upper gastrointestinal studies are more sensitive than endoscopy in detecting subtle esophageal strictures; sensitivity further improves with solid bolus swallows, such as a marshmallow or a 13-mm barium pill.[33,34] Barium studies also have an advantage in patients with Zenker's diverticulum, epiphrenic diverticula, and para-esophageal hernias. Barium studies provide a "road map" for subsequent endoscopy in patients with complex esophageal strictures, where the length and tightness of

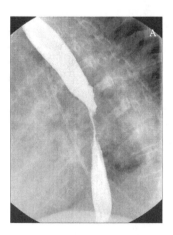
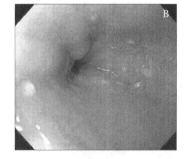

FIGURE 3.2   Esophageal stricture: (A) A tight midesophageal stricture on a barium swallow in an elderly patient who had undergone radiation therapy for lung cancer. The barium study has provided a road map for subsequent endoscopic stricture dilation. (B) Upper endoscopy demonstrates significant narrowing of the esophageal lumen. Since the barium swallow showed a relatively straight strictured segment, a guide wire could be positioned through the stricture and bougie dilation was successfully performed. Also note the rare patches of whitish exudates representing esophageal candidiasis.

the stenosed segment can be easily assessed (Figure 3.2).[30] Barium studies are less expensive than endoscopy for the diagnosis of esophageal disorders, but the cost benefit is lost if therapeutic endoscopy is subsequently performed. Barium studies performed under fluoroscopy can demonstrate certain esophageal motility disorders, particularly achalasia and diffuse esophageal spasm.[35]

3.2.2.3 Esophageal Manometry

Esophageal manometry is used for the evaluation of unexplained dysphagia, after luminal or obstructive lesions have been excluded with a negative endoscopy or barium swallow.[36] In this setting, esophageal motor abnormalities were detected in 90% of patients in one series, but a change in management based on manometric findings is reported in only half the patients referred for this procedure.[37] Advances in this technique include the use of multiple recording sites with computerized data acquisition and topographic display, a technological advance termed high resolution manometry that improves the sensitivity and diagnostic accuracy.[38] The procedure is well tolerated with no serious side effects.[19] Esophageal manometry is the gold standard for the diagnosis of esophageal motor disorders, particularly achalasia, diffuse esophageal spasm, and esophageal hypomotility associated with connective tissue disorders.[36,37] Manometry is less useful in the diagnosis of disordered UES function, but special pharyngeal recording leads can sometimes assist in the characterization of oropharyngeal dysfunction.

3.2.2.4 Imaging Studies

Cross-sectional imaging studies (CT, MRI) are useful in evaluating extrinsic compression of the esophagus and esophageal neoplasia. Positron emission tomography (PET) and endoscopic ultrasound (EUS) are useful in the staging of esophageal neoplasia.

3.3 MANAGEMENT

3.3.1 Oropharyngeal Dysphagia

General measures that can be implemented prior to establishing a diagnosis include assessment of feeding and nutritional needs.[1] Specific pharmacologic, endoscopic, and surgical therapy are only available for a limited number of conditions. Management decisions regarding timing of feeding intervention and route of administration require consideration of the degree of swallowing dysfunction, outcome of swallowing therapy, course of underlying disease process, and patient preferences.[8] The aims of management are to establish oral intake if possible without aspiration using compensatory swallowing techniques, and to concurrently build strength and coordination in oropharyngeal musculature toward eventual unhindered oral intake.[39]

3.3.1.1 Swallowing Therapy and Feeding

Videofluoroscopic analysis is an important tool in assessing swallowing dysfunction and implementing swallowing therapy techniques that may reduce the risk of aspiration.[8,19] These techniques include swallowing maneuvers, postural adjustments, facilitatory techniques, and dietary modifications.[8] Indirect swallowing therapy methods include exercises to enhance the tone and function of muscles involved in swallowing and the swallowing reflex. These methods are more effective when used in conjunction with direct swallowing therapy, consisting of compensatory techniques, such as head and neck positioning during swallowing, supraglottic swallowing, effortful swallowing, and the chin-tuck maneuver.[8,40,41] Despite only modest changes in end-of-trial dysphagia rates, these nonspecific interventions may significantly improve the nutritional state as well as the chances of successful oral feeding in stroke patients. When correctly applied, these measures may allow reversion to oral feeding and removal of gastrostomy feeding tubes thus improving the quality of life in these patients.[42–44]

Oropharyngeal dysphagia is common among patients with stroke, wherein first-year mortality from aspiration pneumonia approaches 20% and subsequent annual mortality remains elevated at 10 to 15%.[45] Formal dysphagia screening of acute stroke patients reduces pneumonia rates.[46] Early behavioral swallowing intervention (e.g., suprahyoid muscle strengthening exercises) improves their ability to resume normal diet and regain swallowing function.[47,48] Aspiration of thin liquids observed videofluorographically can be eliminated in the short term with postural adjustments and thickened liquids.[49] Furthermore, fluid intake may be deficient in stroke patients with dysphagia, and the use of prethickened fluids may help maintain adequate fluid intake while simultaneously addressing nutritional needs.[50] One trial suggests a nonsignificant trend toward lower case fatality with nutritional supplementation in the management of acute stroke.[42] However, it is unclear if postural adjustments or dietary modifications translate into a reduced incidence of aspiration pneumonia.[51] Despite the paucity of data supporting the reduction of mortality or pneumonia risk, potential benefits at relatively low cost drive recommendations for continued use of these postural and dietary adjustments.[8,45,52]

Early initiation of enteral feeding through an endoscopically placed feeding tube (percutaneous endoscopic gastrostomy, PEG) may be superior to nasogastric (NG) tube feeding in the management of acute stroke and dysphagia.[42,53,54] Intolerance of an orally administered pureed diet 14 days after an acute stroke may predict the necessity for enteral feeding using PEG,[55] thereby improving nutritional status as assessed by weight, midarm circumference, and serum albumin when compared to NG tube feeding.[42,54] Further, PEG feeding may prolong survival and reduce treatment failures when compared to NG tube feeding.[42,53,54] However, the reported PEG-related survival benefit may potentially only reflect a higher proportion of survivors with poor outcomes.[56] An alternative to traditional swallowing therapy, neuromuscular electrical stimulation (NMES) is available, but results are variable.[57] Vitamin deficiencies may occur in patients with oropharyngeal dysphagia treated with oral feedings,[58] which can remain undiagnosed unless specific vitamin levels are assessed, particularly cobalamin. Tube-fed patients are less likely to develop these vitamin deficiencies.

3.3.1.2 Surgical Therapy

Surgical intervention is available for Zenker's diverticulum, cricopharyngeal bars, and cricopharyngeus muscle dysfunction. Cricopharyngeal myotomy combined with resection of the diverticulum is a safe and effective procedure that can be performed with relative ease for Zenker's diverticulum.[59,60] Endoscopic diverticulostomy of a moderate-sized Zenker's diverticulum with an endoscopic stapling device or CO_2 laser are effective therapies with good patient results.[61] Patients with manometric evidence of defective upper esophageal stricture opening or elevated cricopharyngeus muscle tone benefit from cricopharyngeal myotomy, particularly in the presence of a symptomatic response to a botulinum toxin injection.[62,63] When aspiration of oropharyngeal secretions and saliva is intractable and continues despite enteral feeding through a PEG tube, laryngotracheal separation or total laryngectomy are options.[64] Relocation of salivary ducts or resection of submandibular salivary glands are rarely performed for hypersalivation.[64]

3.3.1.3 Dilation

Benign proximal esophageal webs and stenoses are effectively disrupted with large caliber (18 to 20 mm) bougie dilation, typically performed over a guide wire.[65] This approach can also be used for elevated UES resting pressures or impaired UES relaxation during swallowing, allowing resumption of oral feeding.[66]

3.3.1.4 Pharmacotherapy

Drug therapy of the causative disorder may improve symptoms in certain myopathic disorders, especially myasthenia gravis and inflammatory myopathies. Myasthenia gravis is amenable to therapy with anticholine esterase agents, oral immunosuppressives, and plasmapheresis.[67] Inflammatory myopathies, such as polymyositis and dermatomyositis also respond to anti-inflammatory and immunosuppressive agents.[68] Conditions associated with excessive salivation and drooling may benefit from anticholinergic medication, especially transdermal scopolamine.[69] There are no data to evaluate the impact of these therapies on dysphagia as a symptom. Cricopharyngeus muscle spasm or hypertonicity and cricopharyngeal achalasia may improve with botulinum toxin injection into the cricopharyngeus.[70] This approach may also provide long-term benefit in neurogenic dysphagia from altered upper esophageal sphincter opening in the presence of preserved pharyngeal contraction.[71] A response to botulinum toxin injection helps confirm the diagnosis in these patients.[70,72]

3.3.2 ESOPHAGEAL DYSPHAGIA

General measures recommended for all patients with esophageal dysphagia include advice to chew food well and to avoid hurried meals. Patients with esophageal narrowing from strictures or neoplasia benefit from a soft or pureed diet. Nutritional supplementation is recommended when dysphagia results in weight loss, in the form of liquid nutritional supplements, enteral tube feedings, or even parenteral nutrition. Specific management depends on the etiology of dysphagia.[1,21]

3.3.2.1 Esophageal Strictures

Intermittent endoscopic dilation is effective in the therapy of peptic esophageal strictures, esophageal webs, and rings.[73,74] Approximately 35% of strictures require repeated dilation within one year.[75] Injection of steroids (triamcinolone 40 to 80 mg) into mucosal rents created by stricture dilation can sometimes prolong the intervals between repeat dilations.[74,76] Benign idiopathic and congenital distal esophageal rings, such as Schatzki rings, can be treated with electrosurgical incision or bougie dilation. Both are safe and effective options, but long-term outcome data are lacking.[77–80] Rings require less frequent dilation; initial dilation with larger caliber dilators and rubber bougies is a common practice.[21,81,82]

Peptic esophageal strictures are treated with intermittent esophageal dilation and aggressive management of reflux disease.[73,81,83] The addition of proton pump inhibitor therapy improves GERD-related symptoms for both peptic strictures and Schatzki rings.[77,81] The decision to use mercury-filled bougies over stiffer polyvinyl bougies placed over endoscopically placed guide wires or balloon dilators depends on the complexity, length, and tortuosity of the stricture.[74,84] Dilations are usually performed progressively to 40 to 60 Fr (13 to 20 mm), and relief of dysphagia is achieved with residual luminal diameters of >15 mm.[2,85] The "rule of threes" is generally followed, wherein no more than three further sizes of bougies or balloons are employed after resistance is encountered during dilation.[86,87] Perforations occur at a rate of 0.1 to 0.5%, and are most common when blind bougie dilation is attempted for complex strictures.[85,86,88] Repeat dilations are performed as necessary in patients with recurrent symptoms. Endoscopic incision and steroid injections are reserved for strictures refractory to adequate antisecretory therapy and requiring frequent dilation.[74,89]

In addition to aggressive acid suppression, fundoplication has also been used as a mode of definitive reflux therapy for peptic strictures, without a higher risk of residual dysphagia on follow-up.[90] Endoscopic dilation is effective in relieving symptoms in about two-thirds of cases of postfundoplication dysphagia when the fundoplication appears intact on endoscopy or barium studies.[91] The use of a large-caliber esophageal bougie across the gastroespophageal junction during fundoplication appears to reduce the incidence of postoperative dysphagia.[92] Even in the absence of obstruction on upper endoscopy and barium studies, empiric dilation using a 50 Fr bougie may improve dysphagia.[93] Such empiric dilation may be more beneficial for patients with solid food dysphagia than those with both solid and liquid food dysphagia.[94]

3.3.2.2 Food Impaction

Mechanical impediment to the passage of a food bolus can sometimes result in food bolus impaction at the site of obstruction. Symptoms are rapid in onset, usually occur during a meal, and consist of total or near total dysphagia, chest pain, and severe retching. Patients are often unable to swallow their own saliva. A trial of smooth muscle relaxants, such as glucagon or nitroglycerine, can be considered, but impactions rarely resolve spontaneously, and endoscopy with mechanical dislodgement are frequently necessary.[95] The management of food bolus obstruction has changed with the recognition of eosinophilic esophagitis as a frequent cause of food impaction.[96] Dilation can increase the risk of mucosal tearing or perforation in patients with eosinophilic esophagitis. Therefore, in young patients with clinical history or endoscopic findings suggestive of eosinophilic esophagitis, gentle bolus disimpaction and biopsy are recommended, and dilation is considered unsafe. However, dilation at the time of food disimpaction is safe in discrete strictures not related to eosinophilic esophagitis, particularly with Schatzki rings or peptic strictures.[95]

3.3.2.3 Gastroesophageal Reflux Disease

Gastroesophageal reflux disease (GERD) is initially treated with acid suppression.[75] Aggressive acid suppression with proton pump inhibitors improves dysphagia and decreases the need for subsequent esophageal dilation in patients with reflux disease.[81,83,97] Surgery also offers adequate therapy of reflux-induced dysphagia even when a stricture is not found, although a loose fundoplication is performed when esophageal peristalsis is feeble on preoperative esophageal manometry.[94,98]

3.3.2.4 Malignant Dysphagia

Whenever possible, neoplastic disorders are managed with curative surgery. Palliation with radiotherapy or chemotherapy are options when curative measures are not possible.[99] Dilation or stent placement may be necessary to allow oral intake. Endoscopic laser therapy or argon plasma coagulation has a low complication rate in alleviating malignant dysphagia, and is particularly useful when the life expectancy is estimated to be short. This can be combined with the use of plastic and metal stents. Endoscopically placed self-expanding metallic and plastic stents provide comparable relief of dysphagia in patients with esophageal cancer, with benefits at times lasting for over a year.[100–102] Stent placement for esophageal malignancy is a cost-effective treatment option that improves quality of life compared to other palliative alternatives and complications are rare.[103] While plastic stents may be less expensive, metallic stents may contribute to improved quality of life. The safety of these stents is documented at locations as proximally as the upper esophageal sphincter and as distally as the gastroesophageal junction.[104,105] Recurrent ingrowths of tumor through the stent can be effectively treated with endoscopic laser therapy or argon plasma coagulation.[101] Endoluminal stents can also be used in malignant extrinsic compression of the esophagus, though stent migration may be a complication. Newer esophageal stents fitted with an antireflux valve intended to lower gastroesophageal reflux are available, albeit without clear demonstration of a consistent benefit.[106,107] Further stent design modifications are encouraging and the safety of these new class of stents is validated.[108,109] The cost of single-dose brachytherapy and stent placement in the palliative treatment of esophageal cancer are comparable.[110]

3.3.2.5 Eosinophilic Esophagitis

Eosinophilic esophagitis is becoming more recognized as a cause for solid food dysphagia, particularly in young adult males.[111] Eosinophilic infiltration of the esophageal mucosa occurs with mucosal edema and reduced compliance of the esophageal wall. The esophagus may be of small caliber, but may appear normal on barium swallow. Endoscopy may demonstrate edema, erythema, vertical furrows, and whitish exudates. Histopathology typically reveals ≥15 eosinophils/high power field.[111–113] Treatment options include systemic and topical corticosteroids, elimination of dietary allergens when identified, mast cell stablizers, and anti-IL5 antibodies, but there is no consensus on optimal therapy at present.[113,114] Dysphagia refractory to topical corticosteroids may be amenable to endoscopic dilation, which needs to be performed with care to reduce the risk of perforation.[114] Long-term outcome studies are lacking.

3.3.2.6 Achalasia

Therapies for achalasia are aimed at reducing (LES) pressure to facilitate esophageal emptying by gravity.[74,115] Isosorbide dinitrate and calcium channel blockers sublingually or orally immediately prior to meals can transiently relax smooth muscle and facilitate LES opening.[115] Compared to placebo, controlled trials have not demonstrated consistent clinical benefit with these agents, and side effects can be troublesome.[116,117] Botulinum toxin injection into the LES during upper endoscopy reduces LES pressure by inhibiting acetylcholine release from nerve endings.[42,115,118] Although this approach can be remarkably effective in the short term, recurrence of symptoms is greater than surgical myotomy or pneumatic dilation.[7,119,120] Nevertheless, it can effectively improve symptoms when more invasive therapies are contraindicated or it can be used as a short-term bridge to durable therapy.[121]

Disruption of the LES with pneumatic dilation or surgical myotomy are the only definitive treatments that consistently improve esophageal emptying in achalasia. Recommendations for individual patients depends on available institutional expertise. Surgical myotomy is offered to otherwise healthy patients who can tolerate laparoscopic surgery, reserving pneumatic dilation for patients who decline surgery or have other risk factors for surgery.[122,123] Both treatments are safe and effectively abate symptoms.[122–125] Patients who fail pneumatic dilation can subsequently undergo surgical myotomy if necessary.[126] Pneumatic dilation uses a specially designed balloon dilator that distends the LES to a diameter of 3 to 4 cm disrupting LES muscle fibers.[115,120] An important complication is perforation, requiring emergency surgical repair, seen in less than 5% of cases.[115,120] Surgical myotomy is performed laparoscopically with good success and a lasting symptomatic benefit.[120,127] Concurrent fundoplication effectively reduces reflux symptoms; a partial fundoplication (e.g., Dor or Toupet) is associated with less dysphagia compared to 360-degree Nissen fundoplication.[128] Computer-enhanced robotic laparoscopic Heller myotomy holds promise to lower surgical complications, but cost-effectiveness is unclear.[129]

3.3.2.7 Spastic Disorders

Spastic motor processes, such as diffuse esophageal spasm and nonspecific spastic disorders, can have obstructive and/or perceptive symptoms, the latter associated with esophageal hypersensitivity.[130] Smooth muscle relaxants have been used, but conclusive literature supporting this approach are lacking.[115,131] In the absence of other pharmacologic alternatives, a therapeutic trial may be considered using either nifedipine or nitrates.[131] Nifedipine reduces esophageal peristaltic amplitude and may improve chest pain in nonspecific spastic disorders, but efficacy has not been conclusively demonstrated in controlled trials.[131] Nitrates have also been used, but results are inconsistent.[131] Case reports demonstrate symptomatic relief and normalization of spastic motor abnormalities with sildenafil.[132] Pneumatic dilation and surgical myotomy are reserved for refractory obstructive situations, though there are no controlled trials addressing these therapeutic measures. Perceptive symptoms and esophageal hypersensitivity may benefit from therapy with low dose trazodone or tricyclic antidepressants. Concurrent reflux disease needs to be managed with antisecretory therapy, as reflux episodes can trigger perceptive esophageal symptoms in spastic motor disorders.[133]

3.3.3 ODYNOPHAGIA

Odynophagia is encountered less often compared to dysphagia, although it can sometimes coexist with dysphagia.[1] The mechanism of symptom production is thought to relate to deep mucosal infiltration with inflammatory processes or neoplasia, or to sensory stimulation from profound mucosal inflammation or infection. Historical clues to the diagnosis include: immunosuppressive diseases or therapies, radiation exposure, caustic ingestion, and foreign body ingestion. Direct mucosal visualization and tissue biopsies are often required.[1] Infectious esophagitis can be seen in a wide range of patients with immunocompromised states, including AIDS, organ transplants, antibiotic use, malignancy, diabetes mellitus, steroid therapy, and other immunosuppressive therapies.[1,2] Esophageal candidiasis is the most common opportunistic process; other frequently encountered opportunistic infections include herpes simplex and cytomegalovirus infections. Viral esophagitis can rarely be seen in the immunocompetent host, most commonly from herpes simplex virus infection. In immunocompromised states, the presence of oral thrush in the setting of odynophagia can prompt empiric therapy for esophageal candidiasis.[134,135] Therapy with either fluconazole 100 to 200 mg/d or itraconazole 200 mg/d for 14 to 21 days is recommended as initial therapy;[75] however, a poor response requires further investigation.

REFERENCES

1. Gyawali CP, Clouse RE. Approach to the patient with dysphagia, odynophagia, or non-cardiac chest pain. In Yamada T, Alpers DH, Kaplowitz N, Owyang C, Powell DW (eds), *Principles of Clinical Gastroenterology*, Wiley-Blackwell Publishing, West Sussex, UK, 2008:62–74.
2. Lawal A, Shaker R. Esophageal dysphagia. *Phys Med Rehabil Clin N Am* 2008;19:729–745.
3. Castell DO, Donner MW. Evaluation of dysphagia: a careful history is crucial. *Dysphagia* 1987;2:65–71.
4. Richter JE. Practical approach to the diagnosis and treatment of esophageal dysphagia. *Comprehensive Therapy* 1998;24:446–453.
5. Castell JA, Castell DO. Upper esophageal sphincter and pharyngeal function and oropharyngeal (transfer) dysphagia. *Gastroenterol Clin North Am* 1996;25:35–50.
6. González-Fernádez M, Daniels SK. Dysphagia in stroke and neurologic disease. *Phys Med Rehabil Clin N Am* 2008;19:867–888.
7. Richter JE. Osophageal motility disorders. *Lancet* 2001;358:823–828.
8. Cook IJ, Kahrilas PJ. AGA technical review on management of oropharyngeal dysphagia. *Gastroenterology* 1999;116:455–478.
9. Hinds NP, Wiles CM. Assessment of swallowing and referral to speech and language therapists in acute stroke. *QJM* 1998;91:829–835.
10. Daneils SK, Brailey K, Priestly DH, et al. Aspiration in patients with acute stroke. *Arch Phys Med Rehabil* 1998;79:14–19.

11. McCullough GH, Wertz RT, Rosenbek JC. Sensitivity and specificity of clinical/bedside examination signs for detecting aspiration in adults subsequent to stroke. *J Commun Disord* 2001;34:55–72.
12. Leder SB, Espinosa JF. Aspiration risk after acute stroke: comparison of clinical examination and fiberoptic endoscopic evaluation of swallowing. *Dysphagia* 2002;17:214–218.
13. Nilsson H, Ekberg O, Olsson R, Hindfelt B. Dysphagia in stroke: a prospective study of quantitative aspects of swallowing in dysphagic patients. *Dysphagia* 1998;13:32–38.
14. Stand EA, Miller RM, Yorkston KM, et al. Management of oral-pharyngeal dysphagia symptoms in amyotropic lateral sclerosis. *Dysphagia* 1996;11:129–139.
15. Kendall KA, McKenzie S, Leonard RJ, Goncalves MI, Walker A. Timing of events in normal swallowing: a videofluoroscopic study. *Dysphagia* 2000;15:74–83.
16. Eisenhuber E, Schima W, Schober E, et al. Videofluoroscopic assessment of patients with dysphagia: pharyngeal retention is a predictive factor for aspiration. *AJR Am J Roentgenol* 2002;178:393–398.
17. Martin-Harris B, Logemann JA, McMahon S, Schleicher M, Sandidge J. Clinical utility of the modified barium swallow. *Dysphagia* 2000;15:136–141.
18. Aviv JE, Kaplan ST, Thomson JE, Spitzer J, Diamond B, Close LG. The safety of flexible endoscopic evaluation of swallowing with sensory testing (FEESST): an analysis of 500 consecutive evaluations. *Dysphagia* 2000;15:39–44.
19. Aviv JE. Prospective, randomized outcome study of endoscopy versus modified barium swallow in patients with dysphagia. *Laryngoscope* 2000;110:563–574.
20. Ertekin C, Aydogdu I, Yuceyar N, Tarlaci S, Kiylioglu N, Pehlivan M, Celebi G. Electrodiagnostic methods for neurogenic dysphagia. *Electroencephalogr Clin Neurophysiol* 1998;109:331–340.
21. Spechler SJ. AGA technical review on treatment of patients with dysphagia caused by benign disorders of the distal esophagus. *Gastroenterology* 1999;117:233–254.
22. Patterson DJ, Graham DY, Smith JL, Schwartz JT, Alpert E, Lanza FL, Cain GD. Natural history of benign esophageal stricture treated by dilatation. *Gastroenterology* 1983;85:346–350.
23. DeVault KR. Epidemiology and significance of Barrett's esophagus. *Dig Dis* 2000-2001;18:195–202.
24. Nayyar AK, Royston C, Bardhan KD. Oesophageal acid-peptic strictures in the histamine H2 receptor antagonist and proton pump inhibitor era. *Dig Liver Dis* 2003;35:143–150.
25. Lagergren J, Bergstrom R, Lindgren A, et al. Symptomatic gastroesophageal reflux as a risk factor for esophageal adenocarcinoma. *N Engl J Med* 1999;340:825–31.
26. Baehr PH, McDonald GB. Esophageal infections: risk factors, presentation, diagnosis, and treatment. *Gastroenterology* 1994;106:509–532.
27. Maddern JG, Horowitz M, Gamieson GG, et al. Abnormalities of esophageal and gastric emptying in progressive systemic sclerosis. *Gastroenterology* 1984;87:922–926.
28. Layke JC, Lopez PP. Esophageal cancer: a review and update. *Am Fam Physician* 2006;73:2187–2194.
29. Wilcox SM, Alexander LN, Clark WS. Localization of an obstructing esophageal lesion. Is the patient accurate? *Dig Dis Sci* 1995;40:2192–2196.
30. Ott DJ. Radiographic techniques and efficacy in evaluating esophageal dysphagia. *Dysphagia* 1990;5:192–203.
31. Cappell MS, Friedel D. The role of esophagogastroduodenoscopy in the diagnosis and management of upper gastrointestinal disorders. *Med Clin North Am* 2002;86:1165–1216.
32. Esfandyari T, Potter JW, Vaezi MF. Dysphagia: a cost analysis of the diagnostic approach. *Am J Gastroenterol* 2002;97:2733–2737.
33. Ott DJ, Chen YM, Wu WC, Gelfand DW, Munitz HA. Radiographic and endoscopic sensitivity in detecting lower esophageal mucosal ring. *AJR* 1986;147:261–265.

34. Ott DJ, Kelley TF, Chen MY, Gelfand DW, Wu WC. Use of a marshmallow bolus for evaluating lower esophageal mucosal rings. *Am J Gastroenterol* 1991;86:817–820.
35. Ott DJ, Richter JE, Chen YM, Wu WC, Gelfand DW, Castell DO. Esophageal radiography and manometry correlation in 172 patients with dysphagia. *AJR* 1987;149:307–311.
36. Kahrilas PJ, Clouse RE, Hogan WJ. AGA technical review on the clinical use of esophageal manometry. *Gastroenterology* 1994;107:1865–1884.
37. Gambitta P, Indriolo R, Grosso C, Pirone Z, Colombo P, Archdiacono R. Role of oesophageal manometry in clinical practice. *Dis Esophagus* 1999;12:41–46.
38. Clouse RE, Prakash C. Topographic esophageal manometry: an emerging clinical and investigative approach. *Dig Dis* 2000;18:64–74.
39. Logemann JA. Treatment of oral and pharyngeal dysphagia. *Phys Med Rehabil Clin N Am* 2008;19:803–816.
40. Neumann S, Bartolome G, Buchholz D, Prosiegel M. Swallowing therapy of neurologic patients: correlation of outcome with pretreatment variables and therapeutic methods. *Dysphagia* 1995;10:1–5.
41. Bulow M, Olsson R, Ekberg O. Videomanometric analysis of supraglottic swallow, effortful swallow, and chin tuck in healthy volunteers. *Dysphagia* 1999;14:67–72.
42. Bath PM, Bath FJ, Smithard DG. Interventions for dysphagia in acute stroke. *Cochrane Database of Systematic Reviews* 2000;2:CD000323.
43. Klor BM, Milianti FJ. Rehabilitation of neurogenic dysphagia with percutaneous endoscopic gastrostomy. *Dysphagia* 1999;14:162–164.
44. Elmstahl S, Bulow M, Ekberg O, Petersson M, Tegner H. Treatment of dysphagia improves nutritional conditions in acute stroke. *Dysphagia* 1999;14:61–66.
45. Saeian K, Shaker R. Oropharyngeal dysphagia. *Clin Perspect Gastroenterol* 2000;3:69.
46. Hinchey JA, Shephard T, Furie K, et al. Formal dysphagia screening protocols prevent pneumonia. *Stroke* 2005;36:1972–1976.
47. Carnaby G, Hankey GJ, Pizzi J. Behavioural intervention for dysphagia in acute stroke: a randomized controlled trial. *Lancet Neurol* 2006;5:31–37.
48. Shaker R, Easterling C, Kern M, et al. Rehabilitation of swallowing by exercise in tube-fed patients with pharyngeal dysphagia due to abnormal UES opening. *Gastroenterology* 2002;122:1314–1321.
49. Logemann JA, Gensler G, Robbins J, et al. A randomized study of three interventions for aspiration of thin liquids in patients with dementia or Parkinson's disease. *J Speech Lang Hear Res* 2008;51:173–183.
50. Whelan K. Inadequate fluid intakes in dyspahgic acute stroke. *Clin Nutr* 2002;20:423–428.
51. Robbins J, Gensler G, Hind J, et al. Comparison of two interventions for liquid aspiration on pneumonia incidence: a randomized trial. *Ann Intern Med* 2008;148:509–518.
52. Martino R, Pron G, Diamant N. Screening for orpharyngeal dysphagia in stroke: insufficient evidence for guidelines. *Dysphagia* 2000;15:19.
53. Rudberg MA, Egleston BL, Grant MD, Brody JA. Effectiveness of feeding tubes in nursing home residents with swallowing disorders. *J Parenter Enteral Nutr* 2000;24:97–102.
54. Norton B, Homer-Ward M, Donnelly MT, Long RG, Holmes GK. A randomized prospective comparison of percutaneous endoscopic gastrostomy and nasogastric tube feeding after acute dysphagic stroke. *BMJ* 1996;312:13–16.
55. Wilkinson TJ, Thomas K, MacGregor S, Tillard G, Wyles C, Sainsbury R. Tolerance of early diet textures as indicators of recovery from dysphagia after stroke. *Dysphagia* 2002;17:227–232.
56. Dennis M, Lewis S, Cranswick G, et al. FOOD a multicentre randomized trial evaluating feeding policies in patients admitted to hospital with a recent stroke. *Health Technol Assess* 2006;10:1–120.

57. Bülow M, Speyer R, Baijens L, et al. Neuromuscular electrical stimulation (NMES) in stroke patients with oral and pharyngeal dysfunction. *Dysphagia* 2008;23:302–309.
58. Leibovitz A, Sela BA, Habot B, Gavendo S, Lansky R, Avni Y, Segal R. Homocysteine blood level in long-term care residents with oropharyngeal dysphagia: comparison of hand-oral and tube-enteral-fed patients. *JPEN K Parenter Enteral Nutr* 2002;26:94–97.
59. Kelly JH. Management of upper esophageal sphincter disorders: indications and complications of myotomy. *Am J Med* 2000;108 Suppl 4a:43S–46S.
60. Adams J, Sheppard B, Andersen P, Myers B, Deveney C, Everts E, Cohen J. Zenker's diverticulostomy with cricopharyngeal myotomy: the endoscopic approach. *Surg Endosc* 2001;15:34–37.
61. Stoeckli SJ, Schmid S. Endoscopic stapler-assisted diverticulo-esophagostomy for Zenker's diverticulum: patient satisfaction and subjective relief of symptoms. *Surgery* 2002;131:158–162.
62. Mason RJ, Bremner CG, DeMeester TR, Crookes PF, Peters JH, Hagen JA, DeMeester SR. Pharyngeal swallowing disorders: selection for and outcome of myotomy. *Ann Surg* 1998;228:598–608.
63. Zaninotto G, Marchese Ragona R, Briani C, et al. The role of botulinum toxin injection and upper esophageal sphincter myotomy in treating oropharyngeal dysphagia. *J Gastrointest Surg* 2004;8:997–1006.
64. Shama L, Connor NP, Ciucci MR, et al. Surgical treatment of dysphagia. *Phys Med Rehabil Clin N Am* 2008;19:817–835.
65. Anon. AGA medical position statement on management of oropharyngeal dysphagia. *Gastroenterology* 1999;116:452–454.
66. Hatlebakk JG, Castell JA, Spiegel J, Paoletti V, Katz PO, Castell DO. Dilatation therapy for dysphagia in patients with upper esophageal sphincter dysfunction—manometric and symptomatic response. *Dis Esophagus* 1998;11:254–259.
67. Heitmiller RF. Myasthenia gravis: clinical features, pathogenesis, evaluation, and medical management. *Semin Thorac Cardiovasc Surg* 1999;11:41–46.
68. Callen JP. Dermatomyositis. *Lancet* 2000;355:53–57.
69. Talmi YP, Finkelstein Y, Zohar Y. Reduction of salivary flow with transdermal scopolamine: a four-year experience. *Otolaryngol Head Neck Surg* 1990;103:615–618.
70. Ahsan SF, Meleca RJ, Dworkin JP. Botulinum toxin injection of the cricopharyngeus muscle for the treatment of dysphagia. *Otolaryngol Head Neck Surg* 2000;122:691–695.
71. Terre R, Valles M, Panades A, et al. Long-lasting effect of a single botulinum toxin injection in the treatment of oropharyngeal dysphagia secondary to upper esophageal sphincter dysfunction: a pilot study. *Scand J Gastroenterol* 2008;43:1296–1303.
72. Parameswaran MS, Soliman AM. Endoscopic botulinum toxin injection for cricopharyngeal dysphagia. *Ann Otol Rhinol Laryngol* 2002;111:871–874.
73. Pereira-Lima JC, Ramires RP, Zamin I Jr, Cassal AP, Marroni CA, Mattos AA. Endoscopic dilation of benign esophageal strictures: report on 1043 procedures. *Am J Gastroenterol* 1999;94:1497–1501.
74. Spechler SJ. AGA medical position statement on treatment of patients with dysphagia caused by benign disorders of the distal esophagus. *Gastroenterology* 1999;117:229–232.
75. Prakash C. Gastrointestinal diseases. In Cooper (ed), *The Washington Manual of Medical Therapeutics* 32nd ed., Lippincott Williams and Wilkins: Philadelphia 2007:439.
76. Ramage JI, Rumalla A, Baron TH, et al. A prospective, randomized, double-blind, placebo-controlled trial of endoscopic steroid injection therapy for recalcitrant esophageal peptic strictures. *Am J Gastroenterol* 2005;100:2419–2425.

77. Wills JC, Hilden K, Hisario JA, et al. A randomized prospective trial of electrosurgical incision followed by rabeprazole versus bougie dilation followed by rabeprazole for symptomatic esophageal (Schatzki's) rings. *Gastrointest Endsoc* 2008;67:808–813.
78. Sgouros SN, Vassiliadis K, Bergele C, et al. Single-session, graded esophageal dilation without fluoroscopy in outpatients with lower esophageal (Schatzki's) rings: a prospective, long-term follow-up study. *J Gastroenterol Hepatol* 2007;22:653–657.
79. Ibrahim A, Cole RA, Qureshi WA, et al. Schatzki's ring: to cut or break an unresolved problem. *Dig Dis Sci* 2004;49:379–383.
80. Chotiprasidhi P, Minocha A. Effectiveness of single dilation with Maloney dilator versus endoscopic rupture of Schatzki's ring using biopsy forceps. *Dig Dis Sci* 2000;45:281–284.
81. Smith PM, Kerr GD, Cockel R, et al. A comparison of omeprazole and ranitidine in the prevention of recurrence of benign esophageal stricture. *Gastroenterology* 1994;107:1312–1318.
82. Olson JS, Lieberman DA, Sonnenberg A. Practice patterns in the management of patients with esophageal strictures and rings. *Gastrointest Endosc* 2007;66:670–675.
83. Marks RD, Richter JE, Rizzo H, Koehler RE, Spenney JG, Mills TP, Champion G. Omeprazole versus H2-receptor antagonists in treating patients with peptic stricture and esophagitis. *Gastroenterology* 1994;106:907–915.
84. Hernandez LJ, Jacobson JW, Harris MS. Comparison among the perforation rates of Maloney, balloon, and savary dilation of esophageal strictures. *Gastrointest Endosc* 2000;51:460–462.
85. Gyawali CP, Clouse RE. Esophageal strictures and rings: do we practice what we preach. *Gastrointest Endosc* 2007;66:676–678.
87. Boyce HW. Dilation of difficult benign esophageal strictures. *Am J Gastroenterol* 2005;100:744–745.
88. Hernadez LJ, Jacobson JW, Harris MS. Comparision among the perforation rates of Maloney, balloon, and Savary dilation of esophageal strictures. *Gastrointest Endosc* 2000;51:460–462.
89. Kochhar R, Ray JD, Sriram PV, Kumar S, Singh K. Intralesional steroids augment the effects of endoscopic dilation in corrosive esophageal strictures. *Gastrointest Endosc* 1999;49:509–513.
90. Spivak H, Farrell TM, Trus TL, Branum GD, Warring JP, Hunter JG. Laparoscopic fundoplication for dysphagia and peptic esophageal stricture. *J Gastrointest Surg* 1998;2:555–560.
91. Wo JM, Trus TL, Richardson WS, Hunter JG, Branum GD, Mauren SJ, Waring JP. Evaluation and management of postfundoplication dysphagia. *Am J Gastroenterol* 1996;91:2318–2322.
92. Patterson EJ, Herron DM, Hansen PD, Ramzi N, Standage BA, Swanstrom LL. Effect of an esophageal bougie on the incidence of dysphagia following Nissen fundoplication: a prospective blinded, randomized trial. *Arch Surg* 2000;135:1055–1061.
93. Colon VJ, Young MA, Ramirez FC. The short- and long-term efficacy of empirical esophageal dilation in patients with nonobstructive dysphagia: a prospective, randomized study. *Am J Gastroenterol* 2000;95:910–913.
94. Wetscher GJ, Glaser K, Gadenstaetter M, Profanter C, Hinder RA. The effect of medical therapy and antireflux surgery on dysphagia in patients with gastroesophageal reflux disease without esophageal stricture. *Am J Surg* 1999;177:189–192.
95. Longstreth GF, Longstreth KJ, Yao JF. Esophageal food impaction: epidemiology and therapy. A retrospective, observational study. *Gastrointest Endosc* 2001;53:193–198.
96. Kerlin P, Jones D, Remedios M, Campbell C. Prevalence of eosinophilic esophagitis in adults with food bolus obstruction of the esophagus. *J Clin Gastroenterol* 2007;41:356–361.

97. Oda K, Iwakiri R, Hara M, et al. Dysphagia associated with gastroesophageal reflux disease is improved by proton pump inhibitor. *Dig Dis Sci* 2005;50:1921–1926.
98. Patti MG, Feo CV, De Pinto M, Arcerito M, Tong J, Gantert W, Tyrell D, Way LW. Results of laparoscopic antireflux surgery for dysphagia and gastroesophageal reflux disease. *Am J Surg* 1998;176:564–568.
99. Pfau PR, Ginsberg GG, Lew RJ, Faigel DO, Smith DB, Kochman ML. Esophageal dilation for endosonographic evaluation of malignant esophageal strictures is safe and effective. *Am J Gastroenterol* 2000;95:2813–2815.
100. Conio M, Repici A, Battaglia G, et al. A randomized prospective comparison of self-expandable plastic stents and partially covered self-expandable metal stents in the palliation of malignant esophageal dysphagia. *Am J Gastroenterol* 2007;102:2667–2677.
101. Singhvi R, Abbasakoor F, Manson JM. Insertion of self-expanding metal stents for malignant dysphagia: assessment of a simple endoscopic method. *Ann R Coll Surg Engl* 2000;82:243–248.
102. O'Donnell CA, Fullarton GM, Watt E, Lennon K, Murray GD, Moss JG. Randomized clinical trial comparing self-expanding metallic stents with plastic endoprostheses in the palliation of oesophageal cancer. *Br J Surg* 2002;89:985–992.
103. Xinopoulos D, Dimitroulopoulos D, Moschandrea I, et al. Natural course of inoperable esophageal cancer treated with metallic expandable stents: quality of life and cost-effectiveness analysis. *J Gastroenterol Hepatol* 2004;19:1397–1402.
104. Verschuur EM, Kuipers EJ, Siersema PD. Esophageal stents for malignant strictures close to the upper esophageal sphinter. *Gastrointest Endosc* 2007;66:1082–1090.
105. Yang HS, Zhang LB, Wang TW, et al. Clinical application of metallic stents in treatment of esophageal carcinoma. *World J Gastroenterol* 2005;11:451–453.
106. Sabharwal T, Gulati MS, Fotiadis N, et al. Randomised comparison of FerX Ella anti-reflux stent and the ultraflex stent: proton pump inhibitor combination for prevention of post-stent reflux in patients with esophageal carcinoma involving the esophago-gastric junction. *J Gastroenterol Hepatol* 2008;23:723–728.
107. Power C, Byrne PJ, Lim K, et al. Superiority of anti-reflux stent compared with conventional stents in palliative management of patients with cancer of lower esophageal and esophago-gastric junction: results of a randomized clinical trial. *Dis Esophagus* 2007;20:466–470.
108. Shim CS, Jung IS, Cheon YK, et al. Management of malignant stricture of esophago-gastric junction with a newly designed self-expanding metal stent with an antireflux mechanism. *Endoscopy* 2005;37:335–339.
109. Wenger U, Johnsson E, Arnelo U, et al. An antireflux stent versus conventional stents for palliation of distal esophageal or cardia cancer: a randomized clinical study. *Surg Endosc* 2006;20:1675–1680.
110. Polinder S, Homs MY, Siersema PD, et al. Cost study of metal stent placement vs single-dose brachytherapy in palliative treatment of oesophageal cancer. *Br J Cancer* 2004;90:2067–2072.
111. Potter JW, Saeian K, Staff D, et al. Eosinophilic esophagitis in adults: an emerging problem with unique endoscopic features. *Gastrointest Endosc* 2004;59:355–361.
112. Furuta GT, Liacouras CA, Collins MH, et al. Eosinophilic esophagitis in children and adults: a systematic review and consensus recommendations for diagnosis and treatment. *Gastroenterology* 2007;133:1342–1363.
113. Remedios M, Campbell C, Jones D, et al. Eosinophilic esophagitis in adults: clinical, endoscopic, histologic findings and response to treatment with fluticasone proprionate. *Gastrointest Endosc* 2006;63:3–12.
114. Furuta GT, Straumann A. Review article: the pathogenesis and management of eosinophilic oesophagitis. *Aliment Pharmacol Ther* 2006;24:173–182.

115. Kahrilas PJ. Esophageal motility disorders: current concepts of pathogenesis and treatment. *Can J Gastroenterol* 2000;14:221–231.
116. Traube M, Dubovik S, Lange RC, McCallum RW. The role of nifedipine therapy in achalasia: results of a randomized, double-blind, placebo-controlled study. *Am J Gastroenterol* 1989;84:1259–1262.
117. Triadafilopoulos G, Aaronson M, Sackel S, Burakoff R. Medical treatment of esophageal achalasia: double-blind crossover study with oral nifedipine, verapamil, and placebo. *Dig Dis Sci* 1991;36:260–267.
118. Prakash C, Freedland KE, Chan MF, Clouse RE. Botulinum toxin injections for achalasia symptoms can approximate the short term efficacy of a single pneumatic dilation: a survival analysis approach. *Am J Gastroenterol* 1999;94:328–333.
119. Zaninotto G, Annese V, Costanini M, et al. Randomized controlled trial of botulinum toxin versus laparoscopic Heller myotomy for esophageal achalasia. *Ann Surg* 2004;127:1850–1852.
120. Vaezi MF, Richter JE. Current therapies for achalasia: comparison and efficacy. *J Clin Gastroenterol* 1998;27:21–35.
121. Dughera L, Battaglia E, Maggio D, et al. Botulinum toxin treatment of oesophageal achalasia in the old and oldest old: a 1-year follow-up study. *Drugs Aging* 2005;22:779–783.
122. Kostic S, Kjellin A, Ruth M, et al. Pneumatic dilation or laparoscopic cardiomyotomy in the management of newly diagnosed idiopathic achalasia. *World J Surg* 2007;31:470–478.
123. Dobrucali A, Erzin Y, Tuncer M. Long-term results of graded pneumatic dilatation under endoscopic guidance in patients with primary esophageal achalasia. *World J Gastroenterol* 2004;15:3322–3327.
124. Pohl D, Tutuian R. Achalasia: an overview of diagnosis and treatment. *J Gastrointestin Liver Dis* 2007;16:297–303.
125. Boztas G, Mungan Z, Ozdil S, et al. Pneumatic balloon dilatation in primary achalasia: the long-term follow-up results. *Hepatogastroenterology* 2005;52:475–480.
126. Gockel I, Junginger T, Bernhard. Heller myotomy for failed pneumatic dilation in achalasia: how effective is it? *Ann Surg* 2004;239:371–377.
127. Spiess AE, Kahrilas PJ. Treating achalasia: from whalebone to laparoscope. *JAMA* 1998;280:638–642.
128. Rebecchi F, Giaccone C, Farinella E, et al. Randomized controlled trial of laparoscopic Heller myotomy plus dor fundoplication versus nissen fundoplication for achalasia: long-term results. *Ann Surg* 2008;248:1023–1030.
129. Melvin WS, Dundon JM, Talamini M, et al. Computer-enhanced robotic telesurgery minimizes esophageal perforation during Heller myotomy. *Surgery* 2005;138:558–559.
130. Richter JE, Barish CF, Castell DO. Abnormal sensory perception in patients with esophageal chest pain. *Gastroenterology* 1986;91:845–852.
131. Pandolfino JE, Howden CW, Kahrilas PJ. Motility-modifying agents and management of disorders of gastrointestinal motility. *Gastroenterology* 2000;118:S32–S47.
132. Fox M, Sweis R, Wong T, et al. Sildenafil relieves symptoms and normalized motility in patients with esophageal spasm: a report of two cases. *Neurogastroenterol Motil* 2007;19:798–803.
133. Clouse RE, Lustman PJ, Eckert TC, Ferney DM, Griffith LS. Low-dose trazodone for symptomatic patients with esophageal contraction abnormalities. *Gastroenterology* 1987;92:1027–1036.

134. Richter JE, Dalton CB, Bradley LA, Castell DO. Oral nifedipine in the treatment of noncardiac chest pain in patients with the nutcracker esophagus. *Gastroenterology* 1987;93:21–28.

135. Gutschow CA, Hamoir M, Rombaux P, Otte JB, Goncette L, Collard JM. Management of pharyngoesophageal (Zenker's) diverticulum: which technique? *Ann Thorac Surg* 2002;74:1677–1682.

4 Eosinophilic Esophagitis

Alain M. Schoepfer and Alex Straumann

CONTENTS

4.1　INTRODUCTION, DEFINITION, AND DIAGNOSTIC CRITERIA

Eosinophilic esophagitis (EoE) is rapidly emerging as a distinctive disorder in pediatric and adult gastroenterology. EoE is a chronic inflammatory esophageal disease, characterized clinicopathologically by (1) esophagus-related symptoms and (2) a dense esophageal eosinophilia, both of which persist despite prolonged treatment with proton pump inhibitors. Of note, EoE is neither defined by one single marker, e.g., number of eosinophils in the esophagus, nor by endoscopic findings.

Up until now, several different names, such as *primary eosinophilic esophagitis* (PEE), *allergic eosinophilic esophagitis* (AEE), and *idiopathic eosinophilic esophagitis* (IEE), have been used in the literature, but today most researchers favor the simple term *eosinophilic esophagitis* (EoE or EE).

Esophageal eosinophilia is not exclusively found in EoE. Among other diseases that are associated with esophageal eosinophilia are gastroesophageal reflux disease (GERD), Crohn's disease, collagen vascular disease, infectious esophagitis (e.g., herpes, Candida), drug-induced esophagitis, eosinophilic gastroenteritis, and hypereosinophilic syndromes.

Summarized, the diagnostic guidelines for EoE encompass the following four items:

1. Clinical symptoms of esophageal dysfunction
2. Esophageal histology with ≥15 eosinophils in at least one high-power-field
3. Lack of response to high-dose proton pump inhibitors (PPIs) or normal pH-monitoring
4. Exclusion of other conditions that cause esophageal eosinophilia (Table 4.1)

4.2　EPIDEMIOLOGY

EoE affects males two to three times more frequently than women.[1–13] The disease is found mainly in industrialized countries, such as the United States, Canada, Europe, and Australia, although there have been reports from all continents except Africa. Currently there is a lack of data to verify the geographic variations of prevalence and it is unclear whether EoE is associated with an ethnic or racial group. Socioeconomic distribution as well as seasonal variation in EoE have not been systematically examined. EoE is likely to be a relatively "new" disease as there is strong evidence that it had not been seen prior to the early 1980s. Whether the increased recognition

---

TABLE 4.1

Diagnostic Guidelines for Eosinophilic Esophagitis

- Clinically: Symptoms of esophageal dysfunction
- Histologically: ≥15 eosinophils in one high-power field
- Exclusion of GERD = either lack of response to high-dose PPIs or normal pH-monitoring of the distal esophagus
- Exclusion of other conditions that cause esophageal eosinophilia

is due to a true increase of the *incidence* of EoE or to an increased awareness is debatable. However, there is strong evidence to suggest that the prevalence of EoE is increasing. A population-based, long-term study performed in Switzerland revealed an increase in prevalence from 2 per 100,000 to 27 per 100,000 inhabitants over a 16-year period.[14] In accordance with these findings, Noel et al. identified a fourfold increase in the prevalence of EoE in children in the Midwest United States from 2000 to 2003.[15] A few reports have suggested a familial clustering, but it is unclear whether this is due to genetic predisposition or common environmental exposure.[16] In a recently published paper where sporadic EoE patients were compared to familial EoE patients, a familial form was identified in 4 of 26 (15%) of families. The familial EoE characteristics (clinical, endoscopic, pathologic, and global esophageal transcript expression profile analysis) were similar to sporadic EoE, leading to the estimation that both forms share a comparable pathogenesis.[17] The gene encoding the eosinophil-specific chemoattractant eotaxin-3 is the most highly induced gene in EoE patients compared to its expression level in healthy individuals and its presence may indicate genetic predisposition to EoE.[18]

4.3 IMMUNOPATHOGENESIS

The underlying pathogenesis of EoE is not completely understood. Under healthy conditions, the esophagus is devoid of eosinophils. In contrast, eosinophils are residents of the lower sections of the gastrointestinal tract and they establish themselves early during embryonic development. This process is mainly regulated by eotaxin.[19] Eotaxin also has a central role in the antigen-mediated eosinophil recruitment.[20] Eosinophilic infiltration of the gastrointestinal tract can be observed as a consequence of a variety of inflammatory or infectious conditions, such as gastroesophageal reflux disease (GERD), inflammatory bowel disease, or exposure to food allergens.[21] The association of EoE with allergies leads to the hypothesis that the eosinophilic recruitment in EoE patients may be a response to environmental antigens. However, it is unclear whether it is due to food antigens coming in direct contact with the esophageal mucosa or if the antigens exert their effect outside of the esophagus. In a murine model with sensitized airways, Mishra and colleagues have shown that intranasal administration of allergens induced esophageal eosinophilia, whereas oral or intragastric application of the same allergens did not.[22] Besides eotaxin, interleukin-5 (IL-5) has an important role in eosinophil recruitment with subsequent selective Th2 response.[23,24] This is supported by the observation that IL-5-deficient mice are resistant to EoE.[25] However, the variable response to measures aimed at limiting antigen exposure suggests that other mechanisms may be involved. Eosinophils in the esophagus can persist there through the release of eosinophil chemoattractants, such as Interleukin-3 (IL-3), IL-5, and granulocyte macrophage-colony stimulating factor (GM-CSF).[26] The eosinophils themselves may cause local inflammation by release of major basic protein, a cytotoxic cationic protein.[27] Active eosinophilic esophageal inflammation may cause dysphagia due to motility disorders in the absence of an esophageal narrowing. IL-5 appears to mediate eosinophil-induced esophageal remodeling.[28]

4.4 CLINICAL MANIFESTATIONS OF EOSINOPHILIC ESOPHAGITIS

As in many other diseases, there exist some age-related differences in EoE presenting symptoms between children and adults.[1-13]

4.4.1 SYMPTOMS IN CHILDREN

In neonates and infants, food refusal is a common symptom of EoE and may denote dysphagia, which cannot be easily expressed in this age group. Children often complain of GERD-like symptoms, such as heartburn and reflux (range 5 to 82%), vomiting (range 5 to 68%), and abdominal pain (range 8 to 100%). Dysphagia and food impaction are reported increasingly with age. However, children less frequently present with failure to thrive, chest pain, and diarrhea.

4.4.2 SYMPTOMS IN ADULTS

In contrast to children, EoE in adolescents and adults presents with a narrow spectrum of symptoms. The two leading complaints are dysphagia for solids (range 29 to 100%) and food impaction (range 25 to 100%). A minority of patients report GERD-like symptoms, nonswallowing-related chest pain, and upper abdominal pain. Many adults will have a history of recurrent food impaction prior to the diagnosis of EoE. Table 4.2 compares the symptoms in children and adolescents to the adults. In contrast to the very characteristic history, the physical examination is usually normal in patients with EoE.

Therefore, EoE should be considered in young children with GERD-like symptoms and feeding problems, whereas in older children and adults, a history of food impaction, dysphagia for solids, or refractory retrosternal pain should raise suspicion.

4.5 NATURAL HISTORY OF EOSINOPHILIC ESOPHAGITIS

Four studies have been performed to elucidate the natural history of EoE. Straumann and colleagues described the longest follow-up of 30 adults with EoE.[2] The presenting symptom was mostly dysphagia with food impaction and the diagnostic delay

TABLE 4.2
Symptoms Pointing at Eosinophilic Esophagitis

Children	Adults
Feeding aversion/intolerance	Dysphagia
Vomiting/regurgitation	Food impaction
"GERD refractory to therapy"	"GERD refractory to therapy"
Food impaction/foreign body impaction	
Epigastric pain	
Dysphagia	
Failure to thrive	

was on average 4.6 years (range 0 to 17 years). With follow-up of up to 11.5 years, 23% of patients reported increasing dysphagia and 36.7% reported stable symptoms. Potter et al reported on 29 patients, presenting primarily with dysphagia and with "refractory GERD" symptoms.[4] The majority of patients showed evidence of tissue remodeling at endoscopy. In 86% of patients, rings, strictures, or small caliber esophagus were found, whereas radiographic studies showed narrowing in 67%. Of note, the small caliber esophagus that was observed endoscopically was missed radiographically in four patients. Croese et al reported on 31 patients with EoE (24 men, mean age 34 years, range 14 to 77 years), mostly presenting with bolus impaction or dysphagia.[6] Mean diagnostic delay was 54 months (range 0 to 180 months). Strictures were present in 57% and were localized to the proximal esophagus; dilation caused longitudinal tears in 77% of patients, but there was no perforation. Liacouras and colleagues examined the largest longitudinal study of 381 children with EoE (66% male, mean age 9 years).[12] Most patients presented with symptoms of GERD refractory to acid suppression treatment or with dysphagia. Endoscopy showed rings in 12% and one patient required esophageal dilation.

There have been no reports of a causal association between EoE and Barrett's esophagus or esophageal carcinoma. Although long-term data is limited, careful follow-up of what is a chronic disease is recommended.

In summary, EoE is a chronic inflammatory disease that harbors relevant long-term risks and substantially impairs the quality of life of affected individuals. The major long-term complications of chronic eosinophilic esophagitis are esophageal strictures and a narrowed esophageal lumen resulting in food impaction.

4.6 DIAGNOSTIC MEASURES IN EOE

4.6.1 ENDOSCOPY

Although there is neither a pathognomonic endoscopic sign nor a typical pattern of abnormalities related to EoE, upper endoscopy is the first diagnostic step in the evaluation of an individual with suspected EoE. A number of endoscopic features associated with EoE have been described, including longitudinal furrows, white exudates, edema, longitudinal shearing, friability, crêpe paper mucosa, small caliber esophagus, Schatzki ring, corrugated or ringed esophagus, and solitary rings (Figure 4.1a-d).[1–6,11–12,29–31] These findings are suggestive of the diagnosis of EoE, but the endoscopic suspicion needs confirmation by histology. There are some early studies reporting normal appearing mucosa in EoE. With increasing awareness and experience, more endoscopists will recognize subtle mucosal changes that may have been overlooked in the past. However, in any patient with dysphagia or food impaction, esophageal biopsies should be obtained, even if the mucosa appears normal.

4.6.2 BIOPSY PROCUREMENT AND EVALUATION

Histological findings are a cornerstone in establishing the diagnosis of EoE. It is therefore mandatory to take mucosal biopsies, fixed in formalin, from all patients

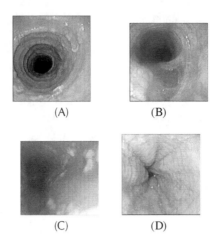

(A)   (B)

(C)   (D)

FIGURE 4.1 (See color insert following Page 112) Endoscopic findings associated with EoE. (A) Mucosal rings representing transient contractions or fixed structures, this aspect is also called trachealization, feline esophagus, or corrugated esophagus. (B) After esophageal dilation a deep mucosal laceration is seen representing a typical finding ("longitudinal shearing"). (C) Whitish exudates scattered across the mucosal surface, representing eosinophilic microabscesses. (D) Esophageal furrowing representing mucosal edema and thickening.

in whom EoE is suspected, e.g., those with dysphagia or food impaction, even if themucosaappears normal. Of note, in a study of 381 children with EoE, 30% had a normal appearing mucosa on endoscopy.[12] Regarding the patchy nature of the eosinophilic infiltration, the question is how many biopsies must be taken to achieve an appropriate sensitivity. Gonsalves and colleagues showed that with a histological cut-off value of 15 eos/HPF, the procurement of one single biopsy specimen had a sensitivity of 55% for diagnosing EoE, whereas the analysis of five biopsy specimens resulted in an almost 100% sensitivity.[32] Areas of gross endosopic abnormalities as well as proximal and distal esophageal mucosa should be assessed histologically. Furthermore, biopsy specimens also should be obtained from stomach and duodenum to rule out other diseases, such as eosinophilic gastroenteritis.

4.6.3 INTRAESOPHAGEAL pH MONITORING

There exists a critical overlap between EoE and GERD. When the diagnosis of gastro-esophageal reflux disease versus EoE is not apparent despite endoscopy and histology, intraesophageal pH monitoring may be of use in excluding pathologic reflux as the reason for esophageal eosinophilia. Alternatively, an upper endoscopy after six to eight weeks of high-dose PPI treatment can help determine the etiology of esophageal eosinophilia.

4.6.4 MOTILITY STUDIES

Nonspecific motor abnormalities have been described in patients with EoE, but these are not diagnostic.

4.6.5 RADIOGRAPHY

In patients with dysphagia, an upper gastrointestinal (GI) contrast study may show a narrowed esophageal lumen. It might also be beneficial for children presenting with vomiting to rule out anatomic etiologies, such as malrotation. The radiographic information is also important for the subsequent upper endoscopy because it may alert the endoscopist to use a smaller caliber endoscope and prepare the endoscopist for the possible need for a dilatation. In contrast to patients presenting with dysphagia, an upper GI contrast study is generally not useful in patients presenting with symptoms typical of GERD, e.g., heartburn.

4.6.6 HISTOPATHOLOGIC FEATURES OF EOSINOPHILIC ESOPHAGITIS

The key diagnostic criterion for diagnosing EoE is an increased number of intraepithelial eosinophils. Values between >5 Eos/HPF up to >30 Eos/HPF have been used by the different research groups. In a consensus conference, a cut-off value of ≥15 Eos/HPF in any biopsy was recommended as diagnostic criterion.[33] The eosinophils are counted under 400 fold magnification. The peak and not the mean number of eosinophils is used for diagnosis. Of note, relevant intraepithelial counts of eosinophils (>20/HPF) have also been reported in adults with GERD.[34]

In addition to their abundance in EoE, eosinophils often form microabscesses[5] and can accumulate in the superficial layers of the squamous epithelium.[10] Most investigators report a basal zone hyperplasia, which occupies more than 20% of the epithelium.[5,11] Papillary lengthening was variably defined and was reported in 50 to 100% of cases of EoE.[10,11,13] Epithelial ulcers were rarely reported, and lamina propria fibrosis is seldom reported, probably due to the absence of lamina propria in most esophageal pinch biopsy specimens.[35] Figure 4.2a,b demonstrates the typical histologic findings of EoE. Beside eosinophils, mast cells and lymphocytes are frequently found in eosinophilic esophagitis.

4.6.7 ALLERGOLOGIC EVALUATION IN EoE

EoE affects mainly patients with preexisting atopic conditions, such as allergic rhino-conjunctivitis, asthma, oral allergy syndrome, and atopic dermatitis.[12] The knowledge of an individual pattern of sensitizations is important, particularly if elimination diet therapy is considered. In some cases, a complementary examination by an allergist regarding other atopic diatheses may be useful (weak evidence).[33]

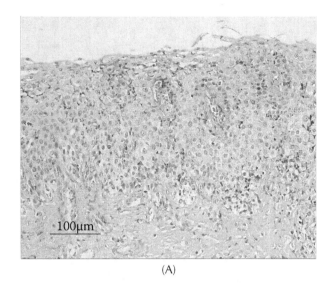

(A)

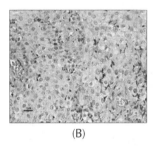

(B)

FIGURE 4.2 (See color insert following Page 112) Eosinophilic esophageal inflammation in EoE. (A) The low-power field (Hemalaun-Eosin, 200-fold magnification) of the epithelium demonstrates an increased number of eosinophils, basal zone hyperplasia, elongated rete papillae, and subepithelial fibrosis. (B) The high-power field (Hemalaun-Eosin, 400-fold magnification) of the epithelium demonstrates a large number of eosinophils, some of them are marked by a green star. (Micrographs courtesy of CH. Bussmann, Kantonhospital, Luzern, Switzerland.)

4.6.8   LABORATORY ANALYSES IN EOSINOPHILIC ESOPHAGITIS

4.6.8.1   Peripheral Eosinophil Count

Between 10 and 50% of adults and 20 to 100% of the children with EoE have a mild eosinophilia on their differential blood count.[2,9] The values seldom exceed 1500 eos/mm^3. The determination of a differential blood count, therefore, may provide supportive evidence for the presence of EoE, but a peripheral eosinophilia is not diagnostic nor does it correlate with the disease activity.

4.6.8.2 Total IgE, Aeroallergen-Specific IgE, Food-Specific IgE

More than 70% of EoE patients have elevated total immunoglobulin E (IgE) values.[10,13] So far, there is no evidence for the role of total IgE as a surrogate marker for disease progression or resolution; patients with high total IgE levels do not readily respond to corticosteroids compared to patients with normal values.[42]

With our present limited understanding of the pathogenic role of food and aero allergens, the value of measuring specific IgE levels is limited.

4.6.8.3 Skin Prick Testing for Antigen Sensitization and Atopy Patch Testing

The combination of prick skin tests and atopy patch testing has shown promising results with regard to food elimination diets and food reintroduction in patients with EoE. However, its use should be reserved until its role in the diagnosis and management of EoE is determined.[33]

4.6.8.4 Eotaxin-3 Measurements

One study documented twofold elevated eotaxin-3 levels in the peripheral blood of EoE patients compared to normal controls and controls with chronic noneosinophilic esophagitis.[17] Eotaxin-3 expression and its genetic variation seem to be promising markers of distinguishing EoE from other causes of esophagitis. Future research concerning the reversibility of eotaxin-3 levels with therapy and their prognostic significance deserve investigation. Until now, assessment of eotaxin-3 remains a research tool and correlations with disease severity and activity remain to be further evaluated.[33]

4.7 TREATMENT OF EOSINOPHILIC ESOPHAGITIS

The optimal treatment for EoE has not been defined, as experience has been limited largely to case series and small controlled trials.[38] Similarly, it is currently uncertain whether treatment of symptoms alone is sufficient or whether resolution of the eosinophilic inflammation is required. Thus, patients should ideally be treated within the context of a clinical study. Following are the data regarding efficacy and safety of known EoE treatments.

4.7.1 PROTON PUMP INHIBITORS

Acid suppression with PPIs is almost mandatory as a part of fulfilling the diagnostic criteria for EoE.[10,12] In addition, it may be used for patients with established EoE who have symptoms due to concomitant GERD. Nevertheless, PPI treatment should not be considered as a primary treatment for patients with EoE, rather as co-therapy because it sometimes alleviates symptoms in part.

4.7.2 CORTICOSTEROIDS

Several clinical trials and many case series have demonstrated that systemic and topical corticosteroids are highly effective in resolving symptoms and signs of acute flares of EoE in both children and adults.[39–42] A comparison of topical with systemic corticosteroids has shown that there is no significant difference regarding the efficacy of these two different forms. However, when topical or systemic corticosteroids are discontinued, the disease generally recurs within a few weeks. In general, topical corticosteroids are used as first line medications. They are well tolerated and, with the exception of oropharyngeal *Candidiasis*, are almost free of side effects. The use of systemic corticosteroids, therefore, may be limited to emergent cases, such as dysphagia requiring hospitalization, dehydration because of swallowing difficulties, or if the inflammation persists despite adequate dosage and correct application of topical corticosteroids. On the basis of expert opinion and the current literature, suggested starting doses range from 440 to 880 µg/day for children and 880 to 2000 µg/day for adolescence/adults. The drug is administered by mouth and can be given in two or four doses per day.[33] It is very important to familiarize the patient with the method of administration; patients should be instructed to administer the medication without the use of a spacer. The spray or dose inhaler should be inserted into the mouth and sprayed with lips sealed around the device. The spray or powder should then be swallowed and not rinsed. It is important to instruct patients not to eat or drink for 30 minutes after each dose in order to ensure a long contact time of the esophagus with the steroid. Duration of treatment for flares is between 2 to 12 weeks. Afterwards, patients are often treated with a maintenance regimen with lower doses of topical corticosteroids up to one year. There is an urgent need for studies to clarify treatment schedules and pharmacodynamic of topical corticosteroid treatment.[43]

4.7.3 Leukotriene Receptor Antagonists and Mast Cell Stabilizers

Cromolyn sodium has no apparent therapeutic effect for patients with EoE. Leukotriene receptor antagonists have been shown to induce symptomatic relief at high dosages; however, its use has not been shown to have any effect on esophageal eosinophilia. The measurements of mucosal leukotriene levels do not suggest a potential therapeutic benefit. The use of these drugs for the treatment of EoE is not supported by the current literature and, therefore, should be omitted.[33]

4.7.4 Biologicals

Novel biologic agents, such as monoclonal antibodies directed against IL-5 (e.g., mepolizumab) or TNF-alpha blocking agents (e.g., infliximab) present a unique opportunity for certain patients with EoE.[44] These molecules await larger clinical trials and cannot be recommended for routine use at the present time.[33]

4.7.5 Dietary Treatment

Individual adjusted elimination diet, semiadjusted six-food elimination diet (removal of the six most common allergenic foods, such as dairy, eggs, wheat, soy, peanuts, fish/shellfish), and protein-free elemental diet have shown to be effective in the treatment of children and adults diagnosed with EoE.[36,37,45] When deciding on the use of a specific dietary therapy, the patient's lifestyle and family resources also need to be considered. So far, dietary treatment has been more effective in children than in adults. The use of dietary therapy in adults requires further evaluation.[33]

4.7.6 ESOPHAGEAL DILATION

Esophageal dilation is useful for patients with symptoms not responding adequately to medical therapy, mainly patients presenting with a functional narrowing of the esophagus.[46] This condition may occur as a sequela of the chronic, untreated eosinophilic inflammation. There is a substantial risk of mucosal tearing and frank perforation, especially if rigid procedures are performed.[47] Because the responsiveness of strictures cannot be predicted on endoscopic appearance, we recommend whenever possible to perform a therapeutic attempt with topical corticosteroids or with an elimination/elemental diet, prior to dilation. We prefer Savory bougienage because the effect is exerted along the entire length of the esophagus. Respecting the abnormal fragility of the EoE mucosa, an inspection of the esophagus should be done following dilation to assess for laceration. One study has shown that dilations increasing the initial esophageal diameter up to 3 mm per session can be regarded as safe.[48] Therefore, several sessions may be necessary until the EoE patients benefit from dilation therapy.

4.8 MONITORING OF PATIENTS WITH EOSINOPHILIC ESOPHAGITIS

In children, as in adults with EoE, regular visits are recommended focusing on symptoms, adherence to therapy, and adverse effects. The goal is to improve the recognition of complications associated with chronic esophageal eosinophilia. Follow-up endoscopies are indicated in patients with refractory or relapsing symptoms or if therapeutic decisions have to be performed.

4.9 OUTLOOK/FUTURE RESEARCH

Despite the fact that our knowledge of EoE has increased enormously during the last decade, there are still many unresolved issues:

- Our understanding of the natural history is very limited.
- We have no predictive factors to identify patients who are at risk of developing esophageal remodeling.
- We need methods to distinguish between pure EoE and GERD-associated esophageal eosinophilia.
- Noninvasive markers to monitor disease activity must be developed and validated.
- The long-term medical management is still not defined.
- The management of patients' refractory to standard therapies is still controversial.

- The management of asymptomatic patients with esophageal eosinophilia is unclear.

Further joint efforts of clinical researchers and basic scientists addressing these issues are urgently needed in order to improve the lives of affected children and adults with eosinophilic esophagitis.

REFERENCES

1. Ngo P, Furuta GT, Antonioli DA, et al. Eosinophils in the esophagus-peptic or allergic eosinophilic esophagitis? Case series of three patients with esophageal eosinophilia. *Am J Gastroenterol* 2006; 101: 1666–1670.
2. Straumann A., Spichtin HP, Grize L, et al. Natural history of primary eosinophilic esophagitis; a follow-up of 30 adult patients for up to 11.5 years. *Gastroenterology* 2003; 125: 1660–1669.
3. Remedios M, Campbell C, Jones DM, et al. Eosinophilic esophagitis in adults; clinical, endoscopic, histologic findings, and response to treatment with fluticasone proprionate. *Gastrointest Endosc* 2006; 63: 3–12.
4. Potter JW, Saeian K, Staff D, et al. Eosinophilic esophagitis in adults; an emerging problem with unique esophageal features. *Gastrointest Endosc* 2004; 59: 355–361.
5. Desai TK, Stecevic V, Chang CH, et al. Association of eosinophilic inflammation with esophageal food impaction in adults. *Gastrointest Endosc* 2005; 61: 795–801.
6. Croese J, Fairley SK, Masson JW, et al. Clinical and endoscopic features of eosinophilic esophagitis in adults. *Gastrointest Endosc* 2003; 58: 516–522.
7. Baxi S, Gupta SK, Swigonski N, et al. Clinical presentation of patients with eosinophilic inflammation of the esophagus. *Gastrointest Endosc* 2006; 64: 473–478.
8. Arora AS, Perrault J, Smyrk TC. Topical corticosteroid treatment of dysphagia due to eosinophilic esophagitis in adults. *Mayo Clin Proc* 2003; 78: 830–835.
9. Teitelbaum J, Fox V, Twarog F, et al. Eosinophilic esophagitis in children; immunopathological analysis and response to fluticasone propionate. *Gastroenterology* 2002; 122: 1216–1225.
10. Sant'Anna AM, Rolland S, Fournet JC, et al. Eosinophilic esophagitis in children: symptoms, histology, and pH probe results. *J. Pediatr Gastroenterol Nutr* 2004; 39: 373–377.
11. Orenstein SR, Shalaby TM, Di Lorenzo C, et al. The spectrum of pediatric eosinophilic esophagitis beyond infancy: a clinical series of 30 children. *Am J Gastroenterol* 2000; 95: 1422–1430.
12. Liacouras CA, Spergel JM, Ruchelli E, et al. Eosinophilic esophagitis: a 10-year experience in 381 children. *Clin Gastroenterol Hepatol* 2005; 3: 1198–1206.
13. Esposito S, Marinello D, Paracchini R, et al. Long-term follow-up of symptoms and peripheral eosinophil counts in seven children with eosinophilic esophagitis. *J Pediatr Gastroenterol Nutr* 2004; 38: 452–456.
14. Straumann A, Simon HU. Eosinophilic esophagitis: escalating epidemiology? *J Allergy Clin Immunol* 2005; 115: 418–419.
15. Noel RJ, Putnam PE, Rothenberg ME. Eosinophilic esophagitis. *N Engl J Med* 2004; 351: 940–941.
16. Patel SM, Falchuk KR. Three brothers with dysphagia caused by eosinophilic esophagitis. *Gastrointest Endosc* 2005; 61: 165–167.

17. Collins MH, Blanchard C, Abonia JP, et al. Clinical, pathologic, and molecular characterization of familial eosinophilic esophagitis compared with sporadic cases. *Clin Gastroenterol Hepatol* 2008; 6: 621–629.
18. Blanchard C, Wang N, Stringer KF, et al. Eotaxin-3 and a uniquely conserved gene-expression profile in eosinophilic esophagitis. *J Clin Invest* 2006; 116: 536–547.
19. Mishra A, Hogan SP, Lee JJ, et al. Fundamental signals that regulate eosinophil homing to the gastrointestinal tract. *J Clin Invest* 1999; 103: 1719–27.
20. Hogan SP, Mishra A, Brandt EB, et al. A critical role for eotaxin in experimental oral antigen-induced eosinophilic gastrointestinal allergy. *Proc Natl Acad Sci USA* 2000; 97: 6681–6686.
21. Winterkamp S, Raithel M, Hahn EG. Secretion and tissue content of eosinophil cationic protein in Crohn's disease. *J Clin Gastroenterol* 2000; 30: 170–175.
22. Mishra A, Hogan SP, Brandt EB, et al. An etiological role for aeroallergens and eosinophils in experimental esophagitis. *J Clin Invest* 2001; 107: 83–90.
23. Gupta SK, Fitzgerald JF, Kondratyuk T, et al. Cytokine expression in normal and inflamed esophageal mucosa: a study into the pathogenesis of allergic eosinophilic esophagitis. *J Pediatr Gastroenterol Nutr* 2006; 42: 22–26.
24. Straumann A, Bauer M, Fischer B, et al. Idiopathic eosinophilic esophagitis is associated with a TH2-type allergic inflammatory response. *J Allergy Clin Immunol* 2001; 108: 954–61.
25. Mishra A, Hogan SP, Brandt EB, et al. IL-5 promotes eosinophil trafficking to the esophagus. *J Immunol* 2002; 168: 2464–2469.
26. Desreumaux P, Bloget F, Seguy D, et al. Interleukin-3, granulocyte-macrophage colony-stimulating factor, and interleukin-5 in eosinophilic gasroenteritis. *Gastroenterology* 1996; 110: 768–774.
27. Talley NJ, Kephart GM, McGovern TW, et al. Deposition of eosinophil granule major basic protein in eosinophilic gastroenteritis and celiac disease. *Gastroenterology* 1992; 103: 137–145.
28. Mishra A, Wang M, Pemmaraju VR, et al. Esophageal remodeling develops as a consequence of tissue specific IL-5 induced eosinophilia. *Gastroenterology* 2008; 134: 204–214.
29. Straumann A, Spichtin HP, Bucher KA, et al. Eosinophilic esophagitis: red on microscopy, white on endoscopy. *Digestion* 2004; 70: 109–116.
30. Nurko S, Teitelbaum JE, Husain K, et al. Association of Schatzki ring with eosinophilic esophagitis in children. *J Pediatr Gastroenterol Nutr* 2004; 38: 436–441.
31. Gupta SK, Fitzgerald JF, Chong SK, et al. Vertical lines in distal esophageal mucosa (VLEM): a true endoscopic manifestation of esophagitis in children? *Gastrointest Endosc* 1997; 45: 485–489.
32. Gonsalves N, Policarpio-Nicolas M, Zhang Q, et al. Histopathologic variability and endoscopic correlates in adults with eosinophilic esophagitis. *Gastrointest Endosc* 2006; 64: 313–319.
33. Furuta GT, Liacouras CA, Collins MH, et al. Eosinophilic esophagitis in children and adults: a systematic review and consensus recommendations for diagnosis and treatment. *Gastroenterology* 2007; 133: 1342–1363.
34. Rodrigo S, Abboud G, Oh D, et al. High intraepithelial counts in esophageal squamous epithelium are not specific for eosinophilic esophagitis in adults. *Am J Gastroenterol* 2008; 103: 435–442.
35. Straumann A, Rossi L, Simon HU, et al. Fragility of the esophageal mucosa: a pathognomonic endoscopic sign of primary eosinophilic esophagitis? *Gastrointest Endosc* 2003; 57: 407–412.

36. Markowitz JE, Spergel JM, Ruchelli E, et al. Elemental diet is an effective treatment for eosinophilic esophagitis in children and adolescents. *Am J Gastroenterol* 2003; 98: 777–782.
37. Kagalwalla AF, Sentongo TA, Ritz S, et al. Effect of six-food elimination diet on clinical and histologic outcomes in eosinophilic esophagitis. *Clin Gastroenterol Hepatol* 2006; 4: 1097–1102.
38. Kukuruzovic R, Elliott E, O'Loughlin E, et al. Non-surgical interventions for eosinophilic esophagitis. *Cochrane Database Syst Rev* 2004; 3: CD004065.
39. Liacouras C, Wenner W, Brown K, et al. Primary eosinophilic esophagitis in children: successful treatment with oral corticosteroids. *J Pediatr Gastroenterol Nutr* 1998; 26: 380–385.
40. Faubion WA Jr, Perrault J, Burgart LJ, et al. Treatment of eosinophilic esophagitis with inhaled corticosteroids. *J Pediatr Gastroenterol Nutr* 1998; 27: 90–93.
41. Lipworth BJ, Systemic adverse effects of inhaled corticosteroid therapy: a systematic review and meta-analysis. *Arch Intern Med* 1999; 159: 941–955.
42. Konikoff MR, Noel RJ, Blanchard C, et al. A randomized double-blind, placebo-controlled trial of fluticasone proprionate for pediatric eosinophilic esophagitis. *Gastroenterology* 2006; 131: 1381–1391.
43. Aceves SS, Bastian JF, Newbury RO, et al. Oral viscous budesonide: a potential new therapy for eosinophilic esophagitis in children. *Am J Gastroenterol* 2007; 102: 2271–2279.
44. Simon D, Braathen LR, Simon HU. Anti-interleukin-5 antibody therapy in eosinophilic diseases. *Pathobiology* 2005; 72: 287–292.
45. Spergel JM, Andrews T, Brown-Whitehorn TF, et al. Treatment of eosinophilic esophagitis with specific food elimination diet directed by a combination of skin prick and patch tests. *Ann Allergy Asthma Immunol* 2005; 95: 336–343.
46. Schoepfer AM, Gschossmann J, Scheurer U, Seibold F, Straumann A. Esophageal strictures in adult eosinophilic esophagitis: dilation is an effective and safe alternative after failure of topical corticosteroids. *Endoscopy* 2008; 40: 161–164.
47. Straumann A, Bussmann C, Zuber M, Vannini S, Simon HU, Schoepfer A. Eosinophilic esophagitis: analysis of food impaction and perforation in 251 adolescent and adult patients. *Clin Gastroenterol Hepatol* 2008; 6: 598–600.
48. Aceves SS, Newbury RO, Dohil R, et al. Esophageal remodeling in pediatric eosinophilic esophagitis. *J Allergy Clin Immunol* 2007; 119: 206–212.

5 Management of Chronic Nausea and Vomiting

Gregory S. Sayuk and C. Prakash Gyawali

CONTENTS

5.1 INTRODUCTION

Nausea is a subjective awareness of an impending urge to vomit. It is always unpleasant and can either precede vomiting or occur on its own. Patients use terms, such as "sick to the stomach" or "queasy," when describing this symptom. Vomiting or emesis consists of rapid, retrograde, forceful ejection of gastric contents through the mouth. Repetitive contraction of abdominal wall muscles, termed retching, generates the pressure gradient necessary for the retrograde evacuation of stomach contents. Retching can occur without vomiting and, therefore, without evacuation of gastric contents. Vomiting can occur without preceding nausea in certain situations.[1]

Vomiting must be distinguished from regurgitation and rumination. Regurgitation refers to passive retrograde movement of esophageal or gastric contents into the mouth, typically not associated with nausea or retching. Rumination consists of effortless regurgitation of recently ingested food into the mouth, sometimes followed by rechewing and reswallowing or spitting out. This usually occurs soon after a meal, may be repetitive, and may be a voluntary pleasurable experience.[1]

Nausea and vomiting can be classified as acute or chronic based on symptom duration. Acute nausea and vomiting consist of symptoms of <1 month duration. This designation is important, as etiologies and management strategies differ between acute and chronic nausea and vomiting. When encountered in the acute setting, most of the causes of nausea and vomiting usually fall into one of the following categories: medication induced (including chemotherapy-related symptoms), postoperative, acute systemic infections, central nervous system disorders (including raised intracranial tension), gastrointestinal obstruction, gastrointestinal inflammatory disorders, metabolic disorders, and pregnancy. In addition to treatment of the causative disorder, judicious use of antiemetic medications and attention to hydration, electrolytes, and nutrition is typically sufficient in early management.

This chapter will focus on chronic nausea and vomiting encountered in gastroenterology practice. The following conditions will be discussed: functional nausea and vomiting, cyclic vomiting syndrome, and delayed gastric emptying.

5.2 FUNCTIONAL NAUSEA AND VOMITING

5.2.1 Definition and Diagnostic Criteria

Chronic nausea and/or vomiting (experienced on average at least once a week over the preceding several months) in the absence of any structural or metabolic explanation is regarded as functional nausea and vomiting. As defined by the Rome III Diagnostic Criteria for the functional gastrointestinal disorders (FGIDs),[1] functional nausea and vomiting can be further subdivided into: (1) chronic idiopathic nausea, (2) functional vomiting, and (3) cyclic vomiting syndrome. The specific diagnostic criteria as established by the consensus of Rome III Committee are listed below.

Chronic Idiopathic Nausea
1. Bothersome nausea occurring at least several times per week
2. Not usually associated with vomiting

    3. Absence of abnormalities at upper endoscopy or metabolic abnormalities that explain the nausea

Functional Vomiting

    1. On average one or more episodes of vomiting per week

    2. Absence of criteria for an eating disorder, rumination, or major psychiatric disease according to DSM-IV

    3. Absence of self-induced vomiting and chronic cannabinoid use and absence of abnormalities in the central nervous system or metabolic disease to explain the recurrent vomiting

Cyclic Vomiting Syndrome

    1. Stereotypical episodes of vomiting regarding onset (acute) and duration (less than one week)

    2. Three or more discrete episodes in the past year

    3. Absence of nausea and vomiting between episodes

Note: All of the criteria must be fulfilled to satisfy the diagnosis, and must be present for the last three months with symptom onset at least six months prior to diagnosis.

Previously, chronic idiopathic nausea was regarded as having significant overlap with functional dyspepsia (Rome II), but has since been recognized as a separate condition given the lack of responsiveness of this syndrome to typical dyspepsia-specific therapeutic approaches.[1] Historically, functional nausea and vomiting has also been called "psychogenic vomiting" in recognition of the substantial overlap of these conditions with other psychiatric and functional co-morbidities.[2–4] For the purpose of this discussion, cyclic vomiting syndrome will be addressed separately given its unique stereotypical pattern of presentation and responsiveness to specific treatment strategies.

5.2.2 EPIDEMIOLOGY

Functional nausea and vomiting generally is regarded as an uncommon condition. One tertiary care center reported a 5% prevalence of functional nausea and vomiting following an extensive evaluation of other potential explanations of symptoms.[5] No clear gender predominance in seen in these conditions, and most commonly these syndromes present in younger adults in their 20s or 30s, though initial presentations can occur through the sixth decade of life.[6]

5.2.3 PATHOGENESIS

Inherent in the diagnosis of chronic idiopathic nausea and functional vomiting is a lack of any structural abnormalities or biological derangements to explain symptom experiences. Hence, the pathogenesis of functional nausea and vomiting has not been fully elucidated. Early on, these disorders were regarded as being purely psychosomatic in origin, which is almost certainly an oversimplified explanation for these disorders. Epidemiologic evidence supports a likely genetic contribution to these disorders, though attempts to identify specific genes responsible for these disorders to date have been disappointing.[7] This is likely due to an important influence of both early environmental learning and psychosocial factors in the expression of these conditions. The potential for abnormal gastroduodenal motility underlying functional nausea and vomiting has been examined, but unfortunately such abnormalities are not consistently present in either chronic idiopathic nausea or functional vomiting, and moreover these motor abnormalities at best only partially correlate with symptoms.[8,9] Visceral hypersensitivity holds potential in explaining not only functional nausea and vomiting, but other functional gastrointestinal (GI) disorders (i.e., irritable bowel syndrome). Visceral sensitivity implies either a lower threshold to abnormal gastroduodenal stimuli (visceral hyperalgesia) or increased sensitivity to normal foregut stimuli (allodynia).[10,11] This visceral hypersensitivity likely involves the "brain–gut axis," and reflects either an enteric sensitization at the level of the gut or an overamplification of the afferent sensory signaling in the higher brain centers responsible for the emotional, cognitive, and sensory interpreting of these ascending visceral signals.[12]

5.2.4 CLINICAL MANIFESTATIONS

Chronic idiopathic nausea (CIN) typically presents as significant nausea symptoms that occur on several occasions throughout the week. CIN usually is not associated with emesis. Functional vomiting patients typically complain of vomiting symptoms at least once a week. These symptoms should be distinguished from the nausea and vomiting that can occasionally be present with functional dyspepsia, often experienced concomitantly with epigastric abdominal discomfort in the latter case. Chronic idiopathic nausea and functional vomiting are chronic conditions, and are typically present for at least six months. Usually, functional nausea and vomiting symptoms are not associated with historical red flag features, such as weight loss or gastrointestinal bleeding, and often patients do not experience symptoms that awaken them from sleep. The presence of any such features should raise suspicion for another potential cause of the patient's nausea and vomiting (see Section 5.2.1). Importantly, functional nausea and vomiting often co-exist with other functional disorders, both gastrointestinal (irritable bowel syndrome) nongastrointestinal (fibromyalgia, migrane headache), as well as psychiatric conditions (depression, anxiety, somatization). The presence of these co-morbidities should elevate one's suspicion of the potential presence of a functional nausea and vomiting disorder to explain these symptomatic complaints.[13] Moreover, the presence of major depression or a conversion disorder alone may predispose an individual to continuous vomiting symptom experiences.[3]

5.2.5 NATURAL HISTORY

The natural history of chronic idiopathic nausea and functional vomiting has not been examined systematically. Often these conditions follow a waxing and waning course wherein patients experience regular low grade symptoms with periodic exacerbations, typically lasting months to years. In contrast to cyclic vomiting syndrome (Section 5.3), stereotypic asymptomatic periods lasting weeks to months are not typically reported.

5.2.6 DIAGNOSTIC MEASURES

Evaluation should exclude the presence of other important causes of chronic nausea and vomiting, most notably gastroparesis, intestinal obstruction, or pseudo-obstruction, as well as central nervous system processes and metabolic derangements. Appropriate testing usually includes an upper endoscopic examination, and a small bowel x-ray (small bowel follow through, computerized tomography (CT)- or magnetic resonance (MR)-enterography) to exclude small bowel inflammation or obstruction. Scintigraphic gastric emptying study can be performed to assess for gastroparesis. A limited biochemical evaluation should include serum chemistries, thyroid testing, pancreatic enzyme assays, and assessment of adrenal function. Performance of a serum or urinary beta-hCG to exclude pregnancy in women of child-bearing age is warranted. A head CT should be pursued to exclude a central nervous system (CNS) lesion. Further testing should be directed by the presence of additional symptoms. Gastroduodenal manometry can be performed to assess for an underlying enteric neuropathy, but typically must be performed at a tertiary care center with considerable expertise, and as such, it is not routinely performed for functional nausea and vomiting symptoms. In the absence of any overt abnormalities following this focused diagnostic evaluation, a diagnosis of functional nausea and vomiting is likely. It should be explained to the patient that any diagnostic evaluation is not being performed to confirm the cyclic vomiting syndrome (CVS) diagnosis, but rather is undertaken to exclude other less likely diagnoses.[14]

5.2.7 MANAGEMENT

Treatment recommendations for the management of functional nausea and vomiting symptoms derive largely from anecdotal experience and small, nonrandomized retrospective studies.[15] First-line approaches typically implement traditional antiemetic or prokinetic agents, which can be useful for symptom relief. Preferred agents include the dopamine receptor antagonists prochlorperazine (5 to 10 mg PO/IM/IV q6h prn) and chlorpromazine (10 to 50 mg PO/IM/IV q8h prn). These agents are generally well tolerated, but have the potential for the development of side effects, which are a consequence of the action of these agents on CNS dopamine receptors, and include sedation, insomnia, mood lability, confusion, dystonia, and tardive dyskinesia. The prokinetic agent metoclopramide (5 to 20 mg PO/IM/IV q6h prn), via its effects on both 5-HT_4 and peripheral dopamine receptors also can be used for acute symptom relief. While its prokinetic effects may attenuate with continued use, metoclopramide may continue to exert a central antiemetic effect. Similar potential for side effects exist with this agent, particularly with long-term use, and include anxiety, tremor, and Parkinsonian symptoms. The 5-HT_3 receptor antagonists ondansetron (4 to 8 mg PO/IV q8h) and granisetron (1 mg PO q12h) may also be used for acute symptom relief of functional nausea and vomiting. While these agents are associated with fewer side effects, their regular use may be cost-prohibitive. Domperidone, a peripheral dopamine receptor antagonist, is a potent prokinetic agent with overlapping antiemetic properties, and is another therapeutic option. As this drug does not have substantial blood–brain barrier penetration, CNS side effects including mood changes and dystonias are less common.[16] At present, this medication is not available in the United States, necessitating patient acquisition of this agent over the Internet from international pharmacies.

The use of low doses of antidepressants, particularly the tricyclic antidepressants, has been described as a prophylactic regimen for functional nausea and vomiting. Agents, such as amitrityline, nortriptyline, and desipramine, at a maintenance dose of 10 to 50 mg at bedtime, have been shown to be effective at suppressing functional nausea and vomiting symptoms in retrospective analysis.[17] Empirically, the selective serotonin reuptake inhibitors (such as fluoxetine, sertaline, and citalopram), bupropion, an inhibitor of neuronal dopamine and norepinephrine reuptake, and the anxiolytic buspirone may also provide suppressive relief of chronic nausea and vomiting symptoms.[18] However, randomized, controlled studies of these agents in this setting currently are lacking.

Anecdotal and small clinical trial experiences have demonstrated that a host of other alternative therapies, including ginger, hypnosis, psychotherapy, biofeedback, and acupuncture may be of adjunct benefit in functional nausea and vomiting patients.[19–21] In patients who remain medically refractory despite the above measures, the use of a gastric stimulator device (Enterra, Medtronic, Inc.), a pacemaker device that delivers rapid electrical stimulation to the gastric wall via implanted electrodes, can be considered. Recent data suggest that this device may be of benefit to patient quality of life regardless of the presence of underlying delays in gastric emptying.[22] In the United States, placement of this device requires U.S. Food and Drug Administration (FDA) humanitarian use approval and thus is performed only in expert centers.

5.2.8 MONITORING

Monitoring of functional nausea and vomiting patients typically includes a periodic assessment of serum electrolytes via a basic metabolic panel as hypernatremia and elevated blood urea nitrogen (BUN) and creatinine may suggest a state of dehydration. Contraction alkalosis with associated hypokalemia may also be present with more severe, prolonged emesis. Patients should monitor weights at home on a regular basis to allow for early detection of significant fluctuation in weight. Fortunately, these objective features are more unusual in cases of functional nausea and vomiting.

5.3 CYCLIC VOMITING SYNDROME

5.3.1 DEFINITION AND DIAGNOSTIC CRITERIA

Cyclic vomiting syndrome (CVS) is a chronic vomiting syndrome manifested by stereotypical episodes of intractable vomiting, both in terms of onset and duration. At least three such episodes should be documented before a diagnosis of CVS is entertained. Importantly, the diagnosis of CVS implies a complete absence of vomiting symptoms between these acute episodes, typically lasting weeks to months. Following a focused evaluation to assess for other biochemical or structural explanations for these symptoms, no objective explanation is found. As such, CVS is regarded as a functional GI disorder. Diagnostic criteria have been offered by the Rome III Committee[1] (see Section 5.2.1). Similar to other FGIDs, substantial overlap exists with CVS and other psychiatric disorders, such as anxiety and depression.[23]

5.3.2 EPIDEMIOLOGY

Some important epidemiologic distinctions exist in comparing CVS to functional vomiting and chronic idiopathic nausea. First, CVS is reported to affect males and females equally. Whereas functional vomiting and chronic idiopathic nausea almost uniformly are diagnosed in adulthood, a significant proportion of CVS patients are diagnosed in childhood.[24] Indeed, CVS was first described in pediatric populations, and was later recognized in adult gastroenterology populations. When manifesting in an adult population, CVS typically presents at an older age compared to other functional vomiting disorders, often in the third or fourth decade of life. CVS is a rare diagnosis, affecting <1% of individuals seeking gastroenterology consults at referral centers.[25]

5.3.3 PATHOGENESIS

As with chronic idiopathic nausea and functional vomiting, a lack of overt structural or biochemical abnormalities is implicit in the diagnosis. The specific pathophysiologic mechanisms underlying CVS, however, remain poorly understood. This lack of an appreciation of the etiology of this condition derives in part from the lack of large patient cohorts to study. Present thinking implicates similar abnormalities in visceral hypersensitivity and brain–gut function as in the case of chronic idiopathic nausea and functional vomiting. Specific infectious, food product, hormonal (menses), and psychosocial stressors may serve as triggering events that sensitize the individual to such central dysfunction. Both physical and psychiatric factors that trigger acute vomiting episodes have been described in a full two-thirds of pediatric CVS cases.[26,27] A multitude of other mechanisms to explain the pathogenesis of CVS have been proposed, including abnormalities in autonomic neurotransmission[28] and gastric emptying,[29,30] mitochondrial dysfunction,[31] and derangements of the cortisol and prostaglandin pathways.[32–34] No single hypothesis, however, has been sufficient to explain the biological basis of CVS.

5.3.4 CLINICAL MANIFESTATIONS

The hallmark of CVS is stereotypical episodes of vomiting ("emetic phase") with interposed, asymptomatic periods ("well phase"). The acute vomiting episodes experienced during the emetic phase of CVS can be quite intense, and will frequently precipitate a visit to an emergency or urgent care setting for dehydration and intravenous (IV) antiemetics. In contrast to functional vomiting, abdominal pain frequently accompanies the vomiting symptoms in as many as 70% of patients.[25,27,34] Prior to the onset of vomiting symptoms, 30% of CVS patients will describe a prodromal phase, manifested by nausea, anorexia, lethargy, and headache. As with migraineurs (those who experience migraines), a subset of patients with antecedent prodromal symptoms will report aura-like symptoms. These prodromal symptoms may last a few minutes to a few hours, and when present are important to recognize as they provide a window of opportunity to intervene medically, and, in so doing, hopefully preventing more of the full-blown emetic phase of the condition.

Early in the course, CVS patient symptoms are often incorrectly ascribed to an infectious gastroenteritis until a pattern becomes more apparent. On average, these acute vomiting attacks last three to five days, but may range from as short as a day to as long as two weeks.[25,34] The duration of episodes may be longer in adult subjects compared to their pediatric counterparts.[27] Given the relative rarity of this condition and the varying frequency with which CVS patients experience vomiting attacks (average every three months), CVS patients commonly experience a significant delay in diagnosis and incorrect diagnoses prior to recognizing CVS.[27,29] Patients with CVS often are mislabeled as malingerers, psychiatric patients, and drug seekers. In one study, patients had experienced symptoms for 6.3 (±1.8) years before a diagnosis of CVS was made.[25] Other conditions associated with CVS include migraine headaches, mood disorders (anxiety and depression, in particular), and other functional GI disorders. A significant number of CVS patients will have overlapping diabetes mellitus, distinct from the gastroparesis often associated with this condition. Chronic marijuana use is also seen in CVS, with 42% of adult patients using marijuana in one study.[35] It remains unclear whether this is a causative factor or whether CVS patients turn to marijuana for its purported antiemetic properties.

5.3.5 NATURAL HISTORY

No long-term follow-up studies have been performed on CVS patients to establish the expected course of this condition over time. The authors have followed several patients with CVS with symptoms for more than 30 years, suggesting that CVS patients can be intermittently symptomatic over the span of several decades. Given the severity and duration of symptoms experienced during acute attacks, and the cyclical nature of these symptoms, what is clear is the substantial social and financial burdens that are imposed by this diagnosis, and CVS patients are often on disability.

5.3.6 DIAGNOSTIC MEASURES

The differential diagnosis for CVS includes a host of gastrointestinal conditions, including intermittent partial bowel obstruction, chronic intestinal pseudo-obstruction, gastroparesis, cholecystitis, biliary dyskinesia, and peptic ulcer disease. Non-GI conditions that might mimic CVS include CNS abnormalities (CNS lesion or hydrocephalus) as well as metabolic disorders (adrenal insufficiency), and a host of systemic conditions (systemic lupus erythematosis, vasculitis, systemic mastocytosis, hereditary angioedema, for example). The diagnostic evaluation should include the basic evaluation as detailed in Section 5.2.6 above. Additional work-up beyond the scope of this chapter may be indicated based on suspected diagnoses.

5.3.7 Management

The aggressive use of an effective abortive regimen is important in the prodromal and emetic phases of CVS to minimize the severity and duration of symptoms. Patients should have a prescribed antiemetic regimen on hand at all times to use at the earliest signs of symptom onset. If symptoms progress in spite of the use of oral and suppository agents, prompt attention in an urgent care or emergency room setting for IV administration is appropriate. To facilitate this care, a detailed letter describing the nature of the condition, previous evaluation, and the description of an effective abortive regimen is provided by the authors to CVS patients. This is an effective approach in minimizing superfluous testing and unnecessary delays in medical care. The antiemetic agents described above in the management of functional nausea and vomiting are indicated. Also potentially effective are the use of IV benzodiazepines, such as lorazepam 1 to 2 mg IV every two hours as needed. A subset of patients, particularly those with associated migraine headaches will respond well to the use of 5-HT$_{1D}$ agonists (sumatriptan, zolmitriptan).[36] In cases where pain is a predominant symptom, use oral or IV narcotics, such as fentanyl 50 to 100 mcg or dilaudid 0.5 to 1 mg q one to two hours as indicated. Provision of a quiet, stress-free environment is indicated, and, in some cases, a warm bath or shower may be helpful. Supportive care measures to consider in the acute phase include IV hydration with D5 ½ NS and correction of any electrolyte deficits. Empirically, many experts also advocate the use of a PPI (either orally or IV) to decrease gastric secretions and pH during the emetic phase.[37]

Prophylactic therapy is the other important component to the medical management of CVS. A prophylactic agent is worth considering in patients experiencing more than two to three episodes of major vomiting per year. Though perhaps less effective than in functional nausea and vomiting, the tricyclic antidepressants (TCAs) are the authors' first line prophylactic agents for CVS, and have the most data in support of their use.[25,38,39] Typically started at very low doses (25 to 50 mg at bedtime), and slowly titrated over weeks to months to doses in the moderate range (75 to 150 mg at bedtime), 59 to 93% of patients will receive at least a partial response, with a full quarter obtaining remission at higher doses.[25,35] When TCAs are not effective or not tolerated, other agents including the beta blocker propranolol (40 mg twice daily)[40] or the contemporary anticonvulsants zonisamide (100 to 400 mg daily) or leveiracetam (500 to 2000 mg a day in divided doses) can be considered as alternative agents.[41] When acute symptoms are clearly linked to menses, the use of oral contraceptives or leuprolide injections can be used.[42] Given the chronic, and often debilitating nature of this condition, many patients benefit from the education and support resources available through the Cyclic Vomiting Syndrome Association (www.cvsaonline.com).

5.3.8 Monitoring

Careful assessment of volume status and frequent monitoring of electrolytes is necessary during the emetic phase as biochemical derangements are common during periods of intense emesis. As treatment goals often are focused on the decrease of emetic phase duration, severity, and frequency rather than a complete remission of symptoms, it is important that an open line of communication exists between the gastroenterologist so that the CVS course can be documented and closely monitored in order to make objective assessments of therapeutic progress.

5.4 DELAYED GASTRIC EMPTYING

5.4.1 DEFINITION AND DIAGNOSTIC CRITERIA

The term *gastroparesis* is loosely used for all situations of delayed gastric emptying encountered on a solid phase gastric emptying study. Common symptoms include nausea, vomiting, and abdominal pain; patients may also complain of bloating, early satiety, abdominal distension, and weight changes.[43–45] In mild cases, weight and nutrition may be maintained with minor dietary modification with or without medications. In moderate cases, sometimes termed *compensated gastroparesis*, dietary and lifestyle adjustments allow for adequate nutrition with concurrent pharmacologic agents. When severe, patients are symptomatic despite pharmacotherapy and dietary adjustments, and are unable to maintain nutrition and body weight with oral intake. These patients may require frequent hospitalization and enteral feeding distal to the stomach.[43]

5.4.2 EPIDEMIOLOGY

In the absence of mechanical gastric outlet obstruction, symptomatic abnormal delay in emptying of the stomach in the postprandial state can be encountered in up to 4% of the general population, predominantly in females.[43,44] There is considerable overlap between true gastroparesis related to neuromuscular dysfunction of gastric emptying and functional dyspepsia with associated delayed gastric emptying. Therefore, the true prevalence of gastroparesis is difficult to estimate. Dyspeptic symptoms compatible with delayed gastric emptying, including nausea and vomiting, can be encountered in 11 to 18% of diabetics.[46,47] The prevalence of delayed gastric emptying as documented by a gastric emptying study is thought to be much higher, documented in as many as 48 to 65% of diabetics at a tertiary care center.[48] This suggests that a delay in gastric emptying in diabetics, although frequent, may be asymptomatic and not require pharmacologic therapy. Further, nausea and vomiting symptoms correlate poorly with the degree of gastric emptying delay in diabetic patients in both short- and long-term follow-up.[48–50] Therefore, it is likely that the majority of diabetic patients with nausea and vomiting have a functional etiology for symptoms. As many as a third of patients with functional dyspepsia have been demonstrated to exhibit gastric emptying delays, especially in the presence of postprandial fullness and vomiting.[51,52] Heightened visceral sensitivity associated with gastric distension may trigger symptoms in both diabetics and patients with functional dyspepsia.[53,54] For these reasons, clinically significant "gastroparesis" needs to be distinguished from functional dyspeptic symptoms that could potentially improve with neuromodulator therapy. When nutrition, body weight, and fluid balance are impacted by a true mechanical impact of delayed or absent gastric emptying, alternate routes of feeding need to be considered; this is typically achieved with enteral feeding distal to the pylorus by means of a jejunostomy tube.

5.4.3 PATHOGENESIS

Normal gastric emptying requires relaxation and tonic contraction of the gastric fundus to accommodate food and to set gastric tone, coordinated phasic distal gastric and antral contractions to break down food particles to 1- to 2-mm sized particles, pyloric relaxation in between antral contractions to allow these small particles to exit the stomach, and adequate antropyloroduodenal coordination to ensure smooth motor function.[45,55] Migrating motor complexes (MMC) ensure emptying of nondigestible solids, wherein coordinated contraction of the distal stomach is associated with persistent pyloric relaxation.[56] Disruption of these physiologic mechanisms can result from autonomic neuropathy, enteric nerve abnormalities, and dysfunction of the interstitial cells of Cajal (ICC).[57,58] In diabetics, vagal autonomic neuropathy may lead to abnormal postprandial gastric accommodation, incoordinated antroduodenal contractions, and sometimes pylorospasm.[55,59] Fluctuations in blood glucose, especially hyperglycemia can affect gastric motor function.[60,61] Viral illnesses can sometimes trigger acute onset of symptoms, wherein motor abnormalities including antroduodenal incoordination and abnormal fundic accommodation can be demonstrated.[62] Psychosomatic factors have also been associated with gastric motor abnormalities in patients with functional dyspepsia.[63,64] In a subset of patients, no clear precipitating mechanism can be elucidated for similar pathophysiologic alterations when the delayed gastric emptying is designated idiopathic.[65]

5.4.4 CLINICAL MANIFESTATIONS

Presenting symptoms of delayed gastric emptying include nausea, vomiting, postprandial abdominal fullness and bloating, early satiety, abdominal pain, and weight loss. Nausea and vomiting are the most frequently reported presenting symptoms, reported by 92% and 84% of 146 patients with gastroparesis in one series.[65] In the same series, 89% had abdominal pain or discomfort, 75% had abdominal bloating, and 60% had early satiety. These symptoms have considerable overlap with functional dyspepsia. Complications of gastric emptying delay and gastroparesis can include a propensity for gastroesophageal reflux and esophagitis, Mallory–Weiss tears at the gastroesophageal junction from retching and emesis, formation of bezoars in the stomach, fluid and electrolyte abnormalities from associated emesis, and nutritional deficiencies including weight loss and vitamin deficiencies.[45,66]

One of the first steps in the evaluation of the patient with suspected delayed gastric emptying is to rule out mechanical obstruction at the gastric outlet or farther distally. This can be achieved with endoscopic examination or radiographic upper gastrointestinal series, specifically looking for pyloric stenosis, peptic ulcer disease, and neoplasia. Further, the presence of retained gastric food residue or bezoars after an overnight fast suggests delayed emptying.[15,45] A small bowel x-ray series or cross-sectional imaging of the abdomen can exclude small bowel processes associated with proximal small bowel obstruction. Manifestations of functional and cyclic nausea and vomiting can overlap with those from delayed gastric emptying, and a careful history can help distinguish these conditions as described in the sections above.[17,25]

5.4.5 DIAGNOSTIC MEASURES

The finding of food residue in the stomach after an overnight fast on upper endoscopic examination can suggest delayed gastric emptying. Quantification of emptying of a solid phase meal using gastric emptying scintigraphy is considered the gold standard for the diagnosis of delayed gastric emptying.[55,67] However, the value of gastric emptying scintigraphy in directing management remains in question.[68] The test is typically performed using 99 mTc sulfur colloid labeled egg sandwich or egg whites after an overnight fast.[67,69] Scintigraphic imaging is continued for at least 90 to 120 minutes; extending the test to four hours is thought to improve the accuracy and specificity in the identification of delayed gastric emptying.[70]

A 13C-labeled breath test can indirectly estimate gastric emptying. A 13C-labeled medium chain triglyceride (octanoate)-based breath test has been demonstrated to be reproducible, and may correlate with solid phase scintigraphic scans.[55] 13C-labeled spirulina, a protein-rich blue-green algae is being validated as an alternate substrate for breath testing. Antroduodenal manometry can help differentiate between neuropathic and myopathic mechanisms of gastric motor dysfunction, while electrogastrography assesses gastric myoelectrical activity; these techniques have little value in patient management, but may help elucidate pathophysiologic mechanisms leading to delayed gastric emptying.[45,55]

5.4.6 MANAGEMENT

Diabetic patients with delayed gastric emptying benefit from good control of blood sugars, since hyperglycemia may promote gastric motor abnormalities.

5.4.6.1 Nutrition

Liquids leave the stomach quicker than solids, and emptying is passive relative to gastric tone. Dietary fiber and high fat content retard gastric emptying. Therefore, patients with delayed gastric emptying are advised to consume frequent, small meals that have low fat content and minimal fiber. Liquids and soups are beneficial. If weight loss or nutritional deficiencies persist despite maximal dietary and pharmacologic therapy, enteral feeding distal to the pylorus needs to be entertained. This is best achieved through an endoscopically or surgically placed jejunostomy tube. A venting gastrostomy tube may be necessary to relieve gastric retention in these situations. Total parenteral nutrition is rarely indicated, usually when small bowel feeding is not tolerated.[55]

5.4.6.2 Pharmacologic Therapy

Metoclopramide is a dopamine and serotonin receptor antagonist that has both antiemetic and prokinetic properties. While the antiemetic effects are central, prokinetic effects are from local effects on cholinergic neurons, dopamine, and muscarinic receptors in the proximal gut.[55] While short-term efficacy is documented, tachyphylaxis ensues, and long-term utility in the management of delayed gastric emptying has not been proved.[71,72] Central nervous system side effects, particularly jitteriness, tremor and extrapyramidal deficits can be limiting, and can be seen in some form in as many as 40% of patients.[72] Domperidone, an alternate dopamine receptor antagonist, may be better tolerated,[73,74] but is only available in the United States by direct import through an FDA-approved investigational new drug (IND) process.[55] Erythromycin induces gastric emptying by stimulating motilin and cholinergic receptors, and is most effective when used intravenously for short periods.[75] Oral administration is less effective, and may be associated with side effects. Cisapride accelerates gastric emptying and small bowel transit, but has been withdrawn because of the risk of fatal cardiac arrhythmias.[76] Tegaserod was also studied as a potential prokinetic agent in delayed gastric emptying, but has also been withdrawn from the market due to risk of vascular events.[77]

Improvement of chronic vomiting can be expected in 75% of patients with suppressive therapy using low dose tricyclic antidepressants. In an open label study, a similar benefit was achieved regardless of the presence of delayed gastric emptying.[78] The mechanism of action is unknown, but may be related to effects on central neural pathways involved in the process of vomiting.[79]

5.4.6.3 Gastric Electrical Stimulation

High-frequency electrical stimulation of the stomach using an implantable device is reported to improve nausea and vomiting, but does not necessarily accelerate gastric emptying.[80] Open label studies suggest a decreased need for nutritional support with the electrical stimulator, mainly from decreased frequency of emesis and fewer hospitalizations. Improvement in nausea and vomiting was noted in 60 to 75% of subjects in open label trials; a multicenter study with one year follow-up suggested a 50% reduction in nausea and vomiting.[80,81] Diabetics responded more favorably compared to idiopathic gastroparesis in a double-blind cross-over study.[82] However, data are insufficient for a more robust recommendation of this device, and human trials are hampered by inconsistency in diagnosis of gastroparesis and the invasive nature of the device.[80]

5.4.6.4 Other

Intrapyloric injection of botulinum toxin has been reported to improve gastric emptying of solids in open label studies,[83,84] but symptomatic benefit was lacking in a double-blind placebo-controlled cross-over study.[85] Near-total gastrectomy has been rarely performed for patients with significant gastric stasis, with reported symptomatic benefit in 43%, but with a complication rate of 40%.[86]

5.4.6.5 Monitoring

Patients with delayed gastric emptying and gastroparesis need to be monitored for fluid, electrolyte, and nutritional deficiencies. Hospital admissions may be necessary for correction of fluid and electrolyte imbalances. It is estimated that 2 to 5% of patients require multiple hospitalizations for management of refractory or ongoing symptoms.[87] Ongoing management hinges on adequate symptom suppression and maintenance of oral nutrition, without overt attempts to improve gastric motor physiology.[78]

REFERENCES

1. Tack J, Talley NJ, Camilleri M, et al. Functional gastroduodenal disorders. In Drossman DA, Corazziari E, Delvaux M, Spiller RC, Talley NJ, Thompson WG, Whitehead WE, eds, *Rome III: The Functional Gastrointestinal Disorders*, 3rd ed., Degnon Associates, McLean, Virginia, 2006:419–486.
2. Hill OW. Psychogenic vomiting. *Gut* 1968;9:348–352.
3. Muraoka M, Mine K, Matsumoto K, Nakai Y, Nakagawa T. Psychogenic vomiting: the relation between patterns of vomiting and psychiatric diagnoses. *Gut* 1990;31:526–528.
4. Wruble LD, Rosenthal RH, Webb WL, Jr. Psychogenic vomiting: a review. Am *J Gastroenterol* 1982;77:318–321.
5. Tosetti C, Stanghellini V, Corinaldesi R. The Rome II Criteria for patients with functional gastroduodenal disorders. *J Clin Gastroenterol* 2003;37:92–93.
6. Agreus L, Svardsudd K, Nyren O, Tibblin G. The epidemiology of abdominal symptoms: prevalence and demographic characteristics in a Swedish adult population. A report from the Abdominal Symptom Study. *Scand J Gastroenterol* 1994;29:102–109.
7. Adam B, Liebregts T, Holtmann G. Mechanisms of disease: genetics of functional gastrointestinal disorders—searching the genes that matter. *Nat Clin Pract Gastroenterol Hepatol* 2007;4:102–110.
8. Verhagen MA, Samsom M, Jebbink RJ, Smout AJ. Clinical relevance of antroduodenal manometry. *Eur J Gastroenterol Hepatol* 1999;11:523–528.
9. Wilmer A, Van Cutsem E, Andrioli A, Tack J, Coremans G, Janssens J. Ambulatory gastrojejunal manometry in severe motility-like dyspepsia: lack of correlation between dysmotility, symptoms, and gastric emptying. *Gut* 1998;42:235–242.
10. Holtmann G, Gschossmann J, Neufang-Huber J, Gerken G, Talley NJ. Differences in gastric mechanosensory function after repeated ramp distensions in non-consulters with dyspepsia and healthy controls. *Gut* 2000;47:332–336.
11. Vandenberghe J, Vos R, Persoons P, Demyttenaere K, Janssens J, Tack J. Dyspeptic patients with visceral hypersensitivity: sensitisation of pain specific or multimodal pathways? *Gut* 2005;54:914–919.
12. Ladabaum U, Minoshima S, Hasler WL, Cross D, Chey WD, Owyang C. Gastric distention correlates with activation of multiple cortical and subcortical regions. *Gastroenterology* 2001;120:369–376.
13. Sayuk GS, Elwing JE, Lustman PJ, Clouse RE. High somatic symptom burdens and functional gastrointestinal disorders. *Clin Gastroenterol Hepatol* 2007;5:556–562.
14. Olden KW, Chepyala P. Functional nausea and vomiting. *Nat Clin Pract Gastroenterol Hepatol* 2008;5:202–208.
15. Quigley EM, Hasler WL, Parkman HP. AGA technical review on nausea and vomiting. *Gastroenterology* 2001;120:263–286.
16. Reddymasu SC, Soykan I, McCallum RW. Domperidone: review of pharmacology and clinical applications in gastroenterology. *Am J Gastroenterol* 2007;102:2036–2045.
17. Prakash C, Clouse RE. Long-term outcome from tricyclic antidepressant treatment of functional chest pain. *Dig Dis Sci* 1999;44:2373–2379.
18. Clouse RE, Prakash C, Anderson RJ. Antidepressants for functional gastrointestinal symptoms and syndromes: a meta-analysis. *Gastroenterology* 2001;120:A 642.
19. Ernst E, Pittler MH. Efficacy of ginger for nausea and vomiting: a systematic review of randomized clinical trials. *Br J Anaesth* 2000;84:367–371.
20. Rashed H, Cutts T, Abell T, Cowings P, Toscano W, El-Gammal A, Adl D. Predictors of response to a behavioral treatment in patients with chronic gastric motility disorders. *Dig Dis Sci* 2002;47:1020–1026.
21. Takahashi T. Acupuncture for functional gastrointestinal disorders. *J Gastroenterol* 2006;41:408–417.

22. Gourcerol G, Leblanc I, Leroi AM, Denis P, Ducrotte P. Gastric electrical stimulation in medically refractory nausea and vomiting. *Eur J Gastroenterol Hepatol* 2007;19:29–35.

23. Jones MP, Crowell MD, Olden KW, Creed F. Functional gastrointestinal disorders: an update for the psychiatrist. *Psychosomatics* 2007;48:93–102.

24. Abu-Arafeh I, Russell G. Cyclical vomiting syndrome in children: a population-based study. *J Pediatr Gastroenterol Nutr* 1995;21:454–458.

25. Prakash C, Clouse RE. Cyclic vomiting syndrome in adults: clinical features and response to tricyclic antidepressants. *Am J Gastroenterol* 1999;94:2855–2860.

26. Li BU, Issenman RM, Sarna SK. Consensus statement—2nd International Scientific Symposium on CVS. The Faculty of the 2nd International Scientific Symposium on Cyclic Vomiting Syndrome. *Dig Dis Sci* 1999;44:9S–11S.

27. Prakash C, Staiano A, Rothbaum RJ, Clouse RE. Similarities in cyclic vomiting syndrome across age groups. *Am J Gastroenterol* 2001;96:684–688.

28. Rashed H, Abell TL, Familoni BO, Cardoso S. Autonomic function in cyclic vomiting syndrome and classic migraine. *Dig Dis Sci* 1999;44:74S–78S.

29. Abell TL, Kim CH, Malagelada JR. Idiopathic cyclic nausea and vomiting—a disorder of gastrointestinal motility? *Mayo Clin Proc* 1988;63:1169–1175.

30. Pfau BT, Li BU, Murray RD, Heitlinger LA, McClung HJ, Hayes JR. Differentiating cyclic from chronic vomiting patterns in children: quantitative criteria and diagnostic implications. *Pediatrics* 1996;97:364–368.

31. Salpietro CD, Briuglia S, Merlino MV, Di Bella C, Rigoli L. A mitochondrial DNA mutation (A3243G mtDNA) in a family with cyclic vomiting. *Eur J Pediatr* 2003;162:727–728.

32. Tache Y. Cyclic vomiting syndrome: the corticotropin-releasing-factor hypothesis. *Dig Dis Sci* 1999;44:79S–86S.

33. Sato T, Igarashi N, Minami S, Okabe T, Hashimoto H, Hasui M, Kato E. Recurrent attacks of vomiting, hypertension and psychotic depression: a syndrome of periodic catecholamine and prostaglandin discharge. *Acta Endocrinol* (Copenh) 1988;117:189–197.

34. Fleisher DR, Gornowicz B, Adams K, Burch R, Feldman EJ. Cyclic Vomiting Syndrome in 41 adults: the illness, the patients, and problems of management. *BMC Med* 2005;3:20.

35. Namin F, Patel J, Lin Z, Sarosiek I, Foran P, Esmaeili P, McCallum R. Clinical, psychiatric and manometric profile of cyclic vomiting syndrome in adults and response to tricyclic therapy. *Neurogastroenterol Motil* 2007;19:196–202.

36. Li BU, Lefevre F, Chelimsky GG, Boles RG, Nelson SP, Lewis DW, Linder SL, Issenman RM, Rudolph CD. North American Society for Pediatric Gastroenterology, Hepatology, and Nutrition consensus statement on the diagnosis and management of cyclic vomiting syndrome. *J Pediatr Gastroenterol Nutr* 2008;47:379–393.

37. Abell TL, Adams KA, Boles RG, Bousvaros A, Chong SK, Fleisher DR, Hasler WL, Hyman PE, Issenman RM, Li BU, Linder SL, Mayer EA, McCallum RW, Olden K, Parkman HP, Rudolph CD, Tache Y, Tarbell S, Vakil N. Cyclic vomiting syndrome in adults. *Neurogastroenterol Motil* 2008;20:269–284.

38. Sudel B, Li BU. Treatment options for cyclic vomiting syndrome. *Curr Treat Options Gastroenterol* 2005;8:387–395.

39. Mitchelson F. Pharmacological agents affecting emesis. A review (Part II). *Drugs* 1992;43:443–463.

40. Weitz R. Prophylaxis of cyclic vomiting with propranolol. *Drug Intell Clin Pharm* 1982;16:161–162.

41. Clouse RE, Sayuk GS, Lustman PJ, Prakash C. Zonisamide or levetiracetam for adults with cyclic vomiting syndrome: a case series. *Clin Gastroenterol Hepatol* 2007;5:44–48.
42. Mathias JR, Clench MH, Abell TL, Koch KL, Lehman G, Robinson M, Rothstein R, Snape WJ. Effect of leuprolide acetate in treatment of abdominal pain and nausea in premenopausal women with functional bowel disease: a double-blind, placebo-controlled, randomized study. *Dig Dis Sci* 1998;43:1347–1355.
43. Waseem S, Moshiree B, Draganov PV. Gastroparesis: Current diagnostic challenges and management considerations. *World J Gastroenterol* 2009;15:25–37.
44. Hasler WL. Gastroparesis: Symptoms, evaluation and treatment. *Gastroenterol Clin N Am* 2007;36:619–647.
45. Parkman HP, Hasler WL, Fisher RS. American gastroenterological association technical review on the diagnosis and treatment of gastroparesis. *Gastroenterology* 2004;127:1592–1622.
46. Bytzer P, Talley NJ, Leemon M, et al. Prevalence of gastrointestinal symptoms associated with diabetes llitus. *Arch Intern Med* 2001;161:1989–1996.
47. Maleki D, Locke GR, Camilleri M, et al. Gastrointestinal tract symptoms among persons with diabetes mellitus in the community. *Arch Intern Med* 2000;160:2808–2816.
48. Jones KL, Russo A, Stevens JE, et al. Predictors of delayed gastric emptying in diabetics. *Diabetes Care* 2001;24:1264–1269.
49. Kendall BJ, Kendall ET, Soykan I, McCallum RW. Cisapride in the long-term treatment of chronic gastroparesis: a 2-year open label study. *J Int Med Res* 1997;25:182–189.
50. Loo FD, Palmer DW, Soergel KH, Kalbfleisch JH, Wood CM. Gastric emptying in patients with diabetes mellitus. *Gastroenterology* 1984;86:485–494.
51. Stanghellini V, Tosetti C, Paternico A, et al. Risk indicators of delayed gastric emptying of solids in patients with functional dyspepsia. *Gastroenterology* 1996;110:1036–1042.
52. Sarnelli G, Caenepeel P, Geypens B, Janssens J, Tack J. Symptoms associated with impaired gastric emptying of solids in liquids in functional dyspepsia. *Am J Gastroenterol* 2003;98:783–788.
53. Lemann M, Dederding JP, Flourie B, et al. Abnormal perception of visceral pain in response to gastric distension in chronic idiopathic dyspepsia. *Dig Dis Sci* 1991;36:1249–1254.
54. Samsom M, Salet GAM, Roelofs JMM, et al. Compliance of the proximal stomach and dyspeptic symptoms in patients with type 1 diabetes mellitus. *Dig Dis Sci* 1995;40:2037–2042.
55. Park M, Camilleri M. Gastroparesis: clinical update. *Am J Gastroenterol* 2006;101: 1129–1139.
56. Hasler WL. Physiology of gastric motility and gastric emptying. In Yamada T, Alpers DH, Kaplowitz N, Laine L, Owyang C, Powell DW, (eds), *Textbook of Gastroenterology*, 4th ed., Lippincott Williams and Wilkins, Philadelphia, 2003:195–219.
57. Ordog T, Takayama I, Cheung WK, Ward SM, Sanders KM. Remodeling of networks of interstitial cells of Cajal in a murine model of diabetic gastroparesis. *Diabetes* 2000;121:427–434.
58. Vinik AI, Maser RE, Mitchell BD, Freeman R. Diabetic autonomic neuropathy. *Diabetes Care* 2003;26:1553–1579.
59. Mearin F, Camilleri M, Malagelada JR. Pyloric dysfunction in diabetics with recurrent nausea and vomiting. *Gastroenterology* 1986;90:1919–1925.
60. Fraser RJ, Horowitz M, Maddox AF, et al. Hyperglycaemia slows gastric emptying in type 1 (insulin dependent) diabetes mellitus. *Diabetologia* 1990;33:675–680.
61. Horowitz M, Maddox AF, Wishart JM, et al. Relationships between oesophageal transit and solid and liquid gastric emptying in diabetes mellitus. *Eur J Nucl Med* 1991;18:229–234.

62. Tack J, Demedts I, Dehondt G, et al. Clinical and pathophysiological characteristics of acute-onset functional dyspepsia. *Gastroenterology* 2002;122:1738–1747.
63. Tack J, Bisschops R. Mechanisms underlying meal-induced symptoms in functional dyspepsia. *Gastroenterology* 2004;127:1844–1847.
64. Bredenoord AJ, Chial HJ, Camilleri M, et al. Gastric accommodation and emptying in evaluation of patients with upper gastrointestinal symptoms. *Clin Gastroenterol Hepatol* 2003;1:264–272.
65. Soykan I, Sivri B, Sarosiek I, et al. Demography, clinical characteristics, psychological and abuse profiles, treatment, and long-term follow up of patients with gastroparesis. *Dig Dis Sci* 1998;43:2398–2404.
66. Parkman HP, Schwartz SS. Esophagitis and other gastrointestinal disorders associated with diabetic gastroparesis. *Arch Intern Med* 1987;147:1477–1480.
67. Parkman HP, Harris AD, Krevsky B, et al. Gastroduodenal motility and dysmotility: updates on techniques available for evaluation. *Am J Gastroenterol* 1995;90:869–892.
68. Galil MA, Critchley M, Mackie CR. Isotope gastric emptying tests in clinical practice: expectation, outcome and utility. *Gut* 1993;34:916–919.
69. Tougas GH, Eaker EY, Abell TL, et al. Assessment of gastric emptying using a low fat meal: establishment of international control values. *Am J Gastroenterol* 2000;95:1456–1462.
70. Guo JP, Maurer AH, Fisher RS, Parkman HP. Extending gastric emptying scintigraphy from two to four hours detects more patients with gastroparesis. *Dig Dis Sci* 2001;46:24–29.
71. Snape WJ, Battle WM, Schwartz SS, et al. Metoclopramide to treat gastroparesis due to diabetes mellitus: a double blind, controlled trial. *Ann Intern Med* 1982;96:444–446.
72. Lata PF, Pigarelli DL. Chronic metoclopramide therapy for diabetic gastroparesis. *Ann Pharmacother* 2003;37:122–126.
73. Silvers D, Kipnes M, Broadstone V, et al. Domperidone in the management of symptoms of diabetic gastroparesis: efficacy, tolerability, and quality-of-life outcomes in a multicenter controlled trial. Dom-USA-5 Study Group. *Clin Ther* 1998;20:438–453.
74. Patterson D, Abell T, Rothstein R, et al. A double-blind multicenter comparison of domperidone and metoclopramide in the treatment of diabetic patients with symptoms of gastroparesis. *Am J Gastroenterol* 1999;94:1230–1234.
75. Coulie B, Tack J, Peeters T, et al. Involvement of two different pathways in the motor effects of erythromycin on the gastric antrum in humans. *Gut* 1998;43:395–400.
76. Wang SH, Lin CY, Huang TY, et al. QT interval effects of cisapride in the clinical setting. *Int J Cardiol* 2001;80:179–183.
77. Tougas G, Chen Y, Luo D, et al. Tegaserod improves gastric emptying in patients with gastroparesis and dyspeptic symptoms. *Gastroenterology* 2003;124:A54.
78. Sawhney MS, Prakash C, Lustman PJ, Clouse RE. Tricyclic antidepressants for chronic vomiting in diabetic patients. *Dig Dis Sci* 2007;52:418–424.
79. Clouse RE, Lustman PJ. The use of psychopharmacological agents for functional gastrointestinal disorders. *Gut* 2005;54:1332–1341.
80. Lin J, Chen JDZ. Implantable gastric electrical stimulation: ready for prime time? *Gastroenterology* 2008;134:665–667.
81. Abell T, McCallum R, Hocking M, et al. Gastric electrical stimulation for medically refractory gastroparesis. *Gastroenterology* 2003;125:421–428.
82. Abell TK, Van Cutsem E, Abrahamsson H, et al. Gastric electrical stimulation in intractable symptomatic gastroparesis. *Digestion* 2002;66:204–212.
83. Ezzeddine D, Jit R, Katz N, et al. Pyloric injection of botulinum toxin for the treatment of diabetic gastroparesis. *Gastrointest Endosc* 2002;55:920–923.
84. Lacy BE, Zayat EN, Crowell MD, et al. Botulinum toxin for the treatment of gastroparesis: a preliminary report. *Am J Gastroenterol* 2002;97:1548–1552.

85. Arts J, Caenepeel P, Degreef T, et al. Randomized double blind cross-over study evaluating the effect of intrapyloric injection of botulinum toxin on gastric emptying and symptoms in patients with gastroparesis. *Gastroenterology* 2005;128:A81.
86. Forstner-Barthell AW, Murr MM, Nitecki S, et al. Near-total completion gastrectomy for severe postvagotomy gastric stasis: analysis of early and long-term results in 62 patients. *J Gastrointest Surg* 1999;3:15–21.
87. Syed AA, Rattansingh A, Furtado SD. Current perspectives on the management of gastroparesis. *J Postgrad Med* 2005;51:54–60.

6 Celiac Disease

Peter David Howdle

CONTENTS

6.1 INTRODUCTION AND HISTORY

Physicians have been aware for centuries of a clinical condition that was probably celiac disease. The word *celiac* is derived from a Greek word meaning "belonging to the belly" and it is claimed to have first been used for a medical condition by Aretaeus from Cappadocia (now part of modern Turkey) who practiced in Rome in the second century AD. However, the first accurate description was published in

1888 by Samuel Gee[1] of St. Bartholomew's Hospital in London. His description of the clinical features remains remarkably accurate even when we now know so much about the disease. He was also percipient in that he said that "if the patient can be cured at all, it must be by means of diet."[1] During the subsequent 60 years, few advances were made although many dietary manipulations were tried, including the famous "banana diet." Some of these diets worked because, unknown to the recommending physician, the patients were obtaining carbohydrates from elsewhere and avoiding wheat to a large extent.

In 1950, Willem Dicke, a pediatrician in Holland, showed that wheat was implicated in causing the clinical symptoms of celiac disease (CD).[2] It is said that he formed this opinion partly out of his observation that when wheat and rye were unavailable in Holland during World War II his young patients improved, only to relapse when these cereals became available at the end of the war. Dicke and coworkers went on to show that the gluten fraction of wheat produced evidence of malabsorption in children with CD.[3]

Two other major advances were made during the 1950s. John Paulley provided an accurate description of the typical gastrointestinal lesion from operative specimens from patients with CD.[4] The development of peroral biopsy instruments enabled small intestinal mucosal biopsies to be obtained without abdominal surgery.[5,6]

Since these seminal findings our understanding of CD has increased markedly. Much is known about the genetics of the disease, the moiety in gluten that is involved, the detail of the mucosal abnormality, and the immunopathogenesis.

Celiac disease can be defined as that disorder in predisposed individuals in which there is an abnormality of the small intestinal mucosa manifested by contact with the gluten fraction of wheat and the similar fractions in rye and barley. It is important to note that this definition refers to a predisposition (the genetics of the disease), to an abnormality of the small intestinal mucosa (but does not state the degree or type of abnormality since we now know this is very variable), and to fractions of three cereals: wheat, rye, and barley (but not a specific "toxic" peptide). Some explanation of all these caveats will be given in Section 6.3 and Section 6.4.

6.2 EPIDEMIOLOGY

Many patients with celiac disease remain undiagnosed, partly because they have minimal symptoms and partly because, unfortunately, many clinicians fail to consider the diagnosis. Hence, the true prevalence is unknown. However, there are many recent studies estimating the prevalence in developed countries using serological tests in normal populations (e.g., blood donors). The estimates range from 1:100 to 1:400;[7–10] these figures are considerably higher than those previously quoted at 1:1000[11] and 1:3000[12] and reflect the fact that many people with minimal or no symptoms are never diagnosed. In the United Kingdom, there is good evidence that the prevalence is 1:100,[7,13] but clinical estimates suggest only 1:800 are diagnosed. These figures have led to the concept of the "celiac iceberg" (Figure 6.1).[14]

At the tip of the iceberg there are diagnosed patients with clinical disease with a known abnormal small intestinal mucosal biopsy. Their symptoms may be gastrointestinal or nongastrointestinal (often called atypical, e.g., anemia, osteopenia).

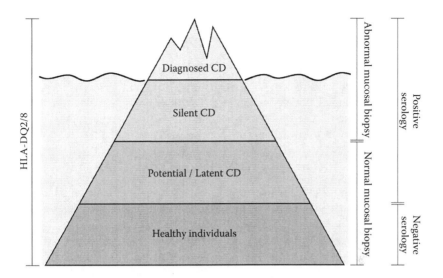

FIGURE 6.1 (See color insert following Page 112) The Celiac Iceberg. (From Maki M, Collin P. Coeliac disease. *Lancet* 1997, 349, 1755–1759. With permission.)

Beneath them, below the waterline, are patients who are undiagnosed; they have few, if any, recognized clinical features, but do have an abnormal mucosa on biopsy (silent CD). Both of these groups of patients would be expected to have a positive serological test. Beneath them, there are individuals who are likely to develop evidence of celiac disease. Those with potential CD have a normal small intestinal mucosal biopsy, but may have a positive serological test and a predisposition to develop the disease, e.g., a blood relative with CD. Those with latent CD constitute a very small number of individuals who have a normal mucosal biopsy while taking a normal (gluten containing) diet, but at some other time, either previously or later, have an abnormal mucosa that responds to gluten withdrawal.[15] They also may have a positive serological test. This latter group provides evidence of the dynamic nature of gluten sensitivity in some individuals. Finally, at the base of the iceberg is a large number of healthy individuals with normal small intestinal mucosa and negative serology who never develop CD, but who have the same predisposing HLA (human leukocyte antigen) genes as the other groups who have CD.

These epidemiological findings are mainly reported for Caucasian populations of European decent, i.e., Europe, Australia, the Americas. The reported prevalences reflect the genetic inheritance, the developed healthcare systems, and the frequency of wheat use in the diet. The prevalence in the United States is said to be variable, which may reflect the diverse racial mix and varying dietary traditions. It certainly seems that from an evolutionary viewpoint the prevalence of the disease reflects the spread of wheat cultivation from the fertile crescent in the Middle East where agriculture began. The disease is rare in countries with traditionally rice or maize-based diets. It is described in those Asian countries where wheat is commonly used in the diet, but rarely, if ever affects those of purely African Caribbean, Chinese, or

Japanese decent. These latter groups presumably inheriting a slightly different HLA genotype irrespective of the traditional cereal component of their diets.

The disease is frequently reported to affect adult females more than males (2:1), although the sex ratio in children is equal. This may reflect the willingness of women to seek medical investigation.

In many developing countries diagnostic facilities are almost nonexistent, malnutrition is common and many gastrointestinal symptoms are due to infectious diseases; hence, CD will not be considered nor regarded as a major medical issue.

6.3   SMALL INTESTINAL PATHOLOGY IN CELIAC DISEASE

The definition of CD given above includes an abnormality of the small intestinal mucosa. It is in the upper portion of the small intestine that the classical abnormalities were described and which are sought in order to make the diagnosis. In modern medical practice biopsies of the upper small intestine (distal duodenum beyond the first part) are easily obtained using a routine gastroscope. Ideally, four mucosal biopsies should be obtained and orientated correctly for histological examination. In CD, it is the mucosa only that is usually affected and when there are major abnormalities these can be seen under the dissecting microscope where, in CD, the surface looks flat, often with a mosaic appearance. There is an absence of villi and the entrances to the crypt vestibules are obvious. A comparison with normal mucosa is seen in Figure 6.2a,b.

Histological sections confirm the absence of villi or loss of villous height with an increase in crypt depth and in inflammatory cells. A comparison with normal mucosa is seen in Figure 6.3a,b. In CD, the surface enterocytes are cuboidal rather than columnar and have a much more immature appearance. The crypt cells have a normal appearance in CD, but have a greatly increased cell turnover with a reduced cell cycle time, as reflected by the crypt hyperplasia.

As well as these villus—crypt changes, the mucosa has a large increase in inflammatory cells. There is an early increase in intraepithelial lymphocytes (IELs) (predominantly CD8+ve) accompanied by increases in lymphocytes (predominantly CD4+ve), plasma cells, macrophages, polymorphs, eosinophils, and mast cells in the lamina propria. Together with the crypt hyperplasia, this means that the mucosal thickness is similar to normal, despite the loss of villous height.

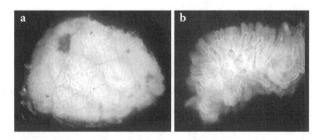

FIGURE 6.2a/b (See color insert following Page 112)   (a) Untreated celiac mucosa at dissecting microscopy (×10); (b) normal mucosa at dissecting microscopy (×10). (From Howdle PD. *Encyclopedia of Food Sciences and Nutrition*, Elsevier, Amsterdam, 2003. With permission.)

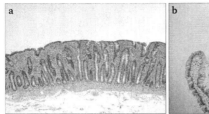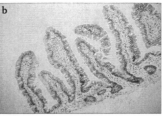

FIGURE 6.3a/b (See color insert following Page 112) (a) Histological section of untreated celiac mucosa (×40); (b) histological section of normal mucosa (×40). (From Howdle PD. *Encyclopedia of Food Sciences and Nutrition*, Elsevier, Amsterdam, 2003. With permission.)

Electron microscopic examination of the enterocytes in CD reveals degenerative changes including shortened and distorted microvilli on the brush boarder (see Figure 6.4a,b for comparison with normal).

Marsh, in a series of elegant studies, showed how dynamic these changes were in the mucosa, particularly in relation to the amount of gluten present.[16] He graded the pathological features on a scale of 0 to 4. Type 0 was "preinfiltrative" where the mucosa is normal, but the patient may have positive serology. Type 1 was "infiltrative" with an increase in IELs but normal architecture. Type 2 was "infiltrative/hyperplasic" with an increase in IELs and LP lymphocytes as well as crypt hyperplasia, but villi of normal height. In Type 3, "flat destructive," there is villous atrophy as well as the other features. Types 2 and 3 represent those features commonly seen in newly diagnosed celiac patients. Type 4 "atrophic hypoplastic" is very rare and irreversible. There is not only villous atrophy but total hypoplasia of the mucosa. It leads to severe malabsorption and is normally untreatable and often fatal.

Routine biopsies of the duodenum in untreated celiac disease do show variability in the mucosal changes. Hence, the lesion is said to be "patchy."[17] This emphasizes the need for several diagnostic biopsies.

The mucosal changes are more severe proximally in the small intestine, so that in most patients there is a length of mid to lower small intestine that is normal. This partly explains the variety and severity of symptoms between patients. Nevertheless, the distal mucosa is gluten sensitive and typical changes occur if gluten is instilled in the ileum.

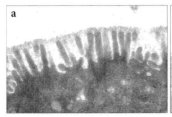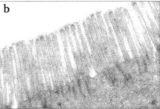

FIGURE 6.4a/b (a) Electron micrograph of microvilli on an untreated celiac enterocyte (×40,000); (b) electron micrograph of microvilli on a normal enterocyte (×40,000). (From Howdle PD. *Your Guide to Coeliac Disease.* Hodder Arnold, London. 2007. With permission.)

Treatment of celiac disease with a gluten-free diet (GFD) results in reversal of the changes described with the mucosa returning toward normal.

6.4 PATHOGENESIS OF CELIAC DISEASE

CD has been a good clinical model allowing a greater understanding of intestinal mucosal immunology. There are three factors involved in the pathogenesis of celiac disease, as suggested in the definition of the disease: the environmental factor (gluten), the genetic predisposition, and the mucosal immune system.[18,19]

6.4.1 THE ENVIRONMENTAL FACTOR

CD can only occur in populations and individuals who consume wheat and related cereals as part of their diet. Dicke and co-workers in the 1950s showed that it was the gluten content of wheat that was responsible for inducing the disease.[3] Gluten is the water-insoluble component of wheat flour and is a complex mixture of proteins. When cooked, gluten gives food the texture that is very palatable. Gliadin is the alcohol-soluble fraction of gluten, whereas glutenin is the insoluble fraction. There are similar fractions in the related cereals rye and barley, the gliadin equivalents being secalin and hordein, respectively. The phylogenic relationships of the cereals are shown in Figure 6.5. The triticeae branch contains the celiac-inducing cereals, and it can be seen that those more distantly related cereals are safe for celiac patients to consume. Most investigations into the relevant pathogenetic fractions have been performed on gliadins. The gliadin genes have large allelic variation so that the gliadins in a single wheat variety comprise a complex mixture.

The gliadins can be separated on the basis of molecular weight into α, β, γ, and ω fractions, and the amino acid structure of several of these proteins has been described. Several peptides from an α-gliadin have been shown to be immunologically active in celiac disease. Interestingly, these are rich in proline and glutamine and are particularly resistant to intestinal peptidases.[18,20]

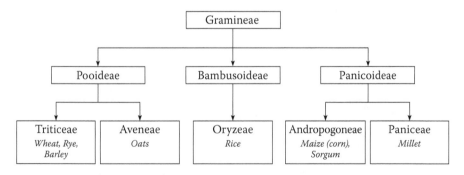

FIGURE 6.5 Taxonomic relationships of cereal grains. Celiac-inducing cereals are in the triticeae group; oats, the most closely related is safe for the vast majority of celiac patients. Other cereals are distantly related and are safe for celiac patients.

6.4.2 GENETIC PREDISPOSITION

Involvement of the human leukocyte antigen region (HLA) on chromosome 6 has been known for some time.[21] More detailed analysis has revealed that almost 95% of celiac patients have the genes that encode for HLA-DQ2 and the remaining 5% for HLA-DQ8.[22] These findings imply that possession of HLA-DQ2 or DQ8 is necessary but not sufficient for the development of celiac disease, since 30% of the healthy population also possess these genes. The genetic basis of CD is supported by the clinical findings that 10% of blood relatives have the disease and that there is at least 70% concordance in monozygotic twins.[23] Several non-HLA genes are also associated with CD, although their role has yet to be determined.[24,25]

6.4.3 THE MUCOSAL IMMUNE RESPONSE

Immune responses to gliadin peptides form the basis of the pathological changes seen in CD, both innate and adaptive immune systems are involved. Certain gliadin peptides (e.g., p31-43 from A-gliadin) have been shown to induce interleukin-15 in enterocytes.[26] IL-15 is involved in T-cell activation, in the activation of IELs expressing the NK-G2D natural killer cell receptor, and in the expression of the stress molecule MIC-A on enterocytes. Interaction between enterocyte MIC-A and lymphocyte NK-G2D results in direct enterocyte killing and is one way in which early damage to the villi occurs.[27,28] Such damage may also enhance the permeability of gliadin peptides into the lamina propria.[29]

IL-15 activation of T-cells also relates to the adaptive immune response. In this system, antigen-presenting cells (APC) expressing HLA DQ2/8 surface receptors preferentially take up gliadin peptides, which have been deamidated by tissue transglutaminase in the lamina propria.[30,31] This deamidation of glutamine to glutamic acid in the gliadin peptides increases their immunogenicity. The APCs process the peptide and present it on the surface bound to the DQ2/8 receptors in order to activate gliadin-sensitive CD4 + T-cells. This results in the release of a variety of cytokines and other mediators involved in the inflammatory response and results in the villous damage and crypt hyperplasia typical of CD (Figure 6.6). As part of this cascade, B-cells are activated into plasma cells specifically producing celiac-relevant antibodies (e.g., antigliadin, antiendomysial, antitissue transglutaminase).[18]

The current understanding of the immune pathogenesis of the disease and its association with other autoimmune diseases, probably via a common genetic predisposition, has led to CD being considered an autoimmune disorder. The specific autoantigen is unknown, but is probably a complex involving elements of a gliadin peptide and tissue transglutaminase, against which specific antibodies are produced.[32]

It is important to note that other factors may have a role in the development of CD by influencing the immune response. For example, breast feeding of infants and the timing of the introduction of gluten into the diet may affect the development of the disease.[33] Certain gastrointestinal infections (e.g., rotavirus) may also increase the risk.[34]

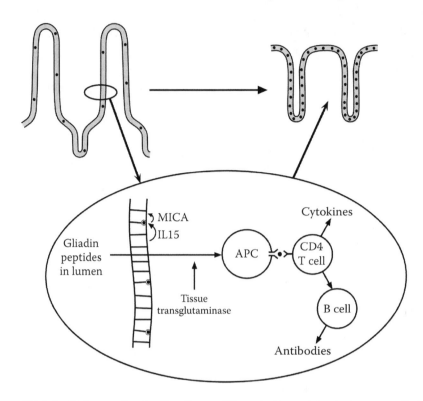

FIGURE 6.6 Pathogenesis of celiac disease. Wheat is digested in the lumen to gliadin peptides. Resistant to further breakdown, they cross the epithelial layer stimulating IL-15 from enterocytes in the innate response. Gliadin peptides in the lamina propria are deaminated by tissue transglutaminase and processed by antigen-presenting cells for presentation via HLA-DQ2/8 molecules to the T-cell receptor of CD4 cells. These initiate the adaptive immune response leading to the characteristic mucosal pathology.

6.5   CLINICAL FEATURES OF CELIAC DISEASE

Since CD is a disease affecting mainly the small intestine with varying severity, this results in a number of clinical effects. There may be gastrointestinal symptoms, or more systemic symptoms believed to result from the malabsorption of a variety of dietary nutrients and from the underlying autoimmune nature of the disease. Thus, patients can have a wide variety of clinical features of varying severity. Those with predominantly gastrointestinal symptoms are said to have "classical" CD, those with more general, mainly nongastrointestinal symptoms, are said to have "atypical" CD, and those with no symptoms have "silent" CD. All of these patients would have the characteristic features in a small intestinal biopsy. These clinical presentations are reflected in the "iceberg" phenomenon described in Section 6.2. Clinical effects can occur at any age, but there are two peaks of incidence, one in early childhood and the other in middle age.[14,19]

6.5.1 Celiac Disease in Childhood

Approximately 30% of all patients who are eventually diagnosed with CD will have had symptoms attributable to the disease in childhood, although not all of them will have had the diagnosis made as children. The majority of children who are diagnosed develop quite marked symptoms early in life between six months and two years of age. Boys and girls are equally affected. Symptoms develop only after the introduction of cereals to the diet. Longer breast feeding and later introduction of cereals may reduce the risk of developing the disease.[33]

Affected infants develop diarrhea, vomiting, and a swollen abdomen. They are generally unwell and irritable and fail to thrive. This is in marked contrast to their initial progress.

In later childhood (2 to 10 years), children have more minor gastrointestinal symptoms, but may be shorter in height than expected with delayed growth and puberty. They may be lacking in energy and have behavioral or learning difficulties. Anemia and nutritional deficiencies may be detected. Some children are now detected following screening of family members.

It is not known why CD is diagnosed less frequently in teenagers. Those who have been diagnosed as children often find a gluten-free diet very difficult to maintain. However, despite frequently consuming large amounts of gluten, they often have none or few symptoms. Why this is the case is not known.

6.5.2 Celiac Disease in Adults

The clinical features of newly diagnosed adults with CD have changed considerably in the past 25 years. Previously patients presented with marked gastrointestinal symptoms and major weight loss. Nowadays, the majority of patients have few symptoms and are frequently diagnosed because of anemia or an incidental deficiency on a routine blood test. This is mainly because clinicians are more aware of the disease, there is a sensitive serological test and it is being diagnosed earlier.[35,36]

The peak age for diagnosing CD in adults is 40 to 55 years, although it can be diagnosed at any age. More patients are being diagnosed over 65 years of age for the first time. General lethargy is a common, and sole, presentation. The ratio of diagnosed female to male adult patients is 2:1 and, although the reason for this is unknown, it may reflect men's reluctance to seek medical attention. Thirty percent will have had symptoms in childhood, which could be attributable to the disease and 10% will have a family history.

Gastrointestinal symptoms are now seen less frequently at diagnosis, these are the "classical" symptoms of diarrhea, abdominal bloating, and weight loss (Table 6.1). Of people diagnosed with irritable bowel syndrome, at least 5% will have CD.[37] Rather than being underweight, 30% of patients will be clinically overweight when first diagnosed.[38]

More usually patients will present with "atypical" features (Table 6.1). Usually these will be lethargy and a finding of anemia. Chronic symptoms with no clinical diagnosis can lead to depression and anxiety. Patients may present with muscle and joint pains, ataxia, and peripheral neuropathy. These neurological findings, although

TABLE 6.1

Classical and Atypical Presenting Clinical Features in CD

Classical	Atypical
Diarrhea	Fatigue
Abdominal discomfort	Anemia
Abdominal swelling	Vitamin deficiencies
Weight loss	Osteopenia/osteoporosis
Indigestion	Arthritis/arthralgia/myalgia
Mouth ulcers	Ataxia
Nausea/vomiting	Peripheral neuropathy
Constipation	Epilepsy
Irritable bowel syndrome	Reduced fertility
Delayed development	Obesity
Childhood history suggestive of CD	Depression/anxiety
	Family history of CD
	Incidentally positive serology or duodenal biopsy

rare are increasingly recognized. Epilepsy and cerebral calcification have been reported, particularly in children, but these are rare. Osteopenia and osteoporosis are common findings in untreated celiac disease, and, conversely, in patients with "idiopathic" osteoporosis, 5 to 10% will be found to have CD.[39]

Problems with fertility have been reported in CD. In adolescent girls, puberty may be delayed and women with a chronic disease have reduced fertility and an early menopause. Well-treated female patients should have none of these problems and fertility is normal in such patients, although celiac women tend to have their children at a slightly later age than average.[40]

On clinical examination very few abnormal physical signs will be found in the celiac patient, reflecting the nonspecific nature of many of the presenting symptoms. For these reasons there are still many patients where it takes a long time for the diagnosis to be made; this delay contributes to the psychological features of chronic ill health.

6.6 ASSOCIATED DISEASES

There are several diseases or conditions that are associated with CD and which occur more commonly in celiac patients than would normally be expected. These are listed in Table 6.2. The more common of these are dermatitis herpetiformis, insulin-dependent diabetes mellitus, thyroid disease, and immunoglobulin A (IgA) deficiency. Many of those listed have an autoimmune basis that perhaps reflects a common genetic basis for the diseases.[41] Five to 10 percent of celiac patients may develop type I diabetes mellitus (DM) or thyroid disease and these should be borne in mind in the follow-up of celiac patients.[42,43]

IgA deficiency occurs in 1:40 of celiac patients compared to 1:400 of the general population. Thus, celiac patients may be prone to more minor infections, but these are not

---

TABLE 6.2

Conditions Associated with CD

Dermatitis herpetiformis
Type I diabetes mellitus
Autoimmune thyroid disease
IgA deficiency
Inflammatory bowel disease and microscopic colitis
Sjogren's syndrome and other connective tissue disorders
Addison's disease
Pulmonary fibrosis
Down's syndrome
Turner's syndrome
Cardiomyopathy
Sarcoidosis
Primary biliary cirrhosis
Persistent abnormal liver function
Chronic thrombocytopenic purpura

---

usually of any practical significance. The main practical problem is that IgA deficiency may have a misleading effect on the antibody tests for CD (see Section 6.7.1 below).

Dermatitis herpetiformis (DH) is a rare skin disease characterized by intensely itchy blisters on elbows, knees, buttocks, and torso.[44] At least 90% of patients have small intestinal mucosal abnormalities identical to those of celiac disease. Patients also have the same HLA genotype and serological profiles as celiac disease. DH patients have few if any gastrointestinal symptoms reflecting the relatively mild nature of the small intestinal mucosal abnormalities normally seen in DH. The skin lesion responds to treatment with dapsone, but also to a gluten-free diet, which is also recommended for the small intestinal disease. DH patients can develop the same complications or associated conditions as those with celiac disease. The pathogenesis of DH is not understood, but there is now evidence that a particular type of tissue transglutaminase, which is specific to the skin, may be involved, presumably rendering gliadin more immunogenic for the skin.

6.7 DIAGNOSIS OF CELIAC DISEASE

In view of the wide variety of symptoms and range of severity (including "silent" disease), clinicians must have a high index of suspicion for CD. Routine blood tests may show anemia, evidence of vitamin and mineral deficiency, or features of a hyposplenic blood film, but none of these are specific for CD.

6.7.1 CELIAC ANTIBODY TESTS

Serological tests have been available for some years, but have become more reliable recently. Such tests usually measure IgA antibodies, but it should be remembered

TABLE 6.3

Range of Published Sensitivities and Specificities for Serological Tests in CD

Serological Test	Sensitivity	Specificity
IgA antigliadin antibodies (AGA)	75–90%	82–95%
IgA endomysial antibodies (EMA)	85–98%	97–100%
IgA tissue transglutaminase antibodies (tTG)	90–98%	94–97%

that IgA deficiency is more common in CD, so that IgA levels should be measured or IgG antibodies also assayed where there is any doubt. Antigliadin antibodies (AGA) are present in CD, but the sensitivity and specificity are not sufficient for a reliable clinical test.[45] Recently antibodies to deamidated gliadin have been measured that may develop into a more reliable test. Antiendomysial antibodies (EMA) are very specific for CD and have a high sensitivity, hence, this is a reliable clinical test. The endomysium is an element of connective tissue and it is now known that the antigenic component of endomysium against which the antibodies develop is the enzyme tissue transglutamase. Measurement of these antibodies (tTG) is also highly sensitive and specific for CD. Therefore, this is also a reliable clinical test. Anti-tTG antibodies are easily measured in the laboratory and, if positive, a confirmatory EMA is usually also performed.[45,46]

The range of sensitivities and specificities of these tests using IgA antibodies is shown in Table 6.3. Since none of these serological tests is 100% accurate, the diagnosis should always be confirmed by small intestinal biopsy.

6.7.2 SMALL INTESTINAL BIOPSY

As already mentioned, when seeking to diagnose CD, four small intestinal biopsies from the second/third part of the duodenum should be obtained via a routine upper gastrointestinal endoscopy. These should be carefully orientated and the histological sections reported by a pathologist with experience of celiac pathology. The characteristic changes have already been described and are represented in Figure 6.3a.

6.8 DIAGNOSTIC PATHWAY

The diagnostic pathway for CD includes the use of both serological tests and mucosal biopsy. Figure 6.7 shows a logical progression. Before proceeding with this scheme, the clinician should ensure that the patient is taking a diet containing gluten.

When following such a diagnostic scheme, there is always a small number of patients on the borderline. These cases should always be reviewed and investigations repeated if there is doubt or discrepancy. Where other causes of villous atrophy (Table 6.4) are being considered specialist follow-up is necessary.

There are three further points to note. A follow-up biopsy 6 to 12 months after starting a gluten-free diet was previously thought to be mandatory in order to show an

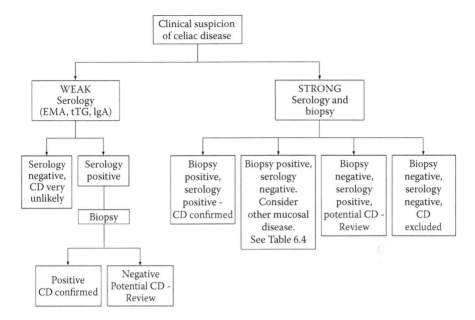

FIGURE 6.7 The diagnostic pathway. If the clinical suspicion of CD is weak (e.g., no suggestive symptoms), serology is performed first. If the suspicion is strong, both serology and a biopsy are performed. In patients with an abnormal biopsy (biopsy positive), but negative serology, other causes of villous atrophy (Table 6.4) must be considered. If excluded or unlikely, the patient should be treated as CD with "false" negative serology. Follow-up biopsies will be needed to assess the mucosal response to gluten withdrawal.

TABLE 6.4
Causes of Villous Atrophy other Than CD

Infections: giardia, tuberculosis, HIV, Whipple's disease, gastroenteritis in children

Tropical sprue

Eosinophilic gastroenteritis

Small bowel bacterial overgrowth syndrome

Crohn's disease

Arterial disease

Drug and radiation damage

Zollinger–Ellison syndrome

Severe malnutrition

Immunodeficiency states, e.g., common variable immunodeficiency

Food intolerance, e.g., cow's milk, soya protein, especially in children improvement in the mucosal abnormalities and, therefore. to confirm the diagnosis. In the majority of patients who respond well clinically and in whom the antibody test becomes negative, a second biopsy is not necessary. Some patients still prefer such a biopsy, however, and some clinicians still regard that as the best means to secure the diagnosis. If symptoms persist or recur, however, further biopsies are always indicated.

In situations where a diagnosis has not been adequately made, for example, where a patient started a GFD prior to investigation, it may be necessary to reintroduce gluten in order to make a diagnosis. This process is called a "gluten challenge" and the situation is probably best managed by a specialist gastroenterologist.

The final point relates to the degree of abnormality in the mucosa, which is necessary to diagnose the disease. In the majority of patients, a Marsh type 2 or 3 lesion is seen, which would be regarded as diagnostic.[16] However, with milder degrees, it is usually advisable to keep the patient under close review and to repeat mucosal biopsies in relation to a gluten-free or a gluten-enhanced diet in order to move toward a definite diagnosis.

6.9   TREATMENT OF CELIAC DISEASE

Once celiac disease has been properly diagnosed, treatment can begin. The cornerstone of treatment is, of course, life-long adherence to a gluten-free diet (GFD). Initially, if patients have severe deficiencies or are seriously malnourished, intravenous replacement may be necessary, but this is very rarely needed. Oral vitamin supplements should be given initially to replenish any deficiency, but eventually normal nutrition can be maintained with an adequate GFD. Such a diet should exclude foods containing products of wheat, rye, or barley. Obviously these cereals form part of the staple diet in many parts of the world and it is a major step in changing to a GFD and it has a substantial impact on the daily life of the patient and his or her family. A GFD can be very healthy, but helping a patient to establish such a diet requires sensitive and sympathetic handling by medical, nursing, and dietetic staff. An experienced dietitian is invaluable to a celiac patient.[47]

It must be stressed that a GFD can be palatable and nutritious. Many natural foods can be eaten, such as vegetables, salads, pulses (legumes), fruits, nuts, meats, fish, poultry, cheese, eggs, and milk. Historically, rice, maize (corn), and potatoes were the substitutes for gluten-containing cereals. A number of grains, seeds, legumes, and nut flours are now available that offer more variety, improved palatability, and higher nutritional quality to a GFD.

There is good evidence that oats are safe for celiac patients to eat.[48] The main practical problem is cross-contamination with other cereals during manufacture.[49] Oats from specialist suppliers should be pure. There is a very small number of celiac patients who are sensitive to oats.[50]

In some European countries, wheat starch is allowed in a GFD, although the very low level of gluten that may be present is strictly limited and this type of starch for use in food manufacturing is called Codex wheat starch. There has also been major European regulation for food labeling, so that now manufactured foods have a clear indication as to whether wheat or gluten is present.

6.10   RESPONSE TO TREATMENT WITH A GFD

The vast majority of patients begin to feel better within weeks of starting a GFD. Even those who had very few or no symptoms initially often report a surprising general feeling of good health.

This clinical improvement is reflected in the histological improvement of the small intestinal mucosa, although this may take several months to improve significantly. Positive serological tests will also become negative over this time if a strict GFD is followed.

There are some clinical problems, however. Weight gain often occurs once absorption has improved in the small intestine. Some patients become constipated because they are eating less fiber in trying to avoid gluten-containing cereals.

6.11   COMPLIANCE WITH A GFD

It can be difficult to comply totally with a GFD. Physicians and dietitians recognize this.[47,51] There are several reasons why patients find it difficult; for example, the diet restricts lifestyle particularly when eating out or traveling. Children and teenagers find it particularly difficult to eat different food from their friends. Patients with "silent" disease may not notice much difference in their few, if any, symptoms and thus there is no incentive to stick to the diet. A GFD is more expensive than a normal diet.

6.12   PROGNOSIS OF CELIAC DISEASE

The prognosis of treated CD is excellent, with at least 90% of patients leading normal healthy lives. Well-treated patients have a normal life expectancy.

A small number of patients do not improve on treatment with a GFD. Most of these have remaining symptoms, but some also have remaining mucosal abnormalities on follow-up biopsies. The reasons for a poor response are listed in Table 6.5.

The most common reason is continuing gluten ingestion, either inadvertently or knowingly. Hence, the need for follow-up by an experienced dietitian. The gastroenterologist should consider the other possibilities, particularly the rare complications that are described below.

6.13   FOLLOW-UP OF CELIAC DISEASE

Regular follow-up of treated celiac patients is recommended by several professional gastroenterological associations.[52] This allows adequate nutritional assessment of the patient, education about the disease, and assessment of the diet. In particular, osteopenia and osteoporosis should be assessed and treated if indicated. Routine vaccination for all age groups should be performed according to national recommendations, but pneumococceal vaccination for celiac patients is also increasingly recommended.

TABLE 6.5

Reasons for a Poor Response to GFD

Continuing gluten ingestion

Incorrect initial diagnosis (see Table 6.4)

Lactose intolerance (primary or secondary)

Other food intolerances

Exocrine pancreatic insufficiency

Microscopic colitis

Co-existent irritable bowel syndrome

Complications of celiac disease: refractory CD, ulcerative jejunitis, small intestinal malignancy

6.14   COMPLICATIONS OF CELIAC DISEASE

There are three major complications of CD affecting the intestinal mucosa, which lead to serious disease.

6.14.1   REFRACTORY CELIAC DISEASE

This condition is rare, and occurs in those patients with a symptomatic severe small intestinal mucosal abnormality, which does not respond either primarily or secondarily to a strict GFD for at least six months and is not explained by other causes of a mucosal abnormality. Other causes of a poor response (Table 6.5) have to be excluded.[53] In primary cases, the mucosa never responds to a GFD, whereas in secondary cases there has been a mucosal response to gluten withdrawal at some stage.

Clinically these patients probably represent about 1% of the celiac population. Some continue for many years with chronic ill health reflected by low body weight and persistent lethargy, presumably due to ongoing malabsorption. Others follow a deteriorating clinical course with severe malnutrition and may require intravenous nutrition.

Refractory CD has now been classified into type 1 where there is a normal intraepithelial lymphocyte phenotype, with IELs exhibiting surface expression of CD3, CD8, and T-cell receptors $\alpha\beta$ and $\gamma\delta$, and type 2 where there is an aberrant IEL population. In this latter type, the IELs express cytoplasmic CD3, but lack surface expression of CD3, CD8, and the T-cell receptors. Immunohistochemical studies can be performed on routine formalin-fixed mucosal biopsy specimens from these patients. This allows differentiation between type 1 and type 2 refractory CD, since in the former, IELs have a normal CD3 + CD8 + phenotype, whereas in type 2, IELs have the abnormal CD3 + CD8- phenotype. The delineation of the two phenotypes is mainly for prognostic purposes because those patients with type 2 and thus aberrant IELs have a high risk of developing ulcerative jejunitis or enteropathy-associated T-cell lymphoma (EATL), whereas type 1 patients, with normal IELs, have a much more benign course.[54–56]

All patients with refractory CD should be investigated and monitored for the development of further complications. Treatment has been tried with limited success using steroids, azathioprine and cyclosporin. More recently, infliximab and cladribine (2-clorodeoxyadenosive) have been used, again with limited success.

6.14.2 ULCERATIVE JEJUNITIS

Rarely patients with refractory CD present in a severe clinical condition, with dehydration, abdominal pain, diarrhea, and malnutrition. Not only do they have an abnormal mucosa on biopsy, but also chronic multiple ulcers throughout the small intestine. These can perforate, bleed, or cause obstructive features. Barium studies, CT scanning, extensive biopsies, and laparotomy may be necessary. Histological examination of the mucosal biopsies shows grossly abnormal features, frequently with the abnormal IELs of type 2 refractory CD. This condition is probably a precursor to lymphoma (see Section 6.14.3 below). Treatment with intravenous feeding and major immunosuppression is usually tried, but with limited success. The prognosis is very poor.

6.14.3 SMALL INTESTINAL MALIGNANCY

There is a longstanding belief that celiac patients have a substantially increased risk of malignancy, particularly small intestinal adenocarcinoma and lymphoma. This resulted from early cohort studies from specialist centers. These results overestimated the risk.[57,58] More recent population studies have shown that there is a moderately increased risk of non-Hodgkin's and small bowel lymphoma and small intestinal adenocarcinoma. However, these tumors are all rare, so that the absolute risk in any one celiac patient is still low. Of particular interest is the EATL, which occurs in celiac disease. This commonly has the CD3 + CD8- phenotype characteristic of the aberrant IELs in type 2 refractory CD, suggesting there is a spectrum of clinical disease encompassing refractory CD, ulcerative jejunitis, and enteropathy-associated T-cell lymphoma.

Patients with small intestinal adenocarcinoma commonly present with weight loss, abdominal pain, abdominal mass, or anemia. They may have treated CD, which appears to have relapsed, or they may present de novo, CD being diagnosed concurrently with the tumor.

Patients with small bowel lymphoma may present with malaise, anorexia, weight loss, abdominal pain, or diarrhea. Once again, CD may be known or be diagnosed concurrently.[59]

Investigation for small bowel malignancy involves barium studies, CT scanning, capsule endoscopy, laparoscopy, or laparotomy, but it is notoriously difficult to diagnose.

Treatment involves surgery and chemotherapy and the prognosis depends upon the stage of the disease, but is generally poor.

There is also a slightly increased risk of cancer of the oropharynx, esophagus, colon, and pancreatobiliary system in CD, although once again it must be stressed that these tumors are rare in CD. Interestingly, breast cancer has a reduced incidence, although the reason for this is as yet unknown.[57,58]

6.15   FUTURE DEVELOPMENTS IN CELIAC DISEASE

As a result of the greater understanding of the pathogenesis of CD, several therapeutic possibilities have been opened up.[18] Bacterial prolyl endopeptidases have been produced that breakdown immunostimulatory gliadin peptides to immunologically inactive peptides and amino acids. Theoretically, these could be used as dietary supplements to prevent low-level gluten exposure in patients. The identification of dominant wheat gliadin epitopes is the initial step in producing a desensitizing vaccine.

It may be possible to produce genetically modified (GM) cereals that have reduced or absent T-cell stimulatory peptides, although this will be a major challenge for plant scientists.

Other therapeutic possibilities include blocking tTG deaminating activity, blocking zonulin-mediated intestinal permeability, and blocking innate or adaptive immune mechanisms.

A useful development will be the development of better screening assays for the gluten content of foods.

6.16   CONCLUSIONS

CD occurs in up to 1% of the population in societies where wheat is a staple in the diet. Modern serological tests have helped to increase the number of patients diagnosed. There is a wide spectrum of clinical presentations and the vast majority of patients respond well to treatment with a GFD. Complications of the disease are rare and the prognosis is good.

Recent developments in genetics, immunology, and molecular biology have unraveled much of the pathogenesis of the disease and opened the way to novel therapeutic possibilities.

REFERENCES

1. Gee S, *On the Coeliac Affection*. St Barts Hospital. Reports, London, 1888, xxiv, 17–20.
2. Dicke W, *Coeliac Disease: Investigations of Harmful Effects of Certain Types of Cereal on Patients with Coeliac Disease*. The Netherlands: University of Utrecht, 1950.
3. Van de Kamer, Weijers HA, Dicke WK. Coeliac Disease IV. An investigation into injurious constituents of wheat in connection with their action in patients with coeliac disease. *Acta. Paediatr.* 1953, 42, 223–231.
4. Paulley JW, Observations on the aetiology of idiopathic steatorhoea. *BMJ.* 1954, 2, 1318–1321.
5. Crosby WH, Kugler HW. Intraluminal biopsy of the small intestine. *Amer. J. Dig. Dis.* 1957, 2, 236–241.
6. Rubin CE, Brandborg LL, Phelps PC et al. Studies of coeliac disease. I. The apparent identical and specific nature of the duodenal and proximal jejunal lesion in celiac disease and idiopathic sprue. *Gastroenterology* 1960, 38, 28–49.
7. West J, Logan RF, Hill PG et al. Seroprevalence, correlates and characteristics of undetected coeliac disease in England. *Gut* 2003, 52, 960–965.

8. Riestra S, Fernandez E, Rodrigo L et al. Prevalence of coeliac disease in the general population of Northern Spain. Strategies of serological screening. *Scad. J. Gastroenterol.* 2000, 35, 398–402.

9. Volta U, Bellentani S, Bianchi FB et al. High prevalence of celiac disease in Italian general population. *Dig. Dis. Sci.* 2001, 46, 1500–1505.

10. Fasano A, Berti I, Gerarduzzi T et al. Prevalence of celiac disease in at-risk and not-at-risk groups in United States: a large multicenter study. *Arch. Intern. Med.* 2003, 163, 286–292.

11. Logan RF, Tucker G, Rifkind EA et al. Changes in clinical features of coeliac disease in adults in Edinburgh and the Lothians 1960–79. *BMJ* 1983, 286, 95–97.

12. Fasano A. Where have all the American celiacs gone? *Acta. Paediatr.* 1996, Suppl., 412, 20.

13. Bingley PJ, Williams AJ, Narcross AJ et al. Undiagnosed coeliac disease at age seven: population based prospective birth cohort study. *BMJ* 2004, 328, 322–323.

14. Maki M, Collin P. Coeliac disease. *Lancet* 1997, 349, 1755–1759.

15. Ferguson A. Coeliac disease research and clinical practice: maintaining momentum into the twenty-first century. *Bailliere's Clin. Gastroenterol.* 1995, 9, 395–412.

16. Marsh MN. Gluten, major histocompatibility complex, and the small intestine: a molecular and immunobiologic approach to the spectrum of gluten sensitivity (celiac sprue). *Gastroenterology* 1992, 102, 330–354.

17. Scott BB, Losowsky MS. Patchiness and duodenal–jejunal variation of the mucosal abnormality in coeliac disease and dermatitis herpetiformis. *Gut* 1976, 17, 984–992.

18. Van Heel D, West J. Recent advances in coeliac disease. *Gut* 2006, 55, 1037–1046.

19. Green PHR, Cellier C. Celiac disease. *NEJM* 2007, 357, 1731–1743.

20. Shan L, Molberg O, Parrot I, et al. Structural basis for gluten intolerance in celiac sprue. *Science* 2002, 297, 2275–2279.

21. Stokes P, Asquith P, Holmes GKT, et al. Histocompatibility antigens associated with adult coeliac disease. *Lancet* 1972, 2, 162–164.

22. Sollid LM, Markussen G, Ek J, et al. Evidence for a primary association of celiac disease to a particular HLA-DQ alpha/beta heterodimer. *J. Exp. Med.* 1989, 169, 345–350.

23. Greco L, Romino R, Coto I. et al. The first large population based twin study of coeliac disease. *Gut* 2002, 50, 624–628.

24. Van Heel D, Lude F, Hunt KA, et al. A celiac disease genome-wide association study identifies a susceptibility variant in the IL2/IL21 region. *Nat. Genet.* 2007, 39, 827–829.

25. Hunt KA, Zhernakova A, Turner G, et al. Newly identified genetic risk variants for celiac disease related to the immune response. *Nat. Genet.* 2008, 40, 395–402.

26. Maiuri L, Ciacci C, Ricciordelli I, et al. Association between innate response to gliadin and activation of pathogenic T-cells in coeliac disease. *Lancet* 2003, 362, 30–37.

27. Hue S, Mention JJ, Monteiro RC et al. A direct role for NKG2D/MICA interaction in villous atrophy during celiac disease. *Immunology* 2004, 21, 367–377.

28. Meresse B, Chen Z, Ciszewski C et al. Coordinated induction of IL15 of a TCR-independent NKG2D signalling pathway converts CTL into lymphokine-activated killer cells in celiac disease. *Immunity* 2004, 21, 357–366.

29. Clemente MG, De Virgiliis S, Kang JS et al. Early effects of gliadins on enterocyte intracellular signalling involved in intestinal barrier function. *Gut* 2003, 52, 218–223.

30. Molberg O, McAdam SN, Korner R et al. Tissue transglutaminase selectively modifies gliadin peptides that are recognised by gut-derived T-cells in celiac disease. *Nat. Med.* 1998, 4, 713–717.

31. Vader LW, de Ru A, van der Wal Y et al. Specificity of tissue transglutaminase explains cereal toxicity in celiac disease. *J. Exp. Med.* 2002, 195, 643–649.

32. Fleckenstein B, Qiao SW, Larsen MR et al. Molecular characterisation of covalent complexes between tissue transglutaminase and gliadin peptides. *J. Biol. Chem.* 2004, 279, 17607–17616.

33. Ivarsson A, Hernell O, Stenlund H et al. Breast-feeding protects against celiac disease. *Am. J. Clin. Nutr.* 2002, 75, 914–921.

34. Sterne LC, Honeyman MC, Hoffenberg BJ et al. Rotavirus infection frequency and risk of celiac disease autoimmunity in early childhood: a longitudinal study. *Am. J. Gastroenterol.* 2006, 101, 2333–2340.

35. Hin H, Bird G, Fisher P et al. Coeliac disease in primary care: case finding study. *BMJ* 1999, 318, 164–167.

36. Rampertab SD, Pooran N, Brar P et al. Trends in the presentation of celiac disease. *Am. J. Med.* 2006, 119, 355 e.9–14.

37. Sanders DS, Carter MJ, Hurlstone DP et al. Association of adult coeliac disease with irritable bowel syndrome: a case-control study in patients fulfilling ROME II criteria referred to secondary care. *Lancet* 2001, 358, 1504–1508.

38. Dickey W, Kearney N. Overweight in celiac disease: prevalence, clinical characteristics, and effect of a gluten-free diet. *Am. J. Gastroenterol.* 2006, 101, 2356–2359.

39. Green PH. The many faces of celiac disease: clinical presentation of celiac disease in the adult population. *Gastroenterology* 2005, 128, Suppl. 1, S74–78.

40. Tata LJ, Card TR, Logan RF et al. Fertility and pregnancy-related events in women with celiac disease: a population-based cohort study. *Gastroenterology* 2005, 128, 849–855.

41. Viljamaa M, Kaukinen K, Huhtala H et al. Coeliac disease, autoimmune diseases and gluten exposure. *Scand. J. Gastroenterol.* 2005, 40, 437–443.

42. Sjoberg K, Eriksson KF, Bredberg A et al. Screening for coeliac disease in adult insulin-dependent diabetes mellitus. *J. Intern. Med.* 1998, 243, 133–140.

43. Counsell CE, Ruddell WS. Association between coeliac disease and autoimmune thyroid disease. *Gut* 1995, 36, 475–476.

44. Fry L. Dermatitis herpetiformis. *Bailliere's Clin. Gastroenterol.* 9, 371–393.

45. Rostom A, Dubé C, Cranney A et al. The diagnostic accuracy of serologic tests for celiac disease: a systematic review. *Gastroenterology* 2005, 128, Suppl. 1, S38–46.

46. Lewis NR, Scott BB. Systematic review: the use of serology to exclude or diagnose coeliac disease (a comparison of the endomysial and tissue transglutaminase antibody tests). *Aliment. Pharmacol. Ther.* 2006, 24, 47–54.

47. Pietzak MM. Follow-up of patients with celiac disease: achieving compliance with treatment. *Gastroenterology* 2005, 128, Suppl. 1, S135–141.

48. Janatuinen EK, Kemppainen TA, Julkunen RJ et al. No harm from five-year ingestion of oats in coeliac disease. *Gut* 2002, 50, 332–335.

49. Thompson T. Gluten contamination of commercial oat products in the United States. *NEJM* 2004, 351, 2021–2022.

50. Lundin KE, Nilsen EM, Scott HG et al. Oats-induced villous atrophy in coeliac disease. *Gut* 2003, 52, 1649–52.

51. Howdle PD. *Your Guide to Coeliac Disease.* Hodder Arnold, London, 2007.

52. AGA Institute. Medical position statement on the diagnosis and management of celiac disease. *Gastroenterology* 2006, 131, 1977–1980.

53. O'Mahony S, Howdle PD, Losowsky MS. Management of patients with non-responsive coeliac disease. *Aliment. Pharmacol. Ther.* 1996, 10, 671–680.

54. Cellier C, Delabesse E, Helmer C et al. Refractory sprue, coeliac disease and enteropathy—associated T-cell lymphoma. *Lancet* 2000, 356, 203–208.

55. Cellier C, Patey N, Mauvieux L et al. Abnormal intestinal intraepithelial lymphocytes in refractory sprue. *Gastroenterology* 1998, 114, 471–481.

56. Patey-Mariand De Serre N, Cellier C, Jabri B et al. Distinction between coeliac disease and refractory sprue: a simple immunohistochemical method. *Histopathology* 2000, 37, 70–77.
57. Askling J, Linet M, Gridley G et al. Cancer incidence in a population-based cohort of individuals hospitalised with celiac disease or dermatitis herpetiformis. *Gastroenterology* 2002, 123, 1428–1435.
58. West J, Logan RF, Smith CJ et al. Malignancy and mortality in people with coeliac disease: population based cohort study. *BMJ* 2004, 329, 716–719.
59. Howdle PD, Jalal PK, Holmes GKT et al. Primary small-bowel malignancy in the UK and its association with coeliac disease. *QJM* 2003, 96, 345–353.

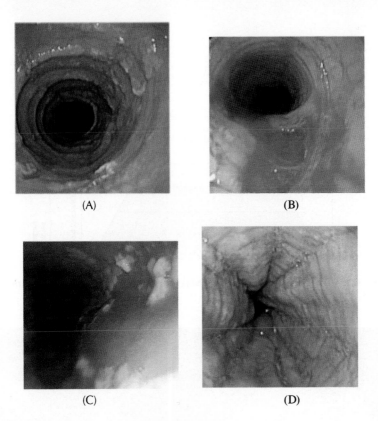

FIGURE 4.1 Endoscopic findings associated with EoE. (A) Mucosal rings representing transient contractions or fixed structures, this aspect is also called trachealization, feline esophagus, or corrugated esophagus. (B) After esophageal dilation a deep mucosal laceration is seen representing a typical finding ("longitudinal shearing"). (C) Whitish exudates scattered across the mucosal surface, representing eosinophilic microabscesses. (D) Esophageal furrowing representing mucosal edema and thickening.

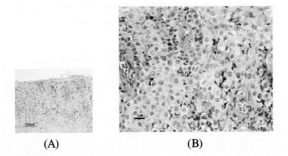

FIGURE 4.2 Eosinophilic esophageal inflammation in EoE. (A) The low-power field (Hemalaun-Eosin, 200-fold magnification) of the epithelium demonstrates an increased number of eosinophils, basal zone hyperplasia, elongated rete papillae, and subepithelial fibrosis. (B) The high-power field (Hemalaun-Eosin, 400-fold magnification) of the epithelium demonstrates a large number of eosinophils, some of them are marked by a green star. (Micrographs courtesy of Ch. Bussmann.)

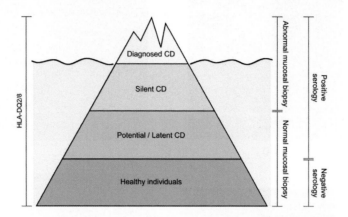

FIGURE 6.1 The Celiac Iceberg. (From Maki M, Collin P. Coeliac disease. *Lancet* 1997, 349, 1755–1759. With permission.)

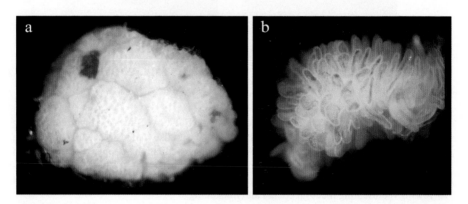

FIGURE 6.2a/b (a) Untreated celiac mucosa at dissecting microscopy (×10); (b) normal mucosa at dissecting microscopy (×10). (From Howdle PD. *Encyclopedia of Food Sciences and Nutrition*, Elsevier, Amsterdam, 2003. With permission.)

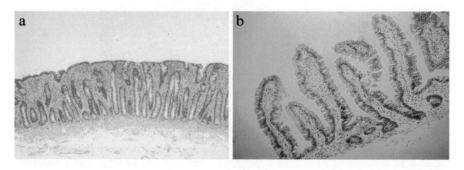

FIGURE 6.3a/b (a) Histological section of untreated celiac mucosa (×40); (b) histological section of normal mucosa (×40). (From Howdle PD. *Encyclopedia of Food Sciences and Nutrition*, Elsevier, Amsterdam, 2003. With permission.)

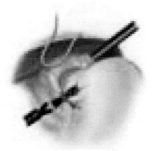

FIGURE 20.1 Dissection of angle of His. (From Jones DB. *Atlas of Minimally Invasive Surgery.* Cine-Med Inc, 2006. With permission.)

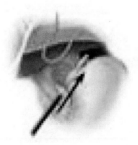

FIGURE 20.2 Pars flaccida approach for creation of retrogastric tunnel. (From Jones DB. *Atlas of Minimally Invasive Surgery.* Cine-Med Inc, 2006. With permission.)

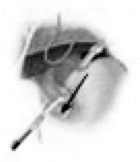

FIGURE 20.3 Lap band placement. (From Jones DB. Atlas of *Atlas of Minimally Invasive Surgery.* Cine-Med Inc, 2006. With permission.)

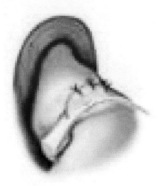

FIGURE 20.4 Completed anterior fundoplication to prevent gastric prolapse. (From Jones DB. *Atlas of Minimally Invasive Surgery.* Cine-Med Inc, 2006. With permission.)

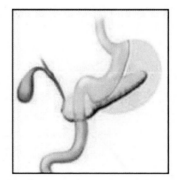

FIGURE 20.5 Completed appearance of a sleeve gastrectomy. (Tucker ON. Indications for sleeve gastrectomy. *J Gastrointest. Surg.* Springer. 4:664, 2008. With permission.)

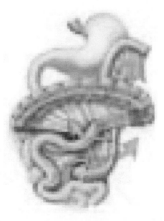

FIGURE 20.6 Completed appearance of a Roux-en-Y gastric bypass. (From Jones DB. *Atlas of Minimally Invasive Surgery.* Cine-Med Inc, 2006. With permission.)

7 Probiotics in Irritable Bowel Syndrome

Eamonn M. M. Quigley and Fergus Shanahan

CONTENTS

7.1 INTRODUCTION

While probiotics and prebiotics have been used for decades on an anecdotal basis to address a variety of the ills that man is prone to suffer from, the scientific study of probiotics in irritable bowel syndrome (IBS) is more recent and its emergence has paralleled an emerging interest in the role of the microbiota in intestinal disorders. The possibility that the enteric flora, or microbiota, could play a role in the pathogenesis of IBS has only begun to attract concerted scientific attention very recently, though evidence to suggest a link has been extant for some time and contains several distinct, and even contradictory, strands:

1. Epidemiological evidence that antibiotic use may predispose to IBS or to exacerbations thereof.
2. Epidemiological, clinical, and experimental evidence for the existence of postinfectious IBS.
3. Evidence, both experimental and clinical, for a role for low-grade inflammation (perhaps triggered by luminal bacteria) in IBS.
4. The suggestion that IBS may be associated with small intestinal bacterial overgrowth (SIBO) or other changes in the gut flora.
5. Evidence to indicate that manipulation of the gut flora, by antibiotics or probiotics, may ameliorate symptoms in IBS.

7.2 ANTIBIOTIC USE AND IBS

In a survey of 421 subjects in a primary care practice in the United Kingdom, antibiotic use was strongly associated with an increased risk of IBS (odds ratio 3.7).[1] Privileged childhood living conditions were also an important risk factor, which, according to the authors, was consistent with an allergic or infectious etiology for IBS. Other epidemiological studies have come to similar conclusions.[2]

7.3 POSTINFECTIOUS IBS

We are now beginning to see real data to directly support the concept of postinfectious IBS.[3] First reported by McKendrick and Read,[4] the occurrence of IBS following episodes of bacteriologically confirmed gastroenteritis has now been documented in several studies.[5–15] Thabane and colleagues concluded that the overall risk for the development of IBS was increased sixfold following an episode of bacterial gastroenteritis with younger subjects, those who have prolonged fever during the episode of gastroenteritis and those who suffer from anxiety or depression being at greatest risk.[16] These symptoms are not transient; in a Scandinavian study in which 12% of their subjects had IBS within three months of gastroenteritis, 9% still had symptoms five years later.[13] Neal and colleagues documented similar recovery rates for postinfectious and nonpostinfectious IBS in a six-year follow-up study.[17]

One study went on to establish a direct link between prior exposure to an infectious agent, persisting low-grade inflammation and IBS.[8] In this study, an increase in the number of chronic inflammatory cells in the rectal mucosa was seen only among those exposed patients who had developed IBS. Others have demonstrated a persisting increase in rectal mucosal enteroendocrine cells, T lymphocytes, and gut permeability in patients with postdysenteric IBS.[9,10] These observations are important as they indicate a relationship between perturbations of the microbiota, mucosal inflammation, and IBS, an hypothesis that is amply supported by data from studies in experimental animal models. The development of IBS has, recently, been linked with non-GI infections,[18] again, perhaps, invoking a role for a systemic inflammatory response in the mediation of symptoms.

A number of parasites, such as *Dientamoeba fragilis*, *Blastocystis hominis*, and giardia have been associated with the development of chronic gastrointestinal symptoms that may mimic IBS;[19–20] whether parasitic infections can trigger IBS, per se, is unknown. Very recently, an outbreak of viral gastroenteritis was associated with the new onset of an IBS-type syndrome in 24% of affected subjects when interviewed three months later; subsequent follow-up suggested that postviral IBS was more transient than its bacterial counterpart.[21]

Postinfectious IBS may explain only a minority of cases of IBS (1 to 6.7% in one recent study),[22] but it does represent a clear link between exposure to an environmental agent, inflammation, and IBS in predisposed individuals.

7.4 INFLAMMATION AND IBS

Direct and compelling evidence for a role for mucosal inflammation in IBS was first provided by Chadwick and colleagues among 77 IBS patients: 31 demonstrated microscopic inflammation and 8 fulfilled criteria for lymphocytic colitis. However, among the group with "normal" histology, immunohistology revealed increased intraepithelial lymphocytes as well as an increase in CD3+ and CD25+ cells in the lamina propria. All, therefore, showed evidence of immune activation.[23] Subsequent studies have provided further evidence of T-lymphocyte[24,25] and mast cell activation[26–29] in the mucosa in IBS; others have demonstrated an extension of inflammation into the myoneural compartments[30] and still others cytokine profiles in peripheral blood mononuclear cells[31,32] and serum[33] compatible with a proinflammatory state.

It is reasonable to suggest that these immunological changes could result from exposure to an exogenous (such as bacterial) antigen challenge.[34,35] That IBS patients may be predisposed to an, albeit contained, inflammatory response to luminal triggers is, indeed, supported by the finding of polymorphisms in genes that encode for the production of anti-inflammatory cytokines among IBS patients [36,37] and by the very recent description of high titers of antiflagellin antibodies in serum derived from IBS patients.[38,39]

While the idea that IBS patients may truly harbor inflammatory changes in the colonic mucosa is increasingly gaining credence,[40] many important questions remain to be answered and it is clear that this is going to be an area of active investigation for some time to come.

7.5 QUALITATIVE OR QUANTITATIVE CHANGES IN THE ENTERIC FLORA (MICROBIOTA)

For some time, various studies have suggested the presence of qualitative changes in the colonic flora in IBS patients; a relative decrease in the population of bifidobacteria being the most consistent finding.[41–46] It should be noted, however, that these findings have not always been reproduced and the methods employed have been subject to question. Nevertheless, qualitative changes in the colonic flora, be they primary or secondary, could lead to the proliferation of species that produce more gas[45,46] and short chain fatty acids and are more avid in the deconjugation of bile acids. With regard to the former, the displacement of gas-forming species could result in local changes in gas production, a development that may be poorly tolerated by IBS subjects who seem to have difficulties with the transport of gas along the intestine and to be overly sensitive to gas-induced distension. The latter could, in turn, lead to clinically significant changes in water and electrolyte transport in the colon and affect colonic motility and/or sensitivity. Similarly, a repopulation of the flora with the deficient commensal could restore homeostasis. Attractive as this concept may be, it belies the challenges posed by attempts at a comprehensive description of the flora in IBS, or in any condition.

Several factors limit the interpretability of prior studies, including the unrepresentative nature of the fecal flora, a failure to describe those bacterial populations that may be adherent to the mucosal surface and, above all, the recognition that a very significant proportion of the colonic microbiota cannot be identified by conventional culture methods. Molecular methods are now being applied to this complex issue and have, indeed, confirmed that IBS patients, regardless of subtype, do exhibit a fecal flora that is clearly different from control subjects.[43,44,47,48] The precise nature of these differences and their potential to disturb mucosal or myoneural function in the gut wall, or induce local or systemic immune responses, remains to be defined.

More recently, the role of the gut flora in IBS has been taken a stage farther with the suggestion that some IBS patients may harbor quantitative changes in the indigenous flora in the small intestine: small intestinal bacterial overgrowth (SIBO).[49–53] The occurrence of SIBO has been associated with abnormalities in small intestinal motor function[54] and its eradication with symptomatic relief.[49,50,53,55,56–58] These striking results have been the target of much criticism on several grounds.[59–65] First, IBS symptoms are nonspecific and may be mimicked by SIBO, regardless of etiology; patient selection, therefore, is an issue. Second, the hydrogen breath test, which has been the test most widely used to make the diagnosis of SIBO in this context, is subject to considerable error, especially in relation to altered small bowel transit,[66,67] and, third, others have failed to confirm these findings.[68–71]

7.6 EFFICACY OF ANTIBIOTICS IN IBS

The principal evidence for a role for antibiotics in IBS comes from studies among the aforementioned IBS patients with associated SIBO.[49,50,53,55,56] In a subsequent study that did not document bacterial overgrowth, Pimentel and his colleagues treated IBS patients with the poorly absorbed antibiotic rifaximin;[72] some IBS patients, at least, demonstrated a prolonged response (up to 10 week) to a short course of this antibiotic. As pointed out in an accompanying editorial, there are, however, several limitations to this study that reduce its impact.[73] In a recently reported multicenter phase II study, 388 diarrhea-associated IBS subjects were randomized to either rifaximin in a dose of 550 mg twice a day or placebo for 14 days, followed by another 14 days on placebo alone and then 2 weeks follow-up. During treatment, at 4 weeks and at 12 weeks, those randomized to rifaximin had a modest 8 to 13% therapeutic gain for adequate relief of global IBS symptoms and a rather diappointing 4 to 8% gain for relief of bloating.[74,75] However, the eradication of SIBO, as proposed by these authors, may not be the sole explanation for these responses, which could also be explained on the basis of a suppression of fermenting bacteria in the colon, as suggested by Dear et al.[46] and supported by the recent report from Sharara et al.[76] Finally, one must remain reluctant, pending long-term studies, to recommend a prolonged course of antibiotic therapy to any population regardless of the safety profile of a given antibiotic.

7.7 EFFICACY OF PROBIOTICS IN IBS

Given their safety profile, probiotics, if effective, would at first sight appear to be more attractive as potential manipulators of the gut flora in IBS. Are probiotics effective in IBS? Several factors complicate the interpretation of clinical trials of probiotics in IBS: many studies have been underpowered and some earlier studies were even uncontrolled and not blinded. Furthermore, results between studies are difficult to compare because of differences in study design, the use of nonvalidated and differing endpoints, and variations in probiotic dose and strain. Nevertheless, there has been some, but by no means consistent, evidence of symptom improvement.[77–97] Hamilton-Miller, in reviewing earlier studies and while drawing attention to the shortcomings of prior trials in terms of study design, concluded that there was, overall, sufficient evidence of efficacy to warrant further evaluation.[98] More recent reviews[99,100] have explored the scientific rationale behind the use of probiotics in IBS and reviewed the clinical results from studies performed over the past two decades. Outcomes continue to be variable, some studies report little evidence of efficacy,[78,82,87,90] while others document responses only for specific symptoms, or in selected populations.[81,85,88,91,92–96] It is noteworthy that flatulence, bloating, and distension, common and distressing symptoms in IBS,[101] seem especially responsive to probiotic therapy, given the sensitivity of IBS subjects to gas-induced distension[102] and their difficulties with moving gas along the intestine.[103] One probiotic combination containing *Bifidobacterium animalis* (lactis) DN-173-010 has been shown to accelerate intestinal transit and reduce abdominal girth,[97] no doubt explaining its ability to increase stool frequency in IBS patients with constipation and providing some objective evidence in support of an effect of probiotics on bloating.[91] Some studies have employed probiotic "cocktails" rather than single isolates, rendering it difficult to deduce what were the active moieties.[85,88,89,91–96] One particular probiotic, *B. infantis* 35624 appears to have more global effects in IBS. In the first of two studies with this organism, this *Bifidobacterium* was found to be superior to both a *Lactobacillus* and placebo for each of the cardinal symptoms of the irritable bowel syndrome (abdominal pain/discomfort, distension/bloating, and difficult defecation) as well as for a composite score.[31] More recently, these results were replicated in a much larger, dose-ranging, primary care-based study involving 360 IBS subjects, where *B. infantis*, in an encapsulated format and in a dose of 10^8, was associated with significant improvements in the cardinal symptoms of IBS as well as in the subjects global assessment of all symptoms; at study end, over 60% of subjects randomized to the *Bifidobacterium* felt better than before therapy, a therapeutic gain of over 20% over placebo.[104] In both studies, a positive impact on IBS symptomatology occurred independent of any effect on stool frequency indicating that the observed effects were not attributable to either a laxative or antidiarrheal effect. These studies with this particular *B. infantis* strain provide, therefore, evidence for a benefit in IBS for a clearly defined single-organism probiotic preparation and, thereby, suggest that some strains may be more effective than others for this indication.

7.8 CONCLUSIONS

Many recent findings add to a growing body of evidence to suggest that IBS, like inflammatory bowel disease (IBD), may, in part at least, result from a dysfunctional interaction between the indigenous flora and the intestinal mucosa, which, in turn, leads to immune activation in the colonic mucosa. This does not place IBS within the spectrum of IBD where the intensity and distribution of the inflammatory process are vastly different.[105] Some propose a role for bacterial overgrowth as a common causative factor in the pathogenesis of symptoms in IBS; other evidence points to more subtle qualitative changes in the colonic flora; both hypotheses remain to be confirmed, but the likelihood that bacterial overgrowth will prove to be a major factor in IBS now seems remote. On the other hand, the advent of molecular techniques for the identification of the composition of the microbiota holds great promise for the identification of distinctive aspects of the flora in IBS. A role for the flora in IBS is further supported by the observation that short-term therapy with either antibiotics or probiotics does seem to reduce symptoms among IBS patients.[106–108] It seems most likely that the benefits of antibiotic therapy are mediated through subtle and, perhaps, localized, quantitative and/or qualitative changes in the colonic flora. How probiotics exert their effects remains to be defined, but an antiinflammatory effect seems likely. While this approach to the management of IBS is in its infancy, it is evident that manipulation of the flora, whether through the administration of antibiotics or probiotics, deserves further attention in IBS.

REFERENCES

1. Mendall MA, Kumar D. Antibiotic use, childhood affluence and irritable bowel syndrome (IBS). *Eur J Gastroenterol Hepatol* 1998; 10: 59–62.
2. Maxwell PR, Rink E, Kumar D, Mendall MA. Antibiotics increase functional abdominal symptoms. *Am J Gastroenterol* 2002; 97: 104–8.
3. Spiller RC. Postinfectious irritable bowel syndrome. *Gastroenterology* 2003; 124: 1662–71.
4. McKendrick MW, Read MW. Irritable bowel syndrome—post-salmonella infection. *J Infect* 1994; 29: 1–3.
5. Neal KR, Hebdon J, Spiller R. Prevalence of gastrointestinal symptoms six months after bacterial gastroenteritis and risk factors for development of the irritable bowel syndrome. *Br Med J* 1997; 314: 779–82.
6. Garcia Rodriguez LA, Ruigomez A. Increased risk of irritable bowel syndrome after bacterial gastroenteritis: cohort study. *Br Med J* 1999; 318: 565–6.
7. Gwee KA, Graham JC, McKendrick MW et al. Psychometric scores and persistence of irritable bowel after infectious diarrhoea. *Lancet* 1996; 347: 150–3.
8. Gwee KA, Leong YL, Graham C et al. The role of psychological and biological factors in post-infective gut dysfunction. *Gut* 1999; 44: 400–6.
9. Spiller RC, Jenkins D, Thornley JP et al. Increased rectal mucosal enteroendocrine cells T lymphocytes and increased gut permeability following acute Campylobacter enteritis and in post-dysenteric irritable bowel syndrome. *Gut* 2000; 47: 804–11.
10. Dunlop SP, Jenkins D, Neal KR, Spiller RC. Relative importance of enterochromaffin cell hyperplasia, anxiety, and depression in postinfectious IBS. *Gastroenterology* 2003; 125: 1651–9.
11. Mearin F, Perez-Oliveras M, Perello A et al. Dyspepsia and irritable bowel syndrome after a Salmonella gastroenteritis outbreak: one-year follow-up cohort study. *Gastroenterology* 2005; 129: 98–104.

12. Marshall JK, Thabane M, Garg AX, Clark WF, Salvadori M, Collins SM; Walkerton Health Study Investigators. Incidence and epidemiology of irritable bowel syndrome after a large waterborne outbreak of bacterial dysentery. *Gastroenterology* 2006; 131: 445–50.

13. Tornblom H, Holmvall P, Svenungsson B, Lindberg G. Gastrointestinal symptoms after infectious diarrhea: a five-year follow-up in a Swedish cohort of adults. *Clin Gastroenterol Hepatol.* 2007; 5: 461–4.

14. Spence MJ, Moss-Morris R. The cognitive behavioural model of irritable bowel syndrome: a prospective investigation of patients with gastroenteritis. *Gut.* 2007; 56: 1066–71.

15. Ruigomez A, Garcia Rodriguez LA, Panes J. Risk of irritable bowel syndrome after an episode of bacterial gastroenteritis in general practice: influence of comorbidities. *Clin Gastroenterol Hepatol.* 2007; 5: 465–9.

16. Thabane M, Kottachchi DT, Marshall JK. Systematic review and meta-analysis: the incidence and prognosis of post-infectious irritable bowel syndrome. *Aliment Pharmacol Ther.* 2007; 26535–44.

17. Neal KR, Barker L, Spiller RC. Prognosis in post-infective irritable bowel syndrome: a six-year follow-up study. *Gut.* 2002; 51: 410–3.

18. McKeown ES, Parry SD, Stansfield R, Barton JR, Welfare MR. Postinfectious irritable bowel syndrome may occur after non-gastrointestinal and intestinal infection. *Neurogastroenterol Motil.* 2006; 18: 839–43.

19. Stark D, van Hal S, Marriott D, Ellis J, Harkness J. Irritable bowel syndrome: a review on the role of intestinal protozoa and the importance of their detection and diagnosis. *Int J Parasitol.* 2007; 37: 11–20.

20. Grazioli B, Matera G, Laratta C, Schipani G, Guarnieri G, Spiniello E, Imeneo M, Amorosi A, Foca A, Luzza F. Giardia lamblia infection in patients with irritable bowel syndrome and dyspepsia: a prospective study. *World J Gastroenterol.* 2006; 12: 1941–4.

21. Marshall JK, Thabane M, Borgaonkar MR, James C. Postinfectious irritable bowel syndrome after a food-borne outbreak of acute gastroenteritis attributed to a viral pathogen. *Clin Gastroenterol Hepatol.* 2007; 5: 457–60.

22. Borgaonkar MR, Ford DC, Marshall JK, Churchill E, Collins SM. The incidence of irritable bowel syndrome among community subjects with previous acute enteric infection. *Dig Dis Sci.* 2006; 51: 1026–32.

23. Chadwick V, Chen W, Shu D et al. Activation of the mucosal immune system in irritable bowel syndrome. *Gastroenterology* 2002; 122: 1778–83.

24. Holmen N, Isaksson S, Simren M, Sjovall H, Ohman L. CD4+CD25+ regulatory T cells in irritable bowel syndrome patients. *Neurogastroenterol Motil.* 2007; 19: 119–25.

25. Ohman L, Isaksson S, Lundgren A, Simren M, Sjovall H. A controlled study of colonic immune activity and beta7+ blood T lymphocytes in patients with irritable bowel syndrome. *Clin Gastroenterol Hepatol.* 2005; 3: 980–6.

26. Barbara G, Stanghellini V, De Giorgio R et al. Activated mast cells in proximity to colonic nerves correlate with abdominal pain in irritable bowel syndrome. *Gastroenterology* 2004; 126: 693–702.

27. Barbara G, Wang B, Stanghellini V, de Giorgio R, Cremon C, Di Nardo G, Trevisani M, Campi B, Geppetti P, Tonini M, Bunnett NW, Grundy D, Corinaldesi R. Mast cell-dependent excitation of visceral-nociceptive sensory neurons in irritable bowel syndrome. *Gastroenterology* 2007; 132: 26–37.

28. Cenac N, Andrews CN, Holzhausen M, Chapman K, Cottrell G, Andrade-Gordon P, Steinhoff M, Barbara G, Beck P, Bunnett NW, Sharkey KA, Ferraz JG, Shaffer E, Vergnolle N. Role for protease activity in visceral pain in irritable bowel syndrome. *J Clin Invest.* 2007; 117: 636–47.

29. Guilarte M, Santos J, de Torres I, Alonso C, Vicario M, Ramos L, Martinez C, Casellas F, Saperas E, Malagelada JR. Diarrhoea-predominant IBS patients show mast cell activation and hyperplasia in the jejunum. *Gut.* 2007; 56: 203–9.
30. Tornblom H, Lindberg G, Nyberg B, Veress B. Full-thickness biopsy of the jejunum reveals inflammation and enteric neuropathy in irritable bowel syndrome. *Gastroenterology* 2002; 123: 1972–9.
31. O'Mahony L, McCarthy J, Kelly P et al. A Randomized, placebo-controlled, double-blind comparison of the probiotic bacteria lactobacillus and bifidobacterium in irritable bowel syndrome (IBS): symptom responses and relationship to cytokine profiles. *Gastroenterology* 2005; 128: 541–51.
32. Liebregts T, Adam B, Bredack C, Roth A, Heinzel S, Lester S, Downie-Doyle S, Smith E, Drew P, Talley NJ, Holtmann G. Immune activation in patients with irritable bowel syndrome. *Gastroenterology* 2007; 132: 913–20.
33. Dinan TG, Quigley EM, Ahmed SM et al. Hypothalamic–pituitary–gut axis dysregulation in irritable bowel syndrome: plasma cytokines as a potential biomarker? *Gastroenterology* 2006; 130: 304–11.
34. Collins SM. A case for an immunological basis for irritable bowel syndrome. *Gastroenterology* 2002; 122: 2078–80.
35. Spiller RC. Role of nerves in enteric infection. *Gut* 2002; 51: 759–62.
36. Gonsalkorale WM, Perrey C, Pravica V, Whorwell PJ, Hutchinson IV. Interleukin 10 genotypes in irritable bowel syndrome: evidence for an inflammatory component? *Gut* 2003; 52: 91–3.
37. van der Veek PP, van den Berg M, de Kroon YE, Verspaget HW, Masclee AA. Role of tumor necrosis factor-alpha and interleukin-10 gene polymorphisms in irritable bowel syndrome. *Am J Gastroenterol.* 2005; 100: 2510–6.
38. Schoepfer AM, Schaffer T, Seibold-Schmid B, Muller S, Seibold F. Antibodies to flagellin indicate reactivity to bacterial antigens in IBS patients. *Neurogastroenterol Motil.* 2008; 20: 1110–8.
39. Ivison SM, Steiner TS. Anti-flagellin antibodies in irritable bowel syndrome: another attack on our commensals! *Neurogastroenterol Motil.* 2008; 20: 1081–5.
40. Kirsch R, Riddell RH. Histopathological alterations in irritable bowel syndrome. *Mod Pathol.* 2006; 19: 1638–45.
41. Bradley HK, Wyatt GM, Bayliss CE, Hunter JO. Instability in the faecal flora of a patient suffering from food–related irritable bowel syndrome. *J Med Microbiol.* 1987; 23: 29–32.
42. Si JM, Yu YC, Fan YJ, Chen SJ. Intestinal microecology and quality of life in irritable bowel syndrome patients. *World J Gastroenterol.* 2004; 10: 1802–5.
43. Malinen E, Rinttila T, Kajander K et al. Analysis of the fecal microbiota of irritable bowel syndrome patients and healthy controls with real-time PCR. *Am J Gastroenterol.* 2005; 100: 373–82.
44. Matto J, Maunuksela L, Kajander K et al. Composition and temporal stability of gastrointestinal microbiota in irritable bowel syndrome—a longitudinal study in IBS and control subjects. *FEMS Immunol Med Microbiol.* 2005; 43: 213–22.
45. King TS, Elia M, Hunter JO. Abnormal colonic fermentation in irritable bowel syndrome. *Lancet* 1998; 352: 1187–9.
46. Dear KL, Elia M, Hunter JO. Do interventions which reduce colonic bacterial fermentation improve symptoms of irritable bowel syndrome? *Dig Dis Sci.* 2005; 50: 758–66.
47. Maukonen J, Satokari R, Matto J, Soderlund H, Mattila-Sandholm T, Saarela M. Prevalence and temporal stability of selected clostridial groups in irritable bowel syndrome in relation to predominant faecal bacteria. *J Med Microbiol.* 2006; 55 (Pt 5): 625–33.

48. Kassinen A, Krogius-Kurikka L, Makivuokko H, Rinttila T, Paulin L, Corander J, Malinen E, Apajalahti J, Palva A. The fecal microbiota of irritable bowel syndrome patients differs significantly from that of healthy subjects. *Gastroenterology*. 2007; 133: 24–33.

49. Pimentel M, Chow EJ, Lin HC. Eradication of small bowel bacterial overgrowth reduces symptoms of irritable bowel syndrome. *Am J Gastroenterol*. 2000; 95: 3503–6.

50. Pimentel M, Chow E, Lin H. Normalization of lactulose breath testing correlates with symptom improvement in irritable bowel syndrome: a double-blind, randomized, placebo-controlled study. *Am J Gastroenterol*. 2003; 98: 412–9.

51. McCallum R, Schultz C, Sostarich S. Evaluating the role of small intestinal bacterial overgrowth (SIBO) in diarrhea predominant IBS (IBS-D) patients utilizing the glucose breath test. *Gastroenterology* 2005; 128: T1118.

52. Nucera G, Gabrielli A, Lupascu A et al. Abnormal breath tests to lactose, fructose and sorbitol in irritable bowel syndrome may be explained by small intestinal bacterial overgrowth. *Aliment Pharmacol Ther*. 2005; 21: 1391–5.

53. Cuoco L, Salvagnini M. Small intestine bacterial overgrowth in irritable bowel syndrome: a retrospective study with rifaximin. *Minerva Gastroenterol Dietol*. 2006; 52: 89–95.

54. Pimentel M, Soffer EE, Chow EJ, Kong Y, Lin HC. Lower frequency of MMC is found in IBS subjects with abnormal lactulose breath test, suggesting bacterial overgrowth. *Dig Dis Sci*. 2002; 47: 2639–43.

55. Majewski M, McCallum RW. Results of small intestinal bacterial overgrowth testing in irritable bowel syndrome patients: clinical profiles and effects of antibiotic trial. *Adv Med Sci*. 2007; 52: 139–42.

56. Esposito I, de Leone A, Di Gregorio G, Giaquinto S, de Magistris L, Ferrieri A, Riegler G. Breath test for differential diagnosis between small intestinal bacterial overgrowth and irritable bowel disease: an observation on non-absorbable antibiotics. *World J Gastroenterol*. 2007; 13: 6016–21.

57. Weinstock LB, Fern SE, Duntley SP. Restless legs syndrome in patients with irritable bowel syndrome: response to small intestinal bacterial overgrowth therapy. *Dig Dis Sci*. 2008; 53: 1252–6.

58. Weinstock LB, Klutke CG, Lin HC. Small intestinal bacterial overgrowth in patients with interstitial cystitis and gastrointestinal symptoms. *Dig Dis Sci*. 2008; 53: 1246–51.

59. Cuoco L, Cammarota G, Jorizzo R et al. Small intestinal bacterial overgrowth and symptoms of irritable bowel syndrome. *Am J Gastroenterol*. 2001; 96: 2281–2.

60. Jones MP, Craig R, Olinger E. Small intestinal bacterial overgrowth is associated with irritable bowel syndrome: the cart lands squarely in front of the horse. *Am J Gastroenterol*. 2001; 96: 3204–5.

61. Mishkin D, Mishkin S. Re: Pimentel et al. Eradication of small intestinal bacterial overgrowth reduces symptoms of irritable bowel syndrome. *Am J Gastroenterol*. 2001; 96: 2505–6.

62. Riordan SM, McIver CJ, Duncombe VM et al. Small intestinal bacterial overgrowth and the irritable bowel syndrome. *Am J Gastroenterol*. 2001; 96: 2506–8.

63. Hasler WL. Lactulose breath testing, bacterial overgrowth, and IBS: just a lot of hot air? *Gastroenterology* 2003; 125: 1898–900.

64. Quigley EM. A 51-year-old with irritable bowel syndrome: test or treat for bacterial overgrowth? *Clin Gastroenterol Hepatol*. 2007; 5: 1140–3.

65. Vanner S. The small intestinal bacterial overgrowth: irritable bowel syndrome hypothesis: implications for treatment. *Gut* 2008; 57: 1315–21.

66. Simrén M, Stotzer P-O. Use and abuse of hydrogen breath tests. *Gut* 2006; 55: 297–393.

67. Vanner S. The lactulose breath test for diagnosing SIBO in IBS patients: another nail in the coffin. *Am J Gastroenterol.* 2008; 103: 964–5.

68. Parisi G, Leandro G, Bottona E et al. Small intestinal bacterial overgrowth and irritable bowel syndrome. *Am J Gastroenterol.* 2003; 98: 2572.

69. Walters B, Vanner SJ. Detection of bacterial overgrowth in IBS using the lactulose H_2 breath test: comparison with ^{14}C-d-Xylose and healthy controls. *Am J Gastroenterol.* 2005; 100: 1566–70.

70. Posserud I, Stotzer PO, Bjornsson E, et al. Small intestinal bacterial overgrowth in patients with irritable bowel syndrome. *Gut* 2006; 56: 802–8.

71. Bratten JR, Spanier J, Jones MP. Lactulose breath testing does not discriminate patients with irritable bowel syndrome from healthy controls. *Am J Gastroenterol.* 2008; 103: 958–63.

72. Pimentel M, Park S, Mirocha J, Kane SV, Kong Y. The effect of a nonabsorbed antibiotic (rifaximin) on the symptoms of the irritable bowel syndrome: a randomized trial. *Ann Intern Med.* 2006; 145: 557–563.

73. Drossman DA. Treatment for bacterial overgrowth in the irritable bowel syndrome. *An Intern Med.* 2006; 145: 626–8.

74. Lembo A, Zakko SF, Ferreira NL, Ringel Y, Bortey E, Courtney K, Corsi E, Forbes WP, Pimentel M. Rifaximin for the treatment of diarrhea-associated irritable bowel syndrome: short-term treatment leading to long term sustained response. *Gastroenterology* 2008; 134: A–545.

75. Ringel Y, Zakko SF, Ferreira NL, Bortey E, Wu T, Courtney K, Forbes WP, Lembo A, Pimentel M. Predictors of clinical response from a phase 2 multi-center efficacy trial using rifaximin, a gut-selective, nonabsorbed antibiotic for the treatment of diarrhea-associated irritable bowel syndrome. *Gastroenterology* 2008; 134: A–550.

76. Sharara AI, Aoun E, Abdul-Baki H, Mounzer R, Sidani S, Ell-Iajj I. A randomized double-blind placebo-controlled trial of rifaximin in patients with abdominal bloating and flatulence. *Am J Gastroenterol.* 2006; 101: 326–33.

77. Halpern GM, Prindiville T, Blankenburg M, Hsia T, Gershwin ME. Treatment of irritable bowel syndrome with lacteol fort: a randomized, double-blind, cross-over trial. *Am J Gastroenterol.* 1996; 91: 1579–85.

78. O'Sullivan MA, O'Morain CA. Bacterial supplementation in the irritable bowel syndrome. A randomised double-blind placebo-controlled crossover study. *Dig Liver Dis.* 2000; 32: 302–4.

79. Nobaek S, Johansson ML, Molin G, Ahrne S, Jeppsson B. Alteration of intestinal microflora is associated with reduction in abdominal bloating and pain in patients with irritable bowel syndrome. *Am J Gastroenterol.* 2000; 95: 1231–8.

80. Brigidi P, Vitali B, Swennen E, Bazzocchi G, Matteuzzi D. Effects of probiotic administration upon the composition and enzymatic activity of human fecal microbiota in patients with irritable bowel syndrome or functional diarrhea. *Res Microbiol.* 2001; 152: 735–41.

81. Niedzielin K, Kordecki H, Birkenfeld B. A controlled, double-blind, randomized study on the efficacy of Lactobacillus plantarum 299V in patients with irritable bowel syndrome. *Eur J Gastroenterol Hepatol.* 2001; 13: 1143–7.

82. Sen S, Mullan MM, Parker TJ, Woolner JT, Tarry SA, Hunter JO. Effect of *Lactobacillus plantarum* 299v on colonic fermentation and symptoms of irritable bowel syndrome. *Dig Dis Sci.* 2002; 47: 2615–20.

83. Bazzocchi G, Gionchetti P, Almerigi PF, Amadini C, Campieri M. Intestinal microflora and oral bacteriotherapy in irritable bowel syndrome. *Dig Liver Dis.* 2002; 34 (Suppl 2): s48–53.

84. Parker P, McNaught CE, Anderson ADG, Mitchell CJ, MacFie J. Synbiotic in irritable bowel syndrome: a double blind prospective randomised controlled trial. *Gut* 2003; 52: A11.
85. Kim HJ, Camilleri M, McKenzie S, Lempke MB, Burton DD. A randomized controlled trail of a probiotic, VSL#3 on gut transit and symptoms in diarrhoea-predominant IBS. *Aliment Pharmacol Ther.* 2003; 17: 895–904.
86. Tsuchiya J, Barreto R, Okura R, Kawakita S, Fesce E, Marotta F. Single-blind follow-up study on the effectiveness of a symbiotic preparation in irritable bowel syndrome. *Chin J Dig Dis.* 2004; 5: 169–74.
87. Bausserman M, Michail S. The use of *Lactobacillus* GG in irritable bowel syndrome in children: a double-blind randomized control trial. *J Pediatr.* 2005; 147: 197–201.
88. Kim HJ, Vazquez Roque MI, Camilleri M et al. A randomized controlled trial of probiotic combination VSL#3 and placebo in IBS with bloating. *Neurogastroenterol Motil.* 2005; 17: 687–96.
89. Kajander K, Hatakka K, Poussa T, Farkkila M, Korpela R. A probiotic mixture alleviates symptoms in irritable bowel syndrome patients: a controlled 6-month intervention. *Aliment Pharmacol Ther.* 2005; 22: 387–94.
90. Niv E, Naftali T, Hallak R, Vaisman N. The efficacy of *Lactobacillus reuteri* ATCC 55730 in the treatment of patients with irritable bowel syndrome—a double blind, placebo-controlled, randomized study. *Clin Nutr.* 2005; 24: 925–31.
91. Guyonnet D, Chassany O, Ducrotte P, et al. Effect of a fermented milk containing *Bifidobacterium animalis* DN-173 010 on the health-related quality of life and symptoms in irritable bowel syndrome in adults in primary acre: a multicentre, randomized, double-blind, controlled trial. *Aliment Pharmacol Ther.* 2007; 26: 475–486.
92. Drouault-Holowacz S, Bieuvelel S, Burckel A, Cazaubiel M, Dray X, Marteau P. A double blind randomized trial of a probiotic combination in 100 patients with irritable bowel syndrome. *Gastroenterol Clin Biol.* 2008; 32: 147–152.
93. Sinn DH, Song JH, Kim HJ, Lee JH, Son HJ, Chang DK, Kim Y-H, Kim JJ, Rhee JC, Rhee P-L. Therapeutic effect of *Lactobacillus acidophilus*-SDC 2012, 2013 in patients with irritable bowel syndrome. *Dig Dis Sci.* 2008; 53: 2714–8.
94. Zeng J, Li Y-Q, Zuo X-L, Zhen Y-B, Yang J, Liu C-H. Clinical trial: effect of active lactic acid bacteria on mucosal barrier function in patients with diarrhoea-predominant irritable bowel syndrome. *Aliment Pharmacol Ther.* 2008; 28: 994–1002.
95. Williams EA, Stimpson J, Wang D, Plummer S, Garaiova I, Barker ME, Corfe BM. Clinical trial: a multistrain probiotic preparation significantly reduces symptoms of irritable bowel syndrome in a double-blind placebo-controlled study. *Aliment Pharmacol Ther.* 2009, epub forthcoming.
96. Kajander K, Myllyluoma E, Rajilić-Stojanović M, Kyrönpalo S, Rasmussen M, Järvenpää S, Zoetendal EG, de Vos WM, Vapaatalo H, Korpela R. Clinical trial: multispecies probiotic supplementation alleviates the symptoms of irritable bowel syndrome and stabilizes intestinal microbiota. *Aliment Pharmacol Ther.* 2008; 27: 48–57.
97. Agarwal A, Houghton LA, Morris J, Reilly B, Guyonnet D, Goupil Feuillerat N, Schlumberger A, Jakob S, Whorwell PJ. Clinical trial: the effects of a fermented milk product containing *Bifidobacterium lactis* DN-173-010 on abdominal distension and gastrointestinal transit in irritable bowel syndrome with constipation. *Aliment Pharmacol Ther.* 2009 epub forthcoming.
98. Hamilton-Miller JMT. Probiotics in the management of irritable bowel syndrome: a review of clinical trials. *Microb Ecol Health Dis.* 2001; 13: 212–6.
99. Quigley EM, Flourie B Probiotics and irritable bowel syndrome: a rationale for their use and an assessment of the evidence to date. *Neurogastroenterol Motil.* 2007; 19: 166–72.

100. Quigley EM. Probiotics in functional gastrointestinal disorders: what are the facts? *Curr Opin Pharmacol*. 2008; 8: 704–8.
101. Quigley EM. Germs, gas and the gut; the evolving role of the enteric flora in IBS. *Am J Gastroenterol*. 2006; 101: 334–5.
102. Galati JS, McKee DP, Quigley EMM. The response to intraluminal gas in the irritable bowel syndrome: motility versus perception. *Dig Dis Sci*. 1995; 40: 1381–1387.
103. Azpiroz F, Malagelada J-R. Abdominal bloating. *Gastroenterology* 2005; 129: 1060–78.
104. Whorwell PJ, Altringer L, Morel J et al. Efficacy of an encapsulated probiotic *Bifidobacterium infantis* 35624 in women with irritable bowel syndrome. *Am J Gastroenterol*. 2006; 101: 326–33.
105. Quigley EM. Irritable bowel syndrome and inflammatory bowel disease: interrelated diseases? *Chin J Dig Dis*. 2005; 6: 122–32.
106. McFarland LV, Dublin S. Meta-analysis of probiotics for the treatment of irritable bowel syndrome. *World J Gastroenterol*. 2008; 14: 2650–61.
107. Nikfar S, Rahimi R, Rahimi F, Derakhshani S, Abdollahi M. Efficacy of probiotics in irritable bowel syndrome: a meta-analysis of randomized, controlled trials. *Dis Colon Rectum*. 2008; 51: 1775–80.
108. Frissora CL, Cash BD. Review article: the role of antibiotics vs conventional pharmacotherapy in treating symptoms of irritable bowel syndrome. *Aliment Pharmacol Ther*. 2007; 25: 1271–81.

8 The Role of Nutrition in Inflammatory Bowel Disease
Food for Thought

Gerard E. Mullin, Melissa Munsell,
and Ashwini Davison

CONTENTS

8.1   INTRODUCTION

Inflammatory bowel disease (IBD) is a chronic illness characterized by unremitting intestinal inflammation caused by increased oxidative and metabolic stress. Increased energy, macronutrient, micronutrient, and electrolyte requirements result from thermodynamic demands of inflammation and tissue losses from intestinal injury. Consequent protein-calorie malnutrition and micronutrient deficiencies are common and require close supervision and corrective supplementation. Food harbors nutrients that play an important role in attenuating the unresolved inflammation of IBD while optimizing healing and immunity. Dietary and nutritional strategies have been studied as primary treatments in IBD. The following chapter reviews the impact of nutrition on the sequelae and treatment of IBD.

8.2   EPIDEMIOLOGY

8.2.1   A Gene Nutrient Interaction

Incidence rates of IBD in the United States have remained stable over the past 30 years with the prevalence of ulcerative colitis estimated at 214 cases per 100,000 and Crohn's disease at 174 per 100,000.[1,2] In parts of the world such as Asia, it is unclear if the increased incidence of IBD is due to improved diagnostic methods or environmental triggers. For example, the increased incidence of IBD in Japan has been concurrent with the integration of Westernized diets into the culture.[3] Diets high in animal fat and sugar, but low in fiber, have been implicated in the development of IBD.[4-6] The exact etiology of IBD has yet to be identified, but it has been proposed that genetically susceptible individuals develop disease when there is an exaggerated immune response to an environmental trigger (i.e., infection, diet) in the gut microbiota. Since IBD is the result of a complex interaction between genetic, immune, microbial, and environmental factors, it is highly plausible that diet, as an environmental factor, may contribute to the pathogenesis. For example, elemental diets have been shown to produce symptomatic relief and objective remission in up to 90% of patients.[7] Elemental diets do not contain intact protein, unlike polymeric diets. In elemental diets, nitrogen is supplied in the form of amino acids and dipeptides. In animal models of IBD, dietary protein has increased intestinal permeability, and elemental diets have led to the resolution of this.[8] Nutrition appears to play an integral role in the pathogenesis and treatment of IBD.

8.3 PATHOPHYSIOLOGY

8.3.1 OVERVIEW OF IBD PRESENTATION

Ulcerative colitis (UC) affects the colonic mucosa in a continuous manner and is characterized by diarrhea, abdominal pain, and hematochezia. Crohn's disease (CD) is characterized by transmural inflammation that is discontinuous and may affect any part of the gastrointestinal tract.[9] The most common location of disease involvement for CD is the small bowel where most nutrients are assimilated and absorbed. Endoscopically, the mucosa is described as cobblestoned with evidence of aphthous ulcerations. Radiographically, evidence of fistulae or stricturing disease may be present. Patients with CD often have symptoms of abdominal pain from stricturing disease, which limits nutrient intake, they also suffer from diarrhea because of severe mucosal injury causing malabsorption of fat and lipid-soluble vitamins. The loss of fluids, electrolytes, and minerals leads to weight loss and overall malnutrition in these patients.

8.3.2 CHRONIC INFLAMMATION

Chronic inflammation in IBD is characterized by the infiltration of monocytes and polymorphonuclear neutrophils into the intestinal wall.[10] The inflammatory response becomes amplified by these cells that recruit and activate more inflammatory cells to the lamina propria. It is believed that mononuclear cells mediate this immune response via secretion of proinflammatory cytokines, such as tumor necrosis factor (TNF), interferon-γ, interleukins, and eicosanoids (prostaglandin class 2, thromboxanes, and leukotriene class 4).[11] Activation of NFκB stimulates expression of these molecules, but also stimulates expression of protective molecules that inhibit inflammation.[12] This mechanism is not completely understood, but is thought to play a key role in the acute and chronic inflammation of IBD.[13] Studies have shown that short chain fatty acids (SCFAs), such as butyrate, polyphenols, and n-3 fatty acids, can reduce NFκB activity, providing hope that these may become nutraceutical therapeutic modalities for IBD.[14-16]

Linoleic acid is an essential polyunsaturated fatty acid (PUFA) and is a substrate for eicosanoids. PUFAs are categorized into two main families: n-6 and n-3. Linoleic acid is the parent compound to proinflammatory n-6 fatty acids and is found in fairly high concentrations in red meat, corn, soybean, and safflower oils. The other class of essential fatty acids are n-3 PUFAs of which the parent compound is α-linoleic acid. These fatty acids play an important role in immunomodulation via the production of prostaglandin class 3 and leukotriene B_5, and the inhibition of arachidonic acid production.[17] The n-3 fatty acids are believed to compete with n-6 fatty acids as precursors for eicosanoid synthesis.[18] N-3 fatty acids also reduce TNFα production by inhibiting protein kinase C activity.[19] N-3 PUFAs are found in flaxseed, canola, walnuts, and oils from deep sea fish. The latter is a more valuable source of n-3 PUFAs because humans do not readily transform α-linoleic acid to eicosapentaenoic acid and docosahexaenoic acid, which are the main precursors for desirable eicosanoids. Fish oil affects the gut immune system by suppressing T cell signaling, inhibiting proinflammatory cytokine synthesis, reducing inflammatory cell recruitment, and enhancing epithelial barrier function.[20,21]

Along with PUFAs, SFCAs are also thought to play a role in IBD pathogenesis. SCFAs are monocarboxylic hydrocarbons produced when endogenous bacterial flora in the colon digest nonabsorbable carbohydrates, such as acetate, propionate, and butyrate.[22] These dietary fibers include nonstarch polysaccharides, resistant starch, cellulose, and pectins.[23] Butyrate is a major source of energy for colonocytes and early studies demonstrate that rectal epithelial cells in patients with UC have impaired oxidation of butyrate, which may be caused by elevated levels of TNFα.[24–26] Other studies have shown that SCFAs, such as butyrate, may have an antiinflammatory effect by down-regulating cytokines.[27,28] Furthermore, SCFAs may promote colonic sodium absorption.[29] The therapeutic potential of SCFAs has been shown in both animal and human studies in IBD.[30]

IBD results from the complex interplay between genetic, immune, and environmental factors, including food and nutrients. Diets high in animal fats or sugar and low in fiber have been implicated in IBD, but studies on the role of diet in IBD are challenging to interpret because other lifestyle and environmental factors also play a role.[1] Dietary microparticles have also been theorized to be involved in the etiology of IBD. Microparticles are bacterial-sized inorganic particles, such as titanium, aluminum, and silicone, which are found in Western diets, often as food additives. They are thought to exacerbate inflammation by increasing intestinal permeability and allowing for increased exposure to antigens.[31,32] Although certain foods aggravate IBD symptoms, there is no evidence linking specific foods as directly causing IBD. The diet for patients with IBD should be a well-varied regimen that includes foods rich in polyphenolsomega-3 fatty acids, and prebiotics. This should be coupled with a healthy lifestyle in patients with IBD to minimize malnutrition, attenuate inflammation, and optimize healing.

8.3.3 Malnutrition

Hospitalized patients with IBD have a higher prevalence of malnutrition than patients hospitalized with other benign conditions.[33] CD patients, in particular, are susceptible to protein-calorie malnutrition, which contributes both to increased length of stay and hospital costs.[34,35] Protein-calorie malnutrition in IBD is often manifested clinically by weight loss.[36] Up to 70% of adult patients with CD are underweight while fewer ambulatory patients with UC experience weight loss, as weight loss is more commonly seen in hospitalized UC patients.[37–39]

Weight loss is also common in outpatients with Crohn's disease and is seen in up to 75% of these patients[40–42] CD patients also have significantly lower lean body mass.[43] Even when they are in remission, 20% of patients remain 10% below their ideal body weight.[44] Male patients with CD have a significantly lower percentage of body fat and hamstring muscle strength compared to healthy controls.[38,45] The reasons for protein-calorie malnutrition in IBD stem from ongoing inflammation and catabolic proinflammatory cytokine production, hypothalamic pituitary adrenal (HPA)-axis dysregulation, malabsorption of nutrients, and diminished intake due to abdominal discomfort.

While weight loss in association with malnutrition is common, obesity can also lead to protein-calorie malnutrition. Fat is often distributed in mesenteric fat, and is independent of body mass index. "Creeping fat" is seen in CD and refers to fat hypertrophy and visceral fat wrapping around the small and large bowel.[1] It was originally thought that creeping fat was simply the result of transmural inflammation. Emerging data shows that mesenteric fat itself is proinflammatory and produces TNFα along with proinflammatory adipocytokines.[46] Hyperinsulinism, cortisol and catecholamine imbalance, as well as enhanced proinflammatory cytokines, can lead to obesity in some patients with IBD. Prednisone therapy can contribute to weight gain by decreasing lipid oxidation and increasing protein oxidation, thereby increasing fat stores and depleting muscle protein.[47,48] The combination of hyperinsulinism, corticosteroid use, and obesity can lead to unique struggles for the patient with IBD.

8.3.4 MECHANISMS OF GROWTH RETARDATION AND MALNUTRITION

Growth impairment in IBD results from poor nutrition, chronic inflammation, and as a complication of medical or surgical therapy.[49,50] Decreased oral intake is frequently seen in those with active disease and may be due to anorexia or sitophobia.[50] Even while in remission, patients may have lower daily intake of nutrients, such as fiber and phosphorus.[44] In addition to reduced dietary intake, malnutrition in patients with Crohn's disease results from malabsorption, enteric loss of nutrients, and rapid GI transit time. Disease activity and extent can markedly influence the prevalence and degree of malnutrition in CD.[51] Patients with diffuse small bowel involvement typically are more at risk for malnutrition. This is due to impaired absorption of nutrients, similar to what is seen in patients with small bowel resection or bacterial overgrowth.[43,52,53] Genetic susceptibility may also play a role as children with NODII/CARD15 variants in CD have lower height and weight percentiles.[54] Insulin-like growth factor (IGF)-1 has also been implicated in metabolic derangements in both children and adults with IBD. Total and free IGF-1 levels are reduced in patients with both Crohn's disease and ulcerative colitis when compared to healthy controls. This may be partially reversed by steroid therapy and TNF inhibitors.[55–57] Once inflammation and disease activity is controlled, the nutritional status of patients with CD usually improves. Biologic therapies improve weight and body mass index (BMI) in children with active CD who respond to treatment.[58] Four to six years after patients with UC undergo total proctocolectomy with ileal pouch-anal anastomosis, muscular strength is increased by 11%, total tissue mass by 4.5%, and bone mineral density by almost 2%.[52]

8.3.5 IMPLICATIONS OF MALNUTRITION

Malnutrition has many detrimental effects including muscle breakdown, impaired immunity, and delayed wound healing.[59] In children, malnutrition leads to stunted growth, and it leads to weight loss in patients of all ages.[60,61] Patients with CD, especially ileal or ileocolonic disease, have a greater loss of muscle than fat.[40] They can develop hypoalbuminemia because of increased protein catabolism and decreased synthesis. Once again this is due to ongoing inflammation, intestinal protein loss, reduced hepatic protein synthesis, malabsorption, and anorexia.[62] Villous atrophy and increased intestinal permeability may occur as a result of malnutrition leading to poor nutrient absorption.[63] Malnutrition on admission to a hospital has been correlated with longer lengths of stay, higher costs, and increased mortality when compared to normally nourished individuals.[64,65] Patients with IBD admitted to the hospital with hypoalbuminemia and evidence of malnutrition require a prompt nutritional evaluation and early intervention. Individuals who undergo an aggressive correction of their underlying malnutrition in the hospital setting have improved outcomes, lower morbidity, lower mortality rates, and shorter hospital stays.[66]

8.3.6   NUTRITION AND BONE HEALTH

Malnutrition, systemic inflammation, and corticosteroid use contribute to decreased bone mineral density in these patients.[67,68] The prevalence of osteopenia in patients with IBD is 50% while the prevalence of osteoporosis is 15%.[69] Though both patients with CD and UC are at risk for decreased bone density, there is a greater risk in CD.[70] One study showed that osteopenia is even seen in newly diagnosed patients with IBD, prior to any steroid therapy.[71] This is in contrast to another study demonstrating that women who developed IBD prior to age 20 are likely to have normal bone mineral density as adults.[72] Though steroid use has often been blamed for reduced bone mineral density in IBD, it has been shown to be a weak predictor of osteopenia in patients with CD. Age, body mass index, serum magnesium, and history of bowel resections appear to be more important predictors for low bone mineral density.[73,74] Calcium and vitamin D supplementation has been shown to maintain and increase bone mineral density in patients with CD.[75,76] Vitamin D can help regulate cytokine responses and dampen inflammatory responses.[77] The ability of vitamin D to influence the immunopathogenesis of IBD has been reviewed elsewhere.[78,79] Biologic therapy with infliximab is associated with increased markers of bone formation without increasing bone resorption.[80] Weight-bearing exercise should be encouraged and smoking should be avoided. All women with IBD should be supplemented with calcium and vitamin D according to the dietary reference intakes (DRIs). However, most experts agree that given the prevalence of vitamin D insufficiency (25(OH) D levels < 32 mcg/mL) in Crohn's disease, supplementation should be individualized to meet individual needs.

8.3.7   NUTRIENT DEFICIENCIES

Vitamin and mineral deficiencies are commonly seen in IBD, especially that of calcium and phosphorous These patients also are deficient in niacin, zinc, copper, and vitamins A and C.[81] Increased oxidative stress along with impaired antioxidant defenses in the form of mucosal zinc, copper, and super oxide dismutase has been shown in studies of serum and diseased intestinal mucosa.[82] Every patient with IBD should be screened at least annually for vitamin and mineral deficiencies. The body

TABLE 8.1
Prospective Studies of Short Chain Fatty Acids for Left-Sided Ulcerative Colitis

Study	Design	No. Patients (Treatment)	Study Duration (wk)	Butyrate Dose	Results
Scheppach	Single-blind	10 (Butyrate enema)	2	100 mM	↓ Stool frequency, hematochezia, ↓ Endoscopic histologic score
Breuer	Crossover Open-label	10 (Placebo) 10 (SCFA enema)	6	100 mL bid 40 mM 100 mL bid	No change with placebo ↓ Disease activity index ↓ Mucosal histology score
Steinhart	Open-label	10 (Butyrate enema)	6	80 mM 60 mL qd	↓ Disease activity index 60% Response 40% Complete remission
Patz	Open-label	10 (SCFA enema)	6	40 mM 100 mL bid	5/10 Endoscopic and clinical improvement
Vernia	Open-label	10 (Butyrate + 5-ASA enema	6	80 mM 100 mL bid	7/9 Endoscopic, clinical, and histologic improvement

Source: Adapted from References 121 to 125.

systems most commonly impacted by nutrient inadequacies in IBD are summarized in Table 8.1.

8.3.8 BONE HEALTH

The relative risk of fractures is 40% greater in IBD patients than in the general population. The risk of fracture is similar in CD and UC, and for both males and females with IBD. The main nutrients involved in bone health are calcium, vitamin D, vitamin K, and magnesium. As discussed earlier, vitamin D appears to have a role in immunomodulation as well and exerts its effects via vitamin D receptors on T-cells and antigen-presenting cells. Vitamin D can antagonize T-helper 1 proinflammatory responses by interfering with antigen presentation and Th1 activation, upregulating Th2 cytokines, and downregulation NFκB in macrophages.[85]

8.3.9 ANEMIA

Anemia is frequently seen in patient with IBD and may be due to iron, B_{12}, or folic acid deficiency. Measurement of serum B_{12} should be performed annually in patients with ileal CD.[83] Methylmalonic acid can be used as a more sensitive test for the diagnosis of cobalamin deficiency.[84] Hyperhomocysteinemia is seen in IBD and is associated with decreased levels of vitamin B_{12} and folate.[85]

TABLE 8.2
Probiotics in IBD

Author	Year	Probiotic	Result
Kruis	1997	*E. coli* Nissle 1917	Equal to mesalamine
Rembacken	1999	*E. coli* Nissle 1917	Equal to mesalamine
Guslandi	2000	*S. boulardii*	Equal to mesalamine
Ishikawa	2003	Bifidobacterium milk	Superior to placebo
Borody	2003	Stool enema	Improved
Kruis	2004	*E. coli* Nissle	Superior to conventional
Kato	2004	Bifidobacterium milk	Superior to placebo
Furrie	2005	Bifidobacterium + fiber	Improved

Source: Adapted from References 150 to 155, 158.

8.4 ROLE OF PARENTERAL NUTRITION

Total parenteral nutrition (TPN) with bowel rest was previously viewed as a primary therapy for Crohn's disease. However, a key study in 1988 demonstrated that complete bowel rest was not a major factor in achieving clinical remission.[86] The practice of bowel rest varies from practitioner to practitioner. TPN carries a risk of sepsis, cholestatic liver disease, and other complications listed in Table 8.2. Overfeeding can also lead to problems in patients with IBD.[87] In animal models, long-term TPN use is associated with small intestinal atrophy and increased intestinal permeability.[88,89] A recent study of nationwide patterns of inpatient TPN utilization showed that usage was associated with higher in-hospital mortality, length of stay, and hospital costs ($51,729 versus $19,563).[90] Enteral nutrition can prevent malnutrition in patients with adequate bowel length and, when feasible, should be favored over TPN due to preservation of mucosal integrity and a favorable adverse effect profile.[91,92]

8.5 ROLE OF ENTERAL NUTRITION

The role of enteral nutrition as primary therapy in IBD remains uncertain, particularly in adults. While enteral nutrition as primary therapy for active CD is less successful in inducing remission than steroid therapy, it has a better response than placebo.[93,94] Meta-analyses have shown that remission rates with enteral feeds in Crohn's disease is approximately 60%.[95,102] Oral diet supplementation with low residue nutrition has been shown to improve nutritional status and decrease disease activity in CD.[96,97] One randomized control study showed that patients obtaining half of their calories from an elemental diet and the remaining half from a polymeric diet had a reduced risk of relapse compared to patients receiving all of their calories from a normal diet.[98] Studies like this are difficult to perform because of large dropout rates from intolerance of the study diet.[18] In terms of the type of enteral feeds, elemental diets have not been shown to be more successful in inducing remission than nonelemental diets.[99,104] In children, enteral nutritional support has a positive effect on growth and development and may help avoid steroid use.[100,101]

Once again, elemental formulations are not palatable and noncompliance becomes a major issue.

8.5.1 Mode of Action of Enteral Nutrition

The mechanism by which enteral nutrition affects the inflammatory process in IBD is not clear. Proposed mechanisms include provision of essential nutrients, reduction of antigenic load, alteration of bowel flora, and improved immune function.[102] The enteral diet may have an antiinflammatory effect on the gastrointestinal mucosa, which may be related to the fatty acids in the feed or alteration of gut flora.[1,103,104] The feeds studied (AL110, Modulen IBD. and ACD004 [Nestlé, Vevey, Switzerland]) all have casein as the protein source, are lactose free. and are rich in the antiinflammatory cytokine, transforming growth factor beta (TGF-beta). They have all been shown to induce clinical remission associated with mucosal healing.[105] Modulen IBD not only led to macroscopic and histological healing of the mucosa, but also decreased mucosal proinflammatory cytokines. This included interleukin-1 mRNA in the colon and ileum, interleukin-8 mRNA in the colon, and interferon gamma mRNA in ileum. It also led to a rise in the regulatory cytokine TGF-beta mRNA in the ileum. Formulas such as this may be influencing the disease process and allowing for clinical remission via a reduction in inflammation.

Clinical response to enteral nutrition is associated with mucosal healing and down regulation of proinflammatory cytokines.[112] Modulen supplementation provided statistically significant protection against weight loss, hypoalbuminemia, acidosis, and GI damage in a rat model of IBD.[106] Future animal research regarding the mechanism of action of Modulen's protective effects is needed before further human trials are considered.

8.5.2 Glutamine

The nonessential amino acid glutamine is a source of energy for intestinal epithelial cells and stimulates proliferation of intestinal epithelial cells.[107] In animal models of IBD, glutamine-enriched parenteral nutrition decreased bacterial translocation and stimulated IgA mucosal secretion.[108,109] New animal data has suggested that parenteral glutamine may have antiinflammatory effects via the NFκB pathway with anti-TNFα properties.[110] These findings led to the hypothesis that glutamine-enriched parenteral nutrition may improve outcomes in patients with CD. However, glutamine-enriched parenteral nutrition has failed to show a clinical benefit in patients with IBD, when compared to standard parenteral nutrition.[111] Intestinal utilization of glutamine appears to be impaired in CD, and this may be why it has not been successful as restorative therapy.[112]

8.6 OTHER DIETARY THERAPY IN IBD

Although diet has been implicated in the pathogenesis of IBD, there is no definitive evidence linking a specific food or additive as a cause of IBD. Therefore, most patients are advised to follow a healthy, well-balanced diet. Alternative dietary strategies, however, do warrant consideration.

8.6.1 POLYUNSATURATED FATTY ACIDS

One proposed mechanism for the efficacy of low-fat elemental diets is that without sufficient n-6 fatty acids, proinflammatory eicosanoids cannot be synthesized.[113] The family of n-3 fatty acids have the parent compound α-linoleic acid, which is synthesized into fatty acids that are important in immunomodulatory and antiinflammatory effects via the production of prostaglandin class 3 and leukotriene B_5, and by inhibiting production of arachidonic acid and TNFα production.[17–19] These findings would suggest that a diet rich in n-3 PUFAs may be protective against IBD, while those rich in n-6 PUFAs may promote inflammation. PUFAs may reduce the risk of recurrence in CD and may also have a role in UC.[114,115] One study evaluated a polymeric enteral diet high in oleate acid (monounsaturated fat) versus an identical diet high in linoleate acid, and demonstrated that remission rates were improved with the linoleate diet.[113] Conversely, elemental diets with increased amounts of long-chain triglycerides (LCTs) resulted in lower remission rates in active Crohn's disease than the same diet with lower LCTs.[116] Soybean oil was used as the LCT with the principal fatty acids being oleic acid and linoleic acid. According to the Cochrane review, omega 3 fatty acids might be effective for maintenance therapy in CD, though this was not supported in UC (Table 8.3).[117,118] Most recently, two randomized, placebo-controlled trials showed omega-3 fatty acids were not effective in the prevention of relapse in CD.[119]

8.6.2 SHORT CHAIN FATTY ACIDS, LOW PARTICLE DIETS, AND POLYPHENOLS

In addition to PUFAs, other dietary strategies in IBD include SCFAs, low particle diets, and polyphenols.[15,27,120,123,124] The majority of studies on SCFAs have been

TABLE 8.3
Prebiotics in Ulcerative Colitis

Author	Year	Fiber	Study	Outcome
Fernandez-Banares	1999	Plantago ovata seed fiber 10 grams BID	Fiber +/- mesalamine in patients in remission	Equal to mesalamine in maintenance of remission
Kanauchi	2002 2003	Barley 20–30 grams	Mild to moderately active UC	Decreased disease activity
Hallert	2003	Oat bran 60 grams (fiber 20 grams)	Patients in remission	Decreased abdominal pain, increased fecal butyrate
Welters	2002	Inulin 24 grams	IPAA	Deceased pouch inflammation

Source: Adapted from References 168 to 171.
Note: IPAA = ileal pouch-anal anastomosis.

conducted in animals, but there is some research on humans. Though the studies,[121,122] were small and of a relatively short duration, they demonstrated clinical response or improvement with SCFA enemas (Table 8.1).[123–125] One small, nonrandomized, open-labeled trial demonstrated a decrease in clinical index activity scores in patients with ulcerative colitis treated with 30 grams of germinated barley, which increased luminal butyrate production.[29]

8.7 PHYTONUTRIENTS IN IBD

8.7.1 Resveratrol

Polyphenols are phytochemicals found in food substances produced from plants, and they are thought to be involved in immunomodulation.[126] Examples of polyphenols include resveratrol, epigallocatechin, and curcumin. Resveratrol is found most abundantly in the skin of red grapes.[127] Resveratrol appears to be antiinflammatory, although its mechanism of action has not been clearly established.[15] In rodent models of inflammatory colitis, resveratrol has been shown to reverse weight loss, increase stool consistency, improve mucosal appearance, improve gut histology, decrease inflammatory infiltrate, and decrease mucosal levels of interleukin-1β, COX-2, and prostaglandin D_2.[128] To date, resveratrol has not been studied in human subjects with IBD.

8.7.2 Catechins

Catechins, such as gallocatechin gallate (EGCG), are abundant in green (nonfermented) tea.[129] Green tea has been studied in the prevention or treatment of cancers, such as breast, lung, ovarian, prostate, and stomach, as well as in diseases, such as hypertension and cardiovascular health.[15] EGCG can modulate and inhibit NFκB activity which may affect inflammation.[130] Similar to resveratrol, green tea has been shown to improve disease activity in murine models of colitis.[131,132] An *in vitro* study involving human colonic tissues showed that EGCG administration resulted in decreased proinflammatory cytokine production, but to date, there are no *in vivo* human studies in IBD.[133]

8.7.3 Curcumin

Another phytonutrient studied for its antiinflammatory role is curcumin, the major chemical component of turmeric. Turmeric, from the herb *Curcuma longa*, is the major spice found in curry.[134] Curcumin is used orally and topically to treat a variety of ailments and has an excellent safety profile.[135,136] It appears to have multiple mechanisms of action including the inhibition of NFκB, which likely leads to the downregulation of proinflammatory genes and cytokines.[137] Overall, in animal models of colitis, curcumin has prevented and ameliorated chemical-induced colonic injury.[138,139] In one randomized, double-blind, placebo-controlled trial, 89 patients with quiescent ulcerative colitis were given 1 gram of curcumin twice daily or placebo for six months. They were followed prospectively for relapse of disease. Of the

44 patients who consumed curcumin, only 2 experienced clinical flares while 8 of the 45 patients taking placebo relapsed (p = 0.049).[140]

8.8 SUPPORTING COLONIC MICROBES

8.8.1 PROBIOTICS

Probiotics are defined as *"live microorganisms, which when administered in adequate amounts, confer a health benefit on the host."*[141] Disturbances in bacterial intestinal flora have been purported as a triggering factor for IBD.[142] Animal models suggest probiotics may be useful in the treatment of UC and CD.[143,144] Based on these animal models, probiotics alter gastrointestinal flora and ameliorate disease.[145,146] Pouchitis (chronic inflammation of the ileo-anal pouch) is a complication of surgery for UC and is typically treated effectively with antibiotics, suggesting a causative role of bacteria.[147] In patients with chronic pouchitis induced to achieve remission with antibiotic therapy, VSL#3 (a high potency probiotic with 450 billion colony=forming units per dose) was successful in maintaining remission.[148] VSL#3 may also have a role as primary prophylaxis of pouchitis in patients with ileal pouch-anal anastomosis.[149]

Probiotics have been shown to be efficacious in maintenance therapy in UC (Table 8.2). Three randomized controlled trials showed that *Escherichia coli* Nissle 1917 equaled conventional 5-aminosalicylic acid treatment, suggesting that probiotics can be used to maintain remission of disease.[150–152] Studies using other probiotic species have yielded mixed results.[153,154] Probiotics have also been studied in the treatment of active ulcerative colitis.[155] When VSL#3 was used in combination with low-dose balsalazide, patients had shorter time to remission than balsalazide alone, suggesting that probiotics can lessen dosage requirements of conventional agents for UC.[156] Of note, the doses of balsalazide used were lower than typically used in a clinical scenario. Additionally, when probiotics have been used as topical therapy with *E. coli* Nissle 1917 enemas, they have led to remission, with the shortest time to remission occurring with the highest dose of enema.[157]

Probiotics have been studied in CD as well. One study showed patients using *Saccharomyces boulardii* plus mesalazine had fewer relapses than those using mesalazine alone.[158] Other studies, however, have not shown probiotics to be effective as a maintenance strategy in CD.[159,160] In treating active CD, probiotics have not been shown to significantly have a role in treatment. One study showed that prebiotics may reduce disease activity in active CD.[161] Research on probiotics and prebiotics is limited for a number of reasons, including enrollment of small number of patients, variability in choice of probiotic or prebiotic used, and variability in patients' diets. Larger randomized controlled trials are needed to determine the role of probiotics and prebiotics in the treatment of IBD.

8.8.2 PREBIOTICS

Prebiotics are compounds that promote intestinal proliferation of probiotic bacteria and are metabolized into SCFAs.[162] Most prebiotics are from the group of dietary fibers found in foods, such as legumes, artichokes, onions, garlic, banana, soya, and other beans.[163] Examples of prebiotics are inulin and oligofructose. When these prebiotics are given in sufficient amounts, they selectively promote the growth of bifidobacteria.[164] Animal models of IBD have shown inulin to reduce inflammatory mediators and reduce histological damage scores.[165] Along with inulin, other prebiotics, such as oligofructose and lactulose, have shown antiinflammatory effects in animal models of IBD.[166,167] In clinical studies, inulin as compared to placebo was associated with improvement in inflammation in UC as well as chronic pouchitis (Table 8.3).[168–171] Combining probiotics and prebiotics as synbiotics may be useful in the treatment of IBD. In mild ulcerative colitis, a synbiotic preparation (oligofructose-enriched inulin and *Bifidobacterium longum*) compared to placebo showed a trend in reduction of mucosal expression of proinflammatory cytokines (TNFα) and improvement in inflammation on a histological level.[172]

8.9   FOOD INTOLERANCE AND IBD

Irritable bowel syndrome (IBS) can be a co-morbid condition in patients with IBD. Healthcare providers need to recognize this association in order to avoid the use of IBD therapy to treat symptoms resulting from IBS.[173] Patients with an IBS overlap may have intolerance to certain foods, such as dairy products, caffeine, fried foods, and high fiber.[174] It is important to note that food intolerance is not a true allergic reaction. If foods cause a true allergic reaction, they need to be *completely* avoided. Patients who have intolerance to certain foods should try to avoid these specific triggers in order to minimize their symptoms.

8.9.1   GLUTEN

Celiac disease has been noted with increased frequency among patients with CD.[175] In general, only those with celiac disease or confirmed gluten-sensitivity should be given a gluten-free diet. There is insufficient data to support or refute a recommendation concerning gluten sensitivity testing for IBD. It is reasonable to suggest that clinicians query patients as to their possible intolerance to gluten and if suspected, IgG_1/IgG_4 and antitransglutaminase/antiendomyseal antibody testing should be considered.

8.9.2   FIBER

IBD, particularly CD, can result in complications of intestinal strictures, fistulae, high-output ostomy as well as short bowel syndrome. Though patients with non-stricturing CD do not benefit universally from a low residue diet, most experts in IBD would recommend a low residue diet in patients who have ongoing intestinal strictures.[176] Insoluble fiber products help serve as prebiotic products to facilitate the population of beneficial enteric bacteria. Thus, continued intake of adequate fiber is helpful for patients with both forms of IBD. Patients with intestinal fistula, high-output ostomy, and short bowel syndrome often are difficult to manage from a nutrition standpoint. Careful management of fluid and electrolyte disturbances is essential, and parenteral nutrition may be necessary in some cases.[177]

8.10 SUMMARY

There is no clear evidence that any specific diet is either the cause or a cure for IBD. Healthcare providers are often faced with the challenge of recommending proper diets for patients with IBD. There is an ongoing struggle between wanting these patients to avoid certain foods while allowing them to enjoy meals as well. In order to prevent food restriction, patients should be encouraged to follow a healthy diet as tolerated; they should be taught about antiinflammatory diets whenever possible. Supplementation with polyphenols, probiotics, and fish oils should be considered as adjuncts to care. Further studies on the role of nutraceuticals used in combination with conventional medical therapies may facilitate improved outcomes and less toxicity.

REFERENCES

1. O'Sullivan M, O'Morain C. Nutrition in inflammatory bowel disease. *Best Practice & Research Clinical Gastroenterology.* 2006;20(3):561–573.
2. Loftus CG, Loftus EV,Jr, Harmsen WS, et al. Update on the incidence and prevalence of Crohn's disease and ulcerative colitis in Olmsted county, Minnesota, 1940–2000. *Inflamm Bowel Dis.* 2007;13(3):254–261.
3. Shoda R, Matsueda K, Yamato S, Umeda N. Epidemiologic analysis of Crohn's disease in Japan: Increased dietary intake of n-6 polyunsaturated fatty acids and animal protein relates to the increased incidence of Crohn's disease in Japan. *Am J Clin Nutr.* 1996;63(5):741–745.
4. Jarnerot G, Jarnmark I, Nilsson K. Consumption of refined sugar by patients with Crohn's disease, ulcerative colitis, or irritable bowel syndrome. *Scand J Gastroenterol.* 1983;18(8):999–1002.
5. Sakamoto N, Kono S, Wakai K, et al. Dietary risk factors for inflammatory bowel disease: A multicenter case-control study in Japan. *Inflamm Bowel Dis.* 2005;11(2):154–163.
6. Kelly DG, Fleming CR. Nutritional considerations in inflammatory bowel diseases. *Gastroenterol Clin North Am.* 1995;24(3):597–611.
7. Akobeng AK, Thomas AG. Enteral nutrition for maintenance of remission in Crohn's disease. *Cochrane Database Syst Rev.* 2007;(3)(3):CD005984.
8. Suzuki H, Hanyou N, Sonaka I, Minami H. An elemental diet controls inflammation in indomethacin-induced small bowel disease in rats: The role of low dietary fat and the elimination of dietary proteins. *Dig Dis Sci.* 2005;50(10):1951–1958.
10. Cho JH. The genetics and immunopathogenesis of inflammatory bowel disease. *Nat Rev Immunol.* 2008 Jun;8(6):458–66.
11. Foell D, Wittkowski H, Ren Z, Turton J, Pang G, Daebritz J, Ehrchen J, Heidemann J, Borody T, Roth J, Clancy R. Phagocyte-specific S100 proteins are released from affected mucosa and promote immune responses during inflammatory bowel disease. *J Pathol.* 2008 Oct;216(2):183–192.
12. Razack R, Seidner DL. Nutrition in inflammatory bowel disease. *Curr Opin Gastroenterol.* 2007;23(4):400–405.
13. Sartor RB. Mechanisms of disease: Pathogenesis of Crohn's disease and ulcerative colitis. *Nat Clin Pract Gastroenterol Hepatol.* 2006;3(7):390–407.

14. Mullin GE, Galinkin D. Anti-IL12 imposes the death sentence on Th1 cells in TNBS colitis: Is there a light at the end of the tunnel for Crohn's disease? *Inflamm Bowel Dis.* 2000;6:261–262.
15. Hodin R. Maintaining gut homeostasis: The butyrate-NF-kappaB connection. *Gastroenterology.* 2000;118(4):798–801.
16. Clarke JO, Mullin GE. A review of complementary and alternative approaches to immunomodulation. *Nutr Clin Pract.* 2008;23(1):49–62.
17. Hudert CA, Weylandt KH, Lu Y, et al. Transgenic mice rich in endogenous omega-3 fatty acids are protected from colitis. *Proc Natl Acad Sci U S A.* 2006;103(30): 11276–11281.
18. Miura S, Tsuzuki Y, Hokari R, Ishii H. Modulation of intestinal immune system by dietary fat intake: Relevance to Crohn's disease. *J Gastroenterol Hepatol.* 1998;13(12):1183–1190.
19. Wild GE, Drozdowski L, Tartaglia C, Clandinin MT, Thomson AB. Nutritional modulation of the inflammatory response in inflammatory bowel disease—from the molecular to the integrative to the clinical. *World J Gastroenterol.* 2007;13(1):1–7.
20. Caughey GE, Mantzioris E, Gibson RA, Cleland LG, James MJ. The effect on human tumor necrosis factor alpha and interleukin 1 beta production of diets enriched in n-3 fatty acids from vegetable oil or fish oil. *Am J Clin Nutr.* 1996;63(1):116–122.
21. Zhang P, Kim W, Zhou L, et al. Dietary fish oil inhibits antigen-specific murine Th1 cell development by suppression of clonal expansion. *J Nutr.* 2006;136(9):2391–2398.
21. Whiting CV, Bland PW, Tarlton JF. Dietary n-3 polyunsaturated fatty acids reduce disease and colonic proinflammatory cytokines in a mouse model of colitis. *Inflamm Bowel Dis.* 2005;11(4):340–349.
22. Kles KA, Chang EB. Short-chain fatty acids impact on intestinal adaptation, inflammation, carcinoma, and failure. *Gastroenterology.* 2006;130(2 Suppl 1):S100–5.
23. James SL, Muir JG, Curtis SL, Gibson PR. Dietary fibre: A roughage guide. *Intern Med J.* 2003;33(7):291–296.
24. Dray X, Marteau P. The use of enteral nutrition in the management of Crohn's disease in adults. *JPEN J Parenter Enteral Nutr.* 2005;29(4 Suppl):S166–9; discussion S169–72, S184–88.
25. Roediger WE. The colonic epithelium in ulcerative colitis: An energy-deficiency disease? *Lancet.* 1980;2(8197):712–715.
26. Yamamoto T, Nakahigashi M, Umegae S, Kitagawa T, Matsumoto K. Impact of elemental diet on mucosal inflammation in patients with active Crohn's disease: Cytokine production and endoscopic and histological findings. *Inflamm Bowel Dis.* 2005;11(6):580–588.
27. Segain JP, Raingeard de la Bletiere, D., Bourreille A, et al. Butyrate inhibits inflammatory responses through NFkappaB inhibition: Implications for Crohn's disease. *Gut.* 2000;47(3):397–403.
28. Tedelind S, Westberg F, Kjerrulf M, Vidal A. Anti-inflammatory properties of the short-chain fatty acids acetate and propionate: A study with relevance to inflammatory bowel disease. *World J Gastroenterol.* 2007 May 28;13(20):2826–2823.
29. Kanauchi O, Suga T, Tochihara M, et al. Treatment of ulcerative colitis by feeding with germinated barley foodstuff: First report of a multicenter open control trial. *J Gastroenterol.* 2002;37(Suppl 14):67–72.
30. Binder HJ, Mehta P. Short-chain fatty acids stimulate active sodium and chloride absorption *in vitro* in the rat distal colon. *Gastroenterology.* 1989;96(4):989–996.
31. Lomer MC, Thompson RP, Powell JJ. Fine and ultrafine particles of the diet: Influence on the mucosal immune response and association with Crohn's disease. *Proc Nutr Soc.* 2002;61(1):123–130.

32. Korzenik JR. Past and current theories of etiology of IBD: Toothpaste, worms, and refrigerators. *J Clin Gastroenterol*. 2005;39(4 Suppl 2):S59–65.

33. Pirlich M, Schutz T, Kemps M, et al. Prevalence of malnutrition in hospitalized medical patients: Impact of underlying disease. *Dig Dis*. 2003;21(3):245–251.

34. O'Sullivan M, O'Morain C. Nutritional therapy in inflammatory bowel disease. *Curr Treat Options Gastroenterol*. 2004;7(3):191–198.

35. Harries AD, Jones L, Heatley RV, Rhodes J, Fitzsimons E. Mid-arm circumference as simple means of identifying malnutrition in Crohn's disease. *Br Med J (Clin Res Ed)*. 1982;285(6351):1317–1318.

36. Silk DB, Payne-James J. Inflammatory bowel disease: Nutritional implications and treatment. *Proc Nutr Soc*. 1989;48(3):355–361.

37. O'Keefe SJ. Nutrition and gastrointestinal disease. *Scand J Gastroenterol Suppl*. 1996;220:52–59.

38. Burke A, Lichtenstein G, Rombeau J. Nutrition and ulcerative colitis. *Bailliére's Clinical Gastroenterology*. 1997;11(1):153–174.

39. Powell-Tuck J. Protein metabolism in inflammatory bowel disease. *Gut*. 1986;27(Suppl 1):67–71.

40. Dyer NH, Dawson AM. Malnutrition and malabsorption in Crohn's disease with reference to the effect of surgery. *Br J Surg*. 1973;60(2):134–140.

41. Lanfranchi GA, Brignola C, Campieri M, et al. Assessment of nutritional status in Crohn's disease in remission or low activity. *Hepatogastroenterology*. 1984;31(3):129–132.

42. Heatley RV. Assessing nutritional state in inflammatory bowel disease. *Gut*. 1986;27(Suppl 1):61–66.

43. Jahnsen J, Falch JA, Mowinckel P, Aadland E. Body composition in patients with inflammatory bowel disease: A population-based study. *Am J Gastroenterol*. 2003;98(7):1556–1562.

44. Harries AD, Jones LA, Heatley RV, Rhodes J. Malnutrition in inflammatory bowel disease: An anthropometric study. *Hum Nutr Clin Nutr*. 1982;36(4):307–313.

45. Geerling BJ, Badart-Smook A, Stockbrugger RW, Brummer RJ. Comprehensive nutritional status in patients with long-standing Crohn disease currently in remission. *Am J Clin Nutr*. 1998;67(5):919–926.

46. Schaffler A, Scholmerich J, Buchler C. Mechanisms of disease: Adipocytokines and visceral adipose tissue—emerging role in intestinal and mesenteric diseases. *Nat Clin Pract Gastroenterol Hepatol*. 2005;2(2):103–111.

47. Al-Jaouni R, Schneider SM, Piche T, Rampal P, Hebuterne X. Effect of steroids on energy expenditure and substrate oxidation in women with Crohn's disease. *Am J Gastroenterol*. 2002;97(11):2843–2849.

48. Cabre E, Gassull MA. Nutritional and metabolic issues in inflammatory bowel disease. *Curr Opin Clin Nutr Metab Care*. 2003;6(5):569–576.

49. Baldassano RN, Piccoli DA. Inflammatory bowel disease in pediatric and adolescent patients. *Gastroenterol Clin North Am*. 1999;28(2):445–458.

50. Reilly J, Ryan J, Strole W, Fischer J. Hyperalimentation in inflammatory bowel disease. *Am J Surg*. 1976;131(2):192–200.

51. Rigaud D, Angel LA, Cerf M, et al. Mechanisms of decreased food intake during weight loss in adult Crohn's disease patients without obvious malabsorption. *Am J Clin Nutr*. 1994;60(5):775–781.

52. Sandstrom B, Davidsson L, Bosaeus I, Eriksson R, Alpsten M. Selenium status and absorption of zinc (65Zn), selenium (75Se) and manganese (54Mn) in patients with short bowel syndrome. *Eur J Clin Nutr*. 1990;44(10):697–703.

53. Jensen MB, Houborg KB, Vestergaard P, Kissmeyer-Nielsen P, Mosekilde L, Laurberg S. Improved physical performance and increased lean tissue and fat mass in patients with ulcerative colitis four to six years after ileoanal anastomosis with a J-pouch. *Dis Colon Rectum*. 2002;45(12):1601–1607.

54. Tomer G, Ceballos C, Concepcion E, Benkov KJ. NOD2/CARD15 variants are associated with lower weight at diagnosis in children with Crohn's disease. *Am J Gastroenterol*. 2003;98(11):2479–2484.

55. Grønbæk H, Thøgersen T, Frystyk J, Vilstrup H, Flyvbjerg A, Dahlerup JF. Low free and total insulin-like growth factor I (IGF-I) and IGF binding protein-3 levels in chronic inflammatory bowel disease: Partial normalization during prednisolone treatment. *Am J Gastroenterol*. 2002;97(3):673–678.

56. Eivindson M, Grønbæk H, Flyvbjerg A, Frystyk J, Zimmermann-Nielsen E, Dahlerup JF. The insulin-like growth factor (IGF)-system in active ulcerative colitis and Crohn's disease: Relations to disease activity and corticosteroid treatment. *Growth Horm IGF Res*. 2007;17(1):33–40.

57. Eivindson M, Gronbaek H, Skogstrand K, et al. The insulin-like growth factor (IGF) system and its relation to infliximab treatment in adult patients with Crohn's disease. *Scand J Gastroenterol*. 2007;42(4):464–470.

58. Walters TD, Gilman AR, Griffiths AM. Linear growth improves during infliximab therapy in children with chronically active severe Crohn's disease. *Inflamm Bowel Dis*. 2007;13(4):424–430.

59. O'Sullivan MA, O'Morain CA. Nutritional therapy in Crohn's disease. *Inflamm Bowel Dis*. 1998;4(1):45–53.

60. Burbige EJ, Shi-Shung Huang, Bayless TM. Clinical manifestations of Crohn's disease in children and adolescents. *Pediatrics*. 1975;55(6):866.

61. McCaffery TD, Nasr K, Lawrence AM, Kirsner JB. Severe growth retardation in children with inflammatory bowel disease. *Pediatrics*. 1970;45(3):386.

62. Stokes MA. Crohn's disease and nutrition. *Br J Surg*. 1992;79(5):391–394.

63. Winter TA, Lemmer ER, O'Keefe SJ, Ogden JM. The effect of severe undernutrition, and subsequent refeeding on digestive function in human patients. *Eur J Gastroenterol Hepatol*. 2000;12(2):191–196.

64. Chima C, Barco K, Dewitt MA, Maeda M, Teran JC, Mullen K. Relationship of nutritional status to length of stay, hospital costs, and discharge status of patients hospitalized in the medicine service. *J Am Diet Assoc*. 1997;97(9):975–978.

65. Nguyen GC, Munsell M, Harris ML. Nationwide prevalence and prognostic significance of clinically diagnosable protein-calorie malnutrition in hospitalized inflammatory bowel disease patients. *Inflamm Bowel Dis*. 2008;14:1105–1111.

66. Brugler L, DiPrinzio MJ, Bernstein L. The five-year evolution of a malnutrition treatment program in a community hospital. *Jt Comm J Qual Improv*. 1999;25(4):191–206.

67. Bjarnason I, Macpherson A, Mackintosh C, Buxton-Thomas M, Forgacs I, Moniz C. Reduced bone density in patients with inflammatory bowel disease. *Gut*. 1997;40(2):228–233.

68. Semeao EJ, Jawad AF, Stouffer NO, Zemel BS, Piccoli DA, Stallings VA. Risk factors for low bone mineral density in children and young adults with Crohn's disease. *J Pediatr*. 1999;135(5):593–600.

69. Bernstein CN, Blanchard JF, Metge C, Yogendran M. The association between corticosteroid use and development of fractures among IBD patients in a population-based database. *Am J Gastroenterol*. 2003;98(8):1797–1801.

70. Jahnsen J, Falch JA, Aadland E, Mowinckel P. Bone mineral density is reduced in patients with Crohn's disease but not in patients with ulcerative colitis: A population based study. *Gut*. 1997;40(3):313–319.

71. Lamb EJ, Wong T, Smith DJ, et al. Metabolic bone disease is present at diagnosis in patients with inflammatory bowel disease. *Aliment Pharmacol Ther*. 2002;16(11): 1895–1902.
72. Bernstein CN, Leslie WD, Taback SP. Bone density in a population-based cohort of premenopausal adult women with early onset inflammatory bowel disease. *Am J Gastroenterol*. 2003;98(5):1094–1100.
73. Habtezion A, Silverberg MS, Parkes R, Mikolainis S, Steinhart AH. Risk factors for low bone density in Crohn's disease. *Inflamm Bowel Dis*. 2002;8(2):87–92.
74. Jong DJ, Corstens FHM, Mannaerts L, Rossum LGM, Naber AHJ. Corticosteroid-induced osteoporosis: Does it occur in patients with Crohn's disease? *Am J Gastroenterol*. 2002;97(8):2011–2015.
75. Vogelsang H, Ferenci P, Resch H, Kiss A, Gangl A. Prevention of bone mineral loss in patients with Crohn's disease by long-term oral vitamin D supplementation. *Eur J Gastroenterol Hepatol*. 1995;7(7):609–614.
76. Siffledeen JS, Fedorak RN, Siminoski K, et al. Randomized trial of etidronate plus calcium and vitamin D for treatment of low bone mineral density in Crohn's disease. *Clin Gastroenterol Hepatol*. 2005;3(2):122–132.
77. Leal JY, Romero T, Ortega P, Amaya D. Serum values of interleukin-10, gamma-interferon and vitamin A in female adolescents. *Invest Clin*. 2007;48(3):317–326.
78. Ginanjar E, Sumariyono, Setiati S, Setiyohadi B. Vitamin D and autoimmune disease. *Acta Med Indones*. 2007;39(3):133–141.
79. Mullin GE, Dobs A. Vitamin D and its role in cancer and immunity: A prescription for sunlight. *Nutr Clin Pract*. 2007;22(3):305–322.
80. Abreu MT, Geller JL, Vasiliauskas EA, et al. Treatment with infliximab is associated with increased markers of bone formation in patients with Crohn's disease. *J Clin Gastroenterol*. 2006;40(1):55–63.
81. Dudrick SJ, Latifi R, Schrager R. Nutritional management of inflammatory bowel disease. *Surg Clin North Am*. 1991;71(3):609–623.
82. Lih-Brody L, Powell SR, Collier KP, et al. Increased oxidative stress and decreased antioxidant defenses in mucosa of inflammatory bowel disease. *Dig Dis Sci*. 1996;41(10):2078–2086.
83. Carter MJ, Lobo AJ, Travis SPL. Guidelines for the management of inflammatory bowel disease in adults. *Gut*. 2004;53(S5):v1–16.
84. Savage DG, Lindenbaum J, Stabler SP, Allen RH. Sensitivity of serum methylmalonic acid and total homocysteine determinations for diagnosing cobalamin and folate deficiencies. *Am J Med*. 1994;96(3):239–246.
85. Romagnuolo J, Fedorak RN, Dias VC, Bamforth F, Teltscher M. Hyperhomocysteinemia and inflammatory bowel disease: Prevalence and predictors in a cross-sectional study. *Am J Gastroenterol*. 2001;96(7):2143–2149.
86. Greenberg GR, Fleming CR, Jeejeebhoy KN, Rosenberg IH, Sales D, Tremaine WJ. Controlled trial of bowel rest and nutritional support in the management of Crohn's disease. *Gut*. 1988;29(10):1309–1315.
87. Jeejeebhoy KN. Enteral and parenteral nutrition: Evidence-based approach. *Proc Nutr Soc*. 2001;60(3):399–402.
88. Rossi TM, Lee PC, Young C, Tjota A. Small intestinal mucosa changes, including epithelial cell proliferative activity, of children receiving total parenteral nutrition (TPN). *Dig Dis Sci*. 1993;38(9):1608–1613.
89. Sedman PC, MacFie J, Palmer MD, Mitchell CJ, Sagar PM. Preoperative total parenteral nutrition is not associated with mucosal atrophy or bacterial translocation in humans. *Br J Surg*. 1995;82(12):1663–1667.

90. Nguyen GC, LaVeist TA, Brant SR. The utilization of parenteral nutrition during the in-patient management of inflammatory bowel disease in the United States: A national survey. *Aliment Pharmacol Ther.* 2007;26(11–12):1499–1507.

91. Dickinson RJ, Ashton MG, Axon AT, Smith RC, Yeung CK, Hill GL. Controlled trial of intravenous hyperalimentation and total bowel rest as an adjunct to the routine therapy of acute colitis. *Gastroenterology.* 1980;79(6):1199–1204.

92. Gonzalez-Huix F, Fernandez-Banares F, Esteve-Comas M, et al. Enteral versus parenteral nutrition as adjunct therapy in acute ulcerative colitis. *Am J Gastroenterol.* 1993;88(2):227–232.

93. Griffiths AM, Ohlsson A, Sherman PM, Sutherland LR. Meta-analysis of enteral nutrition as a primary treatment of active Crohn's disease. *Gastroenterology.* 1995;108(4):1056–1067.

94. Messori A, Trallori G, D'Albasio G, Milla M, Vannozzi G, Pacini F. Defined-formula diets versus steroids in the treatment of active Crohn's disease: A meta-analysis. *Scand J Gastroenterol.* 1996;31(3):267–272.

95. Fernandez-Banares F, Cabre E, Esteve-Comas M, Gassull M. How effective is enteral nutrition in inducing clinical remission in active Crohn's disease? A meta-analysis of the randomized clinical trials. *JPEN J Parenter Enteral Nutr.* 1995;19(5):356–364.

96. Harries AD, Danis V, Heatley RV, et al. Controlled trial of supplemented oral nutrition in Crohn's disease. *The Lancet.* 1983;321(8330):887–890.

97. Koga H, Iida M, Aoyagi K, Matsui T, Fujishima M. Long-term efficacy of low residue diet for the maintenance of remission in patients with Crohn's disease. *Nippon Shokakibyo Gakkai Zasshi.* 1993;90(11):2882–2888.

98. Takagi S, Utsunomiya K, Kuriyama S, et al. Effectiveness of an "half elemental diet" as maintenance therapy for Crohn's disease: A randomized-controlled trial. *Aliment Pharmacol Ther.* 2006;24(9):1333–1340.

99. Verma S, Kirkwood B, Brown S, Giaffer MH. Oral nutritional supplementation is effective in the maintenance of remission in Crohn's disease. *Dig Liver Dis.* 2000;32(9):769–774.

100. Wilschanski M, Sherman P, Pencharz P, Davis L, Corey M, Griffiths A. Supplementary enteral nutrition maintains remission in paediatric Crohn's disease. *Gut.* 1996;38(4):543–548.

101. Newby EA, Sawczenko A, Thomas AG, Wilson D. Interventions for growth failure in childhood Crohn's disease. *Cochrane Database Sys Rev.* 2005;(3):CD003873.

102. Lewis JD, Fisher RL. Nutrition support in inflammatory bowel disease. *Med Clin North Am.* 1994;78(6):1443–1456.

103. Fell JM, Paintin M, Arnaud-Battandier F, et al. Mucosal healing and a fall in mucosal pro-inflammatory cytokine mRNA induced by a specific oral polymeric diet in paediatric Crohn's disease. *Aliment Pharmacol Ther.* 2000;14(3):281–289.

104. Gassull MA, Fernandez-Banares F, Cabre E, et al. Fat composition may be a clue to explain the primary therapeutic effect of enteral nutrition in Crohn's disease: Results of a double blind randomised multicentre European trial. *Gut.* 2002;51(2):164–168.

105. Fell JM. Control of systemic and local inflammation with transforming growth factor beta containing formulas. *JPEN J Parenter Enteral Nutr.* 2005;29(4 Suppl):S126–8; discussion S129–33, S184–8.

106. Harsha WT, Kalandarova E, McNutt P, Irwin R, Noel J. Nutritional supplementation with transforming growth factor-beta, glutamine, and short chain fatty acids minimizes methotrexate-induced injury. *J Pediatr Gastroenterol Nutr.* 2006;42(1):53–58.

107. Bamba T, Kanauchi O, Andoh A, Fujiyama Y. A new prebiotic from germinated barley for nutraceutical treatment of ulcerative colitis. *J Gastroenterol Hepatol.* 2002;17(8):818–824.

108. Kudsk KA, Wu Y, Fukatsu K, et al. Glutamine-enriched total parenteral nutrition maintains intestinal interleukin-4 and mucosal immunoglobulin A levels. *JPEN J Parenter Enteral Nutr*. 2000;24(5):270–274.

109. Chen K, Okuma T, Okamura K, Torigoe Y, Miyauchi Y. Glutamine-supplemented parenteral nutrition improves gut mucosa integrity and function in endotoxemic rats. *JPEN J Parenter Enteral Nutr*. 1994;18(2):167–171.

110. Singleton KD, Beckey VE, Wischmeyer PE. Glutamine prevents activation of NF-κB and stress kinase pathways, attenuate inflammatory cytokine release, and prevents acuter respiratory distress syndrome (ARDS) following sepsis. *Shock*. 2005;24(6):583–589.

111. Ockenga J, Borchert K, Stuber E, Lochs H, Manns MP, Bischoff SC. Glutamine-enriched total parenteral nutrition in patients with inflammatory bowel disease. *Eur J Clin Nutr*. 2005;59(11):1302–1309.

112. Sido B, Seel C, Hochlehnert A, Breitkreutz R, Droge W. Low intestinal glutamine level and low glutaminase activity in Crohn's disease: A rational for glutamine supplementation? *Dig Dis Sci*. 2006;51(12):2170–2179.

113. Fernandez-Banares F, Cabre E, Gonzalez-Huix F, Gassull MA. Enteral nutrition as primary therapy in Crohn's disease. *Gut*. 1994;35(1_Suppl):S55–59.

114. Belluzzi A, Brignola C, Campieri M, Pera A, Boschi S, Miglioli M. Effect of an enteric-coated fish-oil preparation on relapses in Crohn's disease. *N Engl J Med*. 1996;334(24):1557–1560.

115. Shimizu T, Fujii T, Suzuki R, et al. Effects of highly purified eicosapentaenoic acid on erythrocyte fatty acid composition and leukocyte and colonic mucosa leukotriene B4 production in children with ulcerative colitis. *J Pediatr Gastroenterol Nutr*. 2003;37(5):581–585.

116. Bamba T, Shimoyama T, Sasaki M, et al. Dietary fat attenuates the benefits of an elemental diet in active Crohn's disease: A randomized, controlled trial. *Eur J Gastroenterol Hepatol*. 2003;15(2):151–157.

117. Turner D, Zlotkin SH, Shah PS, Griffiths AM. Omega 3 fatty acids (fish oil) for maintenance of remission in Crohn's disease. *Cochrane Database Syst Rev*. 2007;(2): CD006320.

118. Turner D, Steinhart AH, Griffiths AM. Omega 3 fatty acids (fish oil) for maintenance of remission in ulcerative colitis. *Cochrane Database Syst Rev*. 2007;(3):CD006443.

119. Feagan BG, Sandborn WJ, Mittmann U, et al. Omega-3 free fatty acids for the maintenance of remission in Crohn disease: The EPIC randomized controlled trials. *JAMA*. 2008;299(14):1690–1697.

120. Lomer MC, Harvey RS, Evans SM, Thompson RP, Powell JJ. Efficacy and tolerability of a low microparticle diet in a double blind, randomized, pilot study in Crohn's disease. *Eur J Gastroenterol Hepatol*. 2001;13(2):101–106.

121. Scheppach W, Sommer H, Kirchner T, et al. Effect of butyrate enemas on the colonic mucosa in distal ulcerative colitis. *Gastroenterology*. 1992;103(1):51–56.

122. Breuer RI, Buto SK, Christ ML, et al. Rectal irrigation with short-chain fatty acids for distal ulcerative colitis: preliminary report. *Dig Dis Sci*. 1991;36(2):185–187.

123. Steinhart AH, Brzezinski A, Baker JP. Treatment of refractory ulcerative proctosigmoiditis with butyrate enemas. *Am J Gastroenterol*. 1994;89(2):179–183.

124. Patz J, Jacobsohn WZ, Gottschalk-Sabag S, Zeides S, Braverman DZ. Treatment of refractory distal ulcerative colitis with short chain fatty acid enemas. *Am J Gastroenterol*. 1996;91(4):731–734.

125. Vernia P, Cittadini M, Caprilli R, Torsoli A. Topical treatment of refractory distal ulcerative colitis with 5-ASA and sodium butyrate. *Dig Dis Sci*. 1995;40(2):305–307.

126. Shapiro H, Singer P, Halpern Z, Bruck R. Polyphenols in the treatment of inflammatory bowel disease and acute pancreatitis. *Gut*. 2007;56(3):426–435.

127. Athar M, Back JH, Tang X, et al. Resveratrol: A review of preclinical studies for human cancer prevention. *Toxicol Appl Pharmacol.* 2007;224(3):274–283.

128. Martin AR, Villegas I, La Casa C, de la Lastra CA. Resveratrol, a polyphenol found in grapes, suppresses oxidative damage and stimulates apoptosis during early colonic inflammation in rats. *Biochem Pharmacol.* 2004;67(7):1399–1410.

129. Cabrera C, Artacho R, Gimenez R. Beneficial effects of green tea—a review. *J Am Coll Nutr.* 2006;25(2):79–99.

130. Nomura M, Ma W, Chen N, Bode AM, Dong Z. Inhibition of 12-O-tetradecanoylphorbol-13-acetate-induced NF-κB activation by tea polyphenols -epigallocatechin gallate and theaflavins. *Carcinogenesis.* 2000;21(10):1885–1890.

131. Mazzon E, Muia C, Paola RD, et al. Green tea polyphenol extract attenuates colon injury induced by experimental colitis. *Free Radic Res.* 2005;39(9):1017–1025.

132. Oz HS, Chen TS, McClain CJ, de Villiers WJ. Antioxidants as novel therapy in a murine model of colitis. *J Nutr Biochem.* 2005;16(5):297–304.

133. Porath D, Riegger C, Drewe J, Schwager J. Epigallocatechin-3-gallate impairs chemokine production in human colon epithelial cell lines. *J Pharmacol Exp Ther.* 2005;315(3):1172–1180.

134. Nanditha B, Prabhasankar P. Antioxidants in bakery products: A review. *Crit Rev Food Sci Nutr.* 2009 Jan;49(1):1–27.

135. Bengmark S. Curcumin, an atoxic antioxidant and natural NFκB, cyclooxygenase-2, lipooxygenase, and inducible nitric oxide synthase inhibitor: A shield against acute and chronic diseases. *JPEN J Parenter Enteral Nutr.* 2006;30(1):45–51.

136. Cheng AL, Hsu CH, Lin JK, et al. Phase I clinical trial of curcumin, a chemopreventive agent, in patients with high-risk or pre-malignant lesions. *Anticancer Res.* 2001;21(4):2895–2900.

137. Jobin C, Bradham CA, Russo MP, et al. Curcumin blocks cytokine-mediated NF-κ B activation and proinflammatory gene expression by inhibiting inhibitory factor I-κ B kinase activity. *J Immunol.* 1999;163(6):3474–3483.

138. Jian YT, Mai GF, Wang JD, Zhang YL, Luo RC, Fang YX. Preventive and therapeutic effects of NF-κB inhibitor curcumin in rats colitis induced by trinitrobenzene sulfonic acid. *World J Gastroenterol.* 2005;11(12):1747–1752.

139. Deguchi Y, Andoh A, Inatomi O, et al. Curcumin prevents the development of dextran sulfate sodium (DSS)-induced experimental colitis. *Dig Dis Sci.* 2007;52(11):2993–2998.

140. Hanai H, Iida T, Takeuchi K, et al. Curcumin maintenance therapy for ulcerative colitis: Randomized, multicenter, double-blind, placebo-controlled trial. *Clin Gastroenterol Hepatol.* 2006;4(12):1502–1506.

141. FAO/WHO (2001) Health and Nutritional Properties of Probiotics in Food including Powder Milk with Live Lactic Acid Bacteria. Report of a Joint FAO/WHO Expert Consultation on Evaluation of Health and Nutritional Properties of Probiotics in Food Including Powder Milk with Live Lactic Acid Bacteria.

142. Campieri M, Gionchetti P. Probiotics in inflammatory bowel disease: New insight to pathogenesis or a possible therapeutic alternative? *Gastroenterology,.* 1999;116(5):1246–1249.

143. Schultz M, Sartor RB. Probiotics and inflammatory bowel diseases. *Am J Gastroenterol.* 2000;95(1):S19–S21.

144. Shanahan F. Probiotics in inflamatory bowel disease. *Gut.* 2001;48(5):609.

145. Sartor RB. Therapeutic manipulation of the enteric microflora in inflammatory bowel diseases: Antibiotics, probiotics, and prebiotics. *Gastroenterology.* 2004;126(6):1620–1633.

146. Probert HM, Apajalahti JH, Rautonen N, Stowell J, Gibson GR. Polydextrose, lactitol, and fructo-oligosaccharide fermentation by colonic bacteria in a three-stage continuous culture system. *Appl Environ Microbiol.* 2004;70(8):4505–4511.

147. Sandborn W, Waters G, Gregory S, Pemberton J. Ileal pouch anal anastomosis and the problem of pouchitis. *Curr Opin Gastroenterol.* 1997;13(1):34–40.

148. Gionchetti P, Rizzello F, Venturi A, et al. Oral bacteriotherapy as maintenance treatment in patients with chronic pouchitis: A double-blind, placebo-controlled trial. *Gastroenterology,.* 2000;119(2):305–309.

149. Gionchetti P, Rizzello F, Helwig U, et al. Prophylaxis of pouchitis onset with probiotic therapy: A double-blind, placebo-controlled trial. *Gastroenterology,.* 2003;124(5):1202–1209.

150. Kruis W, Schutz E, Fric P, Fixa B, Judmaier G, Stolte M. Double-blind comparison of an oral *Escherichia coli* preparation and mesalazine in maintaining remission of ulcerative colitis. *Aliment Pharmacol Ther.* 1997;11(5):853–858.

151. Kruis W, Fric P, Pokrotnieks J, et al. Maintaining remission of ulcerative colitis with the probiotic *Escherichia coli* Nissle 1917 is as effective as with standard mesalazine. *Gut.* 2004;53(11):1617–1623.

152. Rembacken BJ, Snelling AM, Hawkey PM, Chalmers DM, Axon AT. Non-pathogenic *Escherichia coli* versus mesalazine for the treatment of ulcerative colitis: A randomised trial. *Lancet.* 1999;354(9179):635–639.

153. Ishikawa H, Akedo I, Umesaki Y, Tanaka R, Imaoka A, Otani T. Randomized controlled trial of the effect of bifidobacteria-fermented milk on ulcerative colitis. *J Am Coll Nutr.* 2003;22(1):56–63.

154. Borody TJ, Warren EF, Leis S, Surace R, Ashman O. Treatment of ulcerative colitis using fecal bacteriotherapy. *J Clin Gastroenterol.* 2003;37(1):42–47.

155. Kato K, Mizuno S, Umesaki Y, et al. Randomized placebo-controlled trial assessing the effect of bifidobacteria-fermented milk on active ulcerative colitis. *Aliment Pharmacol Ther.* 2004;20(10):1133–1141.

156. Tursi A, Brandimarte G, Giorgetti GM, Forti G, Modeo ME, Gigliobianco A. Low-dose balsalazide plus a high-potency probiotic preparation is more effective than balsalazide alone or mesalazine in the treatment of acute mild-to-moderate ulcerative colitis. *Med Sci Monit.* 2004;10(11):PI126–131.

157. Matthes H, Krummenerl T, Giensch M, Wolff C, and Schulze J. Treatment of mild to moderate acute attacks of distal ulcerative colitis with rectally-administered *E. coli* Nissle 1917: Dose-dependent efficacy. *Gastroenterol.* 2006;130:A119.

158. Guslandi M, Mezzi G, Sorghi M, Testoni PA. *Saccharomyces boulardii* in maintenance treatment of Crohn's disease. *Dig Dis Sci.* 2000;45(7):1462–1464.

159. Prantera C, Scribano ML, Falasco G, Andreoli A, Luzi C. Ineffectiveness of probiotics in preventing recurrence after curative resection for Crohn's disease: A randomised controlled trial with lactobacillus GG. *Gut.* 2002;51(3):405–409.

160. Schultz M, Timmer A, Herfarth HH, Sartor RB, Vanderhoof JA, Rath HC. Lactobacillus GG in inducing and maintaining remission of Crohn's disease. *BMC Gastroenterol.* 2004;4:5.

161. Lindsay JO, Whelan K, Stagg AJ, et al. Clinical, microbiological, and immunological effects of fructo-oligosaccharide in patients with Crohn's disease. *Gut.* 2006;55(3): 348–355.

162. Gibson GR, Roberfroid MB, Dietary modulation of the human colonic microbiota: introducing the concept of prebiotics. *J Nutr.* 1995;125:1401–1412.

163. Bengmark S. Pre-, pro- and synbiotics. *Curr Opin Clin Nutr Metab Care.* 2001;4(6): 571–579.

164. Roberfroid MB. Introducing inulin-type fructans. *Br J Nutr.* 2005;93 (S1):S13–25.

165. Videla S, Vilaseca J, Antolin M, et al. Dietary inulin improves distal colitis induced by dextran sodium sulfate in the rat. *Am J Gastroenterol.* 2001;96(5):1486–1493.

166. Hoentjen F, Welling GW, Harmsen HJ, et al. Reduction of colitis by prebiotics in HLA-B27 transgenic rats is associated with microflora changes and immunomodulation. *Inflamm Bowel Dis.* 2005;11(11):977–985.

167. Madsen KL, Doyle JS, Jewell LD, Tavernini MM, Fedorak RN. Lactobacillus species prevents colitis in interleukin 10 gene-deficient mice. *Gastroenterology.* 1999;116(5):1107–1114.

168. Fernandez-Banares F, Hinojosa J, Sanchez-Lombrana JL, et al. Randomized clinical trial of plantago ovata seeds (dietary fiber) as compared with mesalamine in maintaining remission in ulcerative colitis: Spanish group for the study of Crohn's disease and ulcerative colitis (GETECCU). *Am J Gastroenterol.* 1999;94(2):427–433.

169. Welters CF, Heineman E, Thunnissen FB, van den Bogaard AE, Soeters PB, Baeten CG. Effect of dietary inulin supplementation on inflammation of pouch mucosa in patients with an ileal pouch-anal anastomosis. *Dis Colon Rectum.* 2002;45(5):621–627.

170. Kanauchi O, Mitsuyama K, Homma T, et al. Treatment of ulcerative colitis patients by long-term administration of germinated barley foodstuff: Multi-center open trial. *Int J Mol Med.* 2003;12(5):701–704.

171. Hallert C, Bjorck I, Nyman M, Pousette A, Granno C, Svensson H. Increasing fecal butyrate in ulcerative colitis patients by diet: Controlled pilot study. *Inflamm Bowel Dis.* 2003;9(2):116–121.

172. Furrie E, Macfarlane S, Kennedy A, et al. Synbiotic therapy (bifidobacterium longum/ Synergy 1) initiates resolution of inflammation in patients with active ulcerative colitis: A randomised controlled pilot trial. *Gut.* 2005;54(2):242–249.

173. Bayless TM, Harris ML. Inflammatory bowel disease and irritable bowel syndrome. *Med Clin North Am.* 1990;74(1):21–28.

174. MacDermott RP. Treatment of irritable bowel syndrome in outpatients with inflammatory bowel disease using a food and beverage intolerance, food and beverage avoidance diet. *Inflamm Bowel Dis.* 2007;13(1):91–96.

175. Tursi A, Giorgetti GM, Brandimarte G, Elisei W. High prevalence of celiac disease among patients affected by Crohn's disease. *Inflamm Bowel Dis.* 2005;11(7):662–666.

176. Levenstein S, Prantera C, Luzi C, D'Ubaldi A. Low residue or normal diet in Crohn's disease: A prospective controlled study in Italian patients. *Gut.* 1985;26(10):989–993.

177. Misiakos EP, Macheras A, Kapetanakis T, Liakakos T. Short bowel syndrome: Current medical and surgical trends. *J Clin Gastroenterol.* 2007;41(1):5–18.

9 Probiotics for Antibiotic-Associated Diarrhea and *Clostridium Difficile*-Associated Disease

Mario Guslandi

CONTENTS

9.1 INTRODUCTION

Antibiotic-associated diarrhea (AAD) is a frequent event, both in outpatients and especially in hospitalized subjects as well as in residents of long-term institutions, with incidence ranging from 5 to 30%.[1] Broad spectrum antibiotics, such as amoxicillin, cephalosporins, clindamycin, and floroquinolones are the most commonly involved among antibacterial agents.[2,3] Between 20 to 30% of cases of AAD are linked to the presence of *Clostridium difficile*,[3] a Gram-positive, anaerobic, spore-forming bacillus that is considered responsible for the large majority of the most severe form of AAD: pseudomembranous colitis. Occasionally other microorganisms, such as *Clostridium perfrigens*, *Klebsiella oxytoca,* and *Staphylococcus aureus* can be implicated.[4,5]

Clostridium difficile-associated disease (CDAD) is especially frequent in elderly people, hospitalized patients, and in subjects on long-term therapy with either immunosuppressive agents or gastric acid inhibitors, particularly proton pump inhibitors.[6]

The incidence of CDAD has been on the rise all over the world.[7,8] A report from the United States shows the incidence of hospitalization due to CDAD doubled from 5.5 cases per 10,000 population in 2000 to 11.2 in 2005[8] with a consequent, obvious economic impact on hospital charges and strain on the healthcare system.

Clinical presentation varies. Uncomplicated diarrhea, which may occur either during antibiotic treatment or up to eight weeks after antibiotics have been discontinued,[9] usually lasts one to seven days both in adults and children.[10,11] In cases in whom antibiotic-associated colitis develops, the diarrhea becomes more severe and is accompanied by abdominal cramps, fever, leukocytosis, and hypoalbuminemia, with more pronounced systemic involvement if pseudomembranous colitis occurs. Diagnosis is based on a positive *C. difficile* assay (culture or, more commonly, finding of toxins A and B in the stools, the latter having a higher sensitivity and specificity) after other causes of diarrhea (*Shigella*, *Giardia*, etc.) have been ruled out.

Toxins A and B are two large molecular weight toxins responsible for induction of proinflammatory cytokines, such as IL-8, with consequent polymorphonuclear leukocyte infiltration, mucosal barrier breakdown. and, ultimately, cell apoptosis.[3] Sigmoidoscopy is performed when CDAD is suspected in spite of a negative stool test or when other intestinal disorders are under consideration.

Identification of pseudomembranes is the main feature of endoscopic diagnosis of CDAD. In up to 35% of cases, CDAD recurs shortly after treatment is stopped.[12]

Treatment of CDAD is initially based on discontinuation of the offending antibiotics (if diarrhea occurs during antibiotic intake). This measure alone promotes disappearance of diarrhea in 20 to 30% of cases over two to four days.[6] Standard pharmacological therapy is carried out by administering either metronidazole or vancomycin. However, both drugs have their drawbacks.

Metronidazole is cheaper, but can be neurotoxic and, recently, high failure rates in severe cases have been reported, while vancomycin, which is considerably more expensive (although apparently more effective in severe cases and in patients resistant to metronidazole), has been shown to promote colonization by vancomincin-resistant enterococci.[13,14]

Understandably, different avenues of action are being pursued in order to manage AAD and, especially, CDAD. In this respect, probiotics constitute a possible, safer alternative.

9.2 PROBIOTICS IN THE PREVENTION OF AAD

The rationale for using probiotics in the treatment and/or prevention of AAD and CDAD is based on the proposed modes of actions of these agents, namely their ability to inhibit pathogens, strengthen intestinal barrier functions, exert anti-inflammatory effect through modulation of cytokine production, and decrease gut permeability. In view of these properties, several probiotic products have been tested.

9.2.1 Lactobacilli

Various randomized controlled studies have investigated the possible effect of *Lactobacilluss spp.* in the prevention of AAD.

Lactobacillus rhamnosus GG was found more effective than placebo in preventing AAD in children taking antibiotics.[15,16] In particular, in a group of 167 children receiving antibiotics to treat respiratory infections, AAD developed in only 5% of cases in the *Lactobacillus* group and in 16% of cases with placebo (p <0.05).[15]

In adults, the results with that particular probiotic have yielded conflicting results. In a small study in erythromycin-treated patients, a *Lactobacillus GG* yogurt was found effective in reducing diarrhea as well as flatulence and abdominal discomfort,[17] whereas, in a large trial enrolling 302 hospitalized, antibiotic-treated patients, no benefit was observed, the incidence of diarrhea being about 29% both in the probiotic and in the placebo group.[18]

Probiotic cocktails have also provided variable, although mostly favorable results. For instance, 63 hospitalized adults taking antibiotics receiving a drink mixture containing *Lactobacillus GG, L. acidophilus*, and *Bifidobacterium bifidus* for 14 days experienced AAD in only 5.9% of cases compared with 27.6% of subjects receiving placebo.[19] Similarly both mixtures of *L. casei* and *L. acidophilus*[20] and of *L. casei, L. bulgaricus,* and *S. thermophilus*[21] were found significantly more effective than placebo in hospitalized patients taking antibiotics.

In the latter study,[21] diarrhea developed in 12% of cases in the probiotic group and in 34% of the placebo group. None of the subjects receiving probiotics became *C. difficile* positive, compared with 17% of patients who were given placebo. The cost to prevent one case of AAD or CDAD was estimated to be $100 to $120, which appears to be quite a saving when considering that the additional cost to treat AAD would have been $3,669.

By contrast, a combination of *L. acidophilus* and *L. bulgaricus* proved to be ineffective both in adults[22] and children[23] treated with oral penicillin. Similarly, in a recent double-blind, placebo-controlled trial carried out in antibiotic-treated children, a probiotic cocktail of *B. longum* PL03, *L. rhamnosus* KL53A, and *L. plantarum* was found to be ineffective in reducing the rate of diarrhea, in spite of a significant reduction of the frequency of stools per day.[24]

9.2.2 Saccharomyces boulardii

Saccharomyces boulardii, a yeast with a complex mode of action, including the inactivation of *C. difficile* toxins[25] has been tested and found significantly superior to placebo in prevention of AAD in at least six controlled trials carried out in large adult populations of both outpatients, hospitalized subjects, and intensive care unit patients.[26–31] The only negative results were obtained in a study employing subtherapeutic doses of *S. boulardii*.[32]

A similar, superior efficacy versus placebo has been observed in several randomized clinical trials performed on children[33,34] taking various oral antibiotics. In particular, in a study including 466 children aged 1 to 15 years, *S. boulardii* significantly reduced the incidence of ampicillin-sulbactam-induced diarrhea (5.7% versus 25.6% with placebo; p <0.05), whereas, rather surprisingly, it was ineffective in azythromicin-treated subjects.[34]

9.2.3 MISCELLANEA

A head-to-head comparison of *Lactobacillus GG*, *S. boulardii* and *L. acidophilus + B. lactis* in the prevention of AAD during *Helicobacter pylori* eradication treatment, found all the above probiotics to be more effective than placebo.[35]

A yogurt preparation with *B. longum* reduced stool frequency during erythro-mycin intake[36] and so did the use of a combination of *B. longum* and *L. acidophilus* in clindamycin-treated patients.[37] On the other hand, *Enterococcus faecium* SF 68 when compared with placebo was shown to be ineffective.[38,39]

9.2.4 META-ANALYSES

The use of probiotics as a group of agents in the prevention of AAD has been the subject of a number of meta-analyses. All found evidence of a benefit for probiot-ics compared with placebo with odds ratios ranging from 0.37 to 0.43.[40–42] Similar conclusions were reached by a meta-analysis considering only studies carried out in children.[43]

A meta-analysis examining only studies employing *S. boulardii* demonstrated a significant preventative effect (o.r. 0.43) (Table 9.1).[44]

9.3   PROBIOTICS IN THE PREVENTION AND TREATMENT OF CDAD

The data on the efficacy of probiotics in the prevention of a first episode of CDAD largely equate those concerning their ability to prevent AAD. A probiotic cocktail shown to be superior to placebo in preventing development of AAD was also found,

TABLE 9.1
Probiotics in the Prevention of AAD

	Meta-Analysis	
	Number of Studies	Results
D'Sousa (40) 2002	9	Probiotics > Placebo
Cremonini (41) 2002	7	Probiotics > Placebo
Szajewska[a] (44) 2005	5	Probiotics > Placebo
Szajewsla[b] (43) 2006	6	Probiotics > Placebo
McFarland[c] (42) 2006	25	Probiotics > Placebo

[a]   Children.
[b]   *S. Boulardii* only.
[c]   Significant for *S. Boulardii, L. rhamnosus*, and probiotic mixtures.

as discussed above, to significantly reduce the appearance of *C. difficile* toxins in antibiotic-treated patients.[21] Similarly, a trial carried out on 150 elderly hospitalized patients treated with antibiotics has compared the effects of a mixture of *L. acidophilus, B. bifidum,* and placebo. After 20 days, *C. difficile* toxin was found in 78% of cases in the placebo group and 46% in the probiotic group.[45]

9.3.1 SACCHAROMYCES BOULARDII

When added to metronidazole and/or vancomycin for four weeks in a group of 124 CDAD patients,[46] 1 g of *S. boulardii* daily failed to induce significant benefits in the treatment of the first episode, although this might have been due to a type II statistical error,[47] but proved to be effective in subjects with recurrent CDAD, in whom relapses during a subsequent four-week follow-up period were reduced by 50%.[46]

In a second study enrolling only subjects with recurrent CDAD, *S. boulardii* was significantly efficacious only in a subgroup of patients treated with high dose vancomycin (the incidence of CDAD being 17 versus 50% with placebo), but not in those treated with either metronidazole (48.1 versus 50% with placebo) or low-dose vancomycin (51.1 versus 44.7% with placebo).[48]

9.3.2 LACTOBACILLI

The possible usefulness of single *Lactobacillus* species in cases of recurrent CDAD has been examined mostly in small, open, uncontrolled studies. Small size, controlled trials versus placebo showed a decrease in recurrence of CDAD in patients receiving *Lactobacillus GG*[49,50] or *L. plantarum*[51] without reaching statistical significance.

9.3.3 MISCELLANEA

Other types of therapies have been tested only in pilot, uncontrolled studies, either administering nontoxigenic *Clostridium* strains[52] or performing rectal instillation of anaerobe mixtures[53] or *Escherichia coli* Nissle 1917.[54] To date the possible efficacy of these unconventional treatments cannot be established.

9.3.4 PREBIOTICS

The ability of prebiotics as nutritional factors for useful components of the intestinal flora (e.g., oligofructose is metabolized by *Bifidobacteria,* thus increasing their number in the colon) may provide a weak rationale for their possible role in AAD prevention, but the experience in this area is even more limited.

A large trial where 450 elderly patients treated with broad spectrum antibiotics were randomized to either oligofructose or placebo, but did not show any significant difference in terms of both incidence of diarrhea and *C. difficile* infection.[55] Risk factors for developing diarrhea were cephalosporins, being female, weight loss, and a long hospital stay.

On the other hand, in a study on 142 in patients with recurrent CDAD,[56] relapses were significantly less frequent with oligofructose (34.3%) than with placebo (8.3%)

TABLE 9.2
Tentative Guidelines for the Use of Probiotics in AAD and CDAD

Aim of Treatment	Probiotic	Evidence	Comment
Prevention of AAD	*S. boulardii* 1 g/day	Good	Adults and children
	Lactobacillus GG $1.2 \times 10_{10}$ CFU/die	Good	Children only
	Probiotic cocktails	Variable	Ideal mixture to be identified
Primary prevention of CDAD	Probiotic cocktails	Variable	Ideal mixture to be identified
Prevention of recurrent CDAD	*S. boulardii* 1 g/day	Moderate	Adults

(p >0.001), although the appearance of *C. difficile* in the stools was similar in the prebiotic group (30%) and in the placebo group (36%). Thus, no definitive conclusions can be drawn by these preliminary studies with oligofructose.

9.4 CONCLUSIONS

As demonstrated in all the published meta-analyses, probiotics, as a group, are significantly effective in preventing AAD both in adults and in children. This is particularly true, according to the largest available meta-analysis[42] for *Saccharomyces boulardii*, *Lactobacillus rhamnosus*, and probiotic cocktails. Which probiotic mixture could be more effective remains to be determined. The extreme variety of the combinations tested in clinical studies makes it impossible to identify the most effective product.

The efficacy of probiotics in the prevention and treatment of CDAD is less straightforward. *S. boulardii* does not appear to be useful in preventing the first episode of CDAD, but was shown to reduce the relapse rate in recurrent CDAD.[46]

Data about *Lactobacilli* are too limited to provide meaningful information.

Clearly, much work remains to be done in this area, but further, larger controlled studies are warranted to better define the therapeutic role of probiotics in AAD and CDAD (Table 9.2).

Probiotics are safer and cheaper that most antibiotics, and their ability to prevent antibiotic-induced diarrhea deserves a wider use, in order to reduce patients' discomfort as well as the costs related to diagnosis, treatment, absence from work, and possible hospitalization.

REFERENCES

1. McFarland LV. Epidemiology, risk factors and treatments for antibiotic-associated diarrhea. *Dig Disease* 1998; 16: 292–307.
2. Owens RCJ, Donskey CJ, Gaynes RP et al. Antimicrobial-associated risk factors for *Clostridium difficile* infection. *Clin Infect Dis* 2008; 46 (suppl 1): S19–31.
3. Barlett JG. Clinical practice: antibiotic-associated diarrhea. *N Engl J Med* 2002; 346: 334–9.

4. Hogenauer C, Langner C, Beubler E et al. *Klebsiella oxytoca* as a causative organism of antibiotic associated hemorrhagic colitis. *N Engl J Med* 2006; 355: 2418–26.

5. Flemming K, Ackermann G. Prevalence of enterotoxin-producing *Staphylococcus aureus* in stools of patients with nosocomial diarrea. *Infection* 2007; 35: 356–8.

6. Aseeri M, Schroeder T, Kramer J, Zackula R. Gastric acid suppression by proton pump inhibitors as a risk factor for *Clostridium difficile*-associated diarrhea in hospitalized patients. *Am J Gastroenterol* 2008; 103: 2308–13.

7. McDonald LC, Owings M, Jernigan DB. *Clostridium difficile* infection in patients discharged from US short-stay hospitals 1996–2003. *Emerg Infect Dis* 2006; 12: 409–15.

8. Zilberberg MD, Shorr AF, Kollef MH. Increase in adult *Clostridium difficile*-related hospitalizations and case-fatality rate, United States 2000–2005. *Emerg Infect Dis* 2008; 14: 929–31.

9. Wistrom J, Norrby SR, Myhre EB et al. Frequency of antibiotic associated diarrhea in 2462 antibiotic-treated hospitalized patients: a prospective study. *J Antimicrob Chemother* 2001; 47: 43–50.

10. Turck D, Bernet JP, Marx J et al. Incidence and risk factors for oral antibiotic associated diarrhoea in an outpatient pediatric population. *J Pediatr Gastroenterol Nutr* 2003; 37: 22–6.

11. Yapar N, Sener A, Karaca B et al. Antibiotic-associated diarrhea in a Turkish outpatient population: investigation of 288 cases. *J Chemother* 2005; 17: 78–81.

12. Maroo S, Lamont JT. Recurrent *Clostridium difficile*. *Gastroenterology* 2006; 130: 1311–6.

13. Fekety R. Guidelines for the diagnosis and management of *Clostridium difficile*-associated diarrhea and colitis. *Am J Gastroenterol* 1997; 92: 739–50.

14. Aslam S, Hamill RJ, Musher DM. Treatment of *Clostridium difficile*-associated disease: old therapies and new strategies. *Lancet Infect Dis* 2005; 5: 549–57.

15. Arvola T, Laiho T, Torkkeli S et al. Prophylactic *Lactobacillus GG* reduces antibiotic-associated diarrhea in children with respiratory infections: a randomized study. *Pediatrics* 1999; 104: 1121–2.

16. Vanderhoof JA, Whitney DB, Antonson DL et al. *Lactobacillus GG* in prevention of antibiotic-associated diarrhea in children. *J Pediatr* 1999; 135: 564–8.

17. Siitonen S, Vapaatalo H, Salminen S et al. Effect of *Lactobacillus GG* yoghurt in prevention of antibiotic-associated diarrhea. *Ann Med* 1990; 22: 57–9.

18. Thomas MR, Litin SC, Osmon DR et al. Lack of effect of *Lactobacillus GG* on antibiotic-associated diarrhea: a randomized, placebo-controlled trial. *Mayo Clin Proc* 2001; 76: 833–9.

19. Wenus C, Goll R, Loken EB et al. Prevention of antibiotic-associated diarrhea by a fermented probiotic. *Eur J Clin Nutr* 2008; 62: 299–301.

20. Beausoleil M, Fortier N, Guénette S et al. Effect of fermented milk combining *Lactobacillus acidophilus* C11385 and *Lactobacillus casei* in the prevention of antibiotic-associated diarrhea: a randomized, double-blind, placebo-controlled trial. *Can J Gastroenterol* 2007; 11: 732–6.

21. Hickson M, D'Souza AL, Muthu N et al. Use of probiotic *Lactobacillus* preparation to prevent diarrhoea associated with antibiotics: randomized double blind placebo controlled trial. *BMJ* 2007; 335: 80.

22. Gotz V, Romankiewicz JA, Moss J et al. Prophylaxis against ampicillin-associated diarrhea with a *Lactobacillus* preparation *Am J Hosp Pharm* 1979; 36: 754–7.

23. Tankanow RM, Ross MB, Ertel IJ et al. A double-blind, placebo-controlled study of the efficacy of Lactinex in the prophylaxis of amoxicillin-induced diarrhea. *DICP Ann Pharmacother* 1990; 24: 382–4.

24. Szymanski H , Malgorzata A, Kowalska-Duplaga K, Szajewska H. *Bifidobacterium longum* PL03, *Lactobacillus rhamnosus* KL53A and *Lactobacillus plantarum* PL02 in the prevention of antibiotic-associated diarrhea in children: a randomized controlled pilot trial. *Digestion* 2008; 78: 13–7.

25. Castagliuolo I, Riegler MF, Valenick L et al. *Saccharomyces boulardii* protease inhibits the effects of *Clostridium difficile* toxins A and B in human colonic mucosa. *Infect Immun* 1999; 67: 302–7.

26. Adam J, Barret C, Barret-Bellet A et al. Essais cliniques controlés en double insu de l'ultra-levure liophilisee. Etude multicentrique par 25 medecins de 388 cas. *Gaz Med France* 1977; 84: 2072–8.

27. Surawicz CM, Elmer GW, Speelman P et al. Prevention of antibiotic-associated diarrhea by *Saccharomyces boulardii*: a prospective study. *Gastroenterology* 1989; 90: 981–8.

28. McFarland LV, Surawicz CM, Greenberg RN et al. Prevention of beta-lactam-associated diarrhea by *Saccharomyces boulardii* compared with placebo. *Am J Gastroenterol* 1995; 90: 439–48.

29. Bleichner G, Blehaut H, Mentec H et al. *Saccharomyces boulardii* prevents diarrhea in critically ill tube-fed patients: a multicenter, randomized, double-blind, placebo-controlled trial. *Intensive care Med* 1997; 23: 517–23.

30. Duman DG, Bor S, Ozutemiz O et al. Efficacy and safety of *Saccharomyces boulardii* in prevention of antibiotic-associated diarrhea due to *Helicobacter pylori* eradication. *Eur J Gastroenterol Hepatol* 2005; 17: 1357–61; *Acta Pediatr* 2005; 94: 1747–51.

31. Can M, Besirbellioglu BA, Avci IY et al. Prophylactic *Saccharomyces boulardii* in the prevention of antibiotic-associated diarrhea: a prospective study. *Med Sci Monit* 2006; 12: 119–22.

32. Lewis SJ, Potts LF, Barry RE. The lack of therapeutic effect of *Saccharomyces boulardii* in the prevention of antibiotic-related diarrhoea in elderly patients. *J Infect* 1998; 36: 171–4.

33. Kotowska M, Albrecht P, Szajewska H. *Saccharomyces boulardii* in the prevention of antibiotic-associated diarrhoea in children: a randomized double-blind placebo-controlled trial. *Aliment Pharmacol Ther* 2005; 21: 583–90.

34. Erdeve O, Tiras U, Dallar Y. The probiotic effect of *Saccharomyces boulardii* in a pediatric age group. *J Trop Pediatrics* 2004; 50: 234–6.

35. Cremonini F, Di Caro S, Covino M et al. Effect of different probiotic preparations on anti-*Helicobacter pilori* therapy-related side effects: a parallel group, triple blind, placebo-controlled study. *Am J Gastroenterol* 2002; 55: 447–52.

36. Colombel JF, Cortot A, Neut C et al. Yoghurt with *Bifidobacterium longum* reduces erythromycin-induced gastrointestinal effects. *Lancet* 1987; 2: 43.

37. Orrhage K, Brignar B, Nord CE. Effects of supplements of *Bifidobacterium longum* and *Lactobacillus acidophilus* on the intestinal microbiota during administration of clindamycin. *Microb Ecol Health Dis* 1994; 7: 17–25.

38. Wunderlich PF, Braun F, Fumagalli I et al. Double-blind report on the efficacy of lactic acid-producing *enterococcus* SF68 in the prevention of antibiotic-associated diarrhoea and in the treatment of acute diarrhoea. *J Int Med Res* 1980; 17: 333–8.

39. Norgia M, Sepe N, Brancato V et al. A controlled clinical study on *Streptococcus faecium* preparation for the prevention of side reactions during long-term antibiotic treatments. *Curr Ther Res* 1982; 31: 266–71.

40. D'Souza AL, Rajkumar C, Cooke J et al. Probiotics in prevention of antibiotic-associated diarrhoea: a meta-analysis. *BMJ* 2002; 324: 1341–5.

41. Cremonini F, Di Caro S, Nista EC et al. Meta-analysis: the effect of probiotic administration on antibiotic-associated diarrhoea. *Aliment Pharmacol Ther* 2002; 16: 1461–7.

42. McFarland LV. Meta-analysis of probiotics for the prevention of antibiotic-associated diarrhea and the treatment of *Clostridium difficile* disease. *Am J Gastroenterol* 2006; 1010: 812–22.

43. Szajewska H, Ruszczynski M, Radzikowski A. Probiotics in the prevention of antibiotic-associated diarrhea in children: a meta-analysis of randomized clinical trials. *J Ped* 2006; 149: 367–72.

44. Szajewska H, Mrukowicz J. Meta-analysis: non-pathogenic yeast *Saccharomyces boulardii* in the prevention of antibiotic-associated diarrhea. *Aliment Pharmacol Ther* 2005; 22: 365–72.

45. Plummer S, Weaver MA, Harris JC et al. *Clostridium difficile* pilot study: effects of probiotic supplementation on the incidence of *C. difficile* diarrhoea. *Int Microbiol* 2004; 7: 59–62.

46. McFarland LV, Surawicz CM, Greenberg RN et al. A randomized placebo-controlled trial of *Saccharomyces boulardii* in combination with standard antibiotics for *Clostridium difficile* disease. *JAMA* 1994; 271: 1913–8.

47. Katz JA. Probiotics for the prevention of antibiotic-associated diarrhea and *Clostridium difficile* diarrhea. *J Clin Gastroenterol* 2006; 40: 249–55.

48. Surawicz CM, McFarland LV, Greenberg RN et al. The search for a better treatment for recurrent *Clostridium difficile* disease: use of high-dose vancomycin combined with *Saccharomyces boulardii*. *Clin Infect Dis* 2000; 31: 1012–17.

49. Pochapin M. The effect of probiotics on *Clostridium difficile* diarrhea. *Am J Gastroenterol* 200; 95 (suppl 1): S11–3.

50. Lawrence SJ, Kirkenik JR, Mundy LM. Probiotics for recurrent *Clostridium difficile* disease. *J Med Microbiol* 2005; 54: 904–6.

51. Wullt M, Hagslatt M, Odenhold I. *Lactobacillus plantarum* 299v for the treatment of recurrent *Clostridium difficile*-associated diarrhea by administration of donated stool directly through a colonscope. *Am J Gastroenterol* 2000; 95: 3283–5.

52. Seal D, Borriello SP, Barclay F et al. Treatment of relapsing *Clostridium difficile* diarrhoea by administration of a non-toxigenic strain. *Eur J Clin Microbiol* 1987; 6: 51–3.

53. Tvede M, Rask-Madsen J. Bacteriotherapy for chronic relapsing *Clostridium difficile* diarrhoea in six patients. *Lancet* 1989; 1: 1156–60.

54. Goerg KJ, Wybierala G, Rauen-Vossloh J et al. A new approach in pseudomembranous colitis: probiotic *Escherichia Coli* Nissle 1917 after intestinal lavage. *Eur J Gastroenterol Hepatol* 2008; 20: 155–6.

55. Lewis S, Burmeister S, Cohen S et al. Failure of dietary oligofructose to prevent antibiotic-associated diarrhoea. *Aliment Pharmacol Ther* 2005; 21: 469–77.

56. Lewis S, Burmeister S, Cohen S et al. Effect of the probiotic oligofructose on relapse of *Clostridium difficile*-associated diarrhea: a randomized, controlled study. *Clin Gastroenterol Hepatol* 2005; 3: 442–8.

10 Endoscopic Enteral Access and Enteral Nutrition

Waqar A. Qureshi and Carol Redel

CONTENTS

10.1 INTRODUCTION

Adequate nutrition is essential in patients who cannot eat and is particularly important for the critically ill patient. Adequate nutrition improves patient outcomes, frequently getting them through a stay in the intensive care units. Nutrition can be provided to a patient either intravenously (parenteral nutrition) or delivered by feeding tubes into the gastrointestinal tract (enteral nutrition). When the gastrointestinal tract is able to function, enteral nutrition (EN) is preferred over parenteral nutrition (PN) because there is less risk of sepsis and metabolic derangements.[1] EN also promotes a healthier gut barrier, an important defense against ingested bacteria.[2] There is growing evidence that EN should be used whenever possible and used early as in severe acute pancreatitis where, until recently, PN or prolonged fasting was commonly recommended. Increasingly a feeding tube or other enteral route is sought when a patient cannot eat in the setting of normal absorptive capability of the digestive tract.

Enteral nutrition can be delivered into the stomach or the proximal small bowel. Endoscopic gastric and enteral access has become the main method of placement of feeding tubes in the gastrointestinal tract. When the need for EN is anticipated to be one month or less, a tube feeding is recommended. If greater that one month, endoscopic percutaneous access is the technique of choice.

10.2   INDICATIONS FOR ENTERAL FEEDING

The most common reason for enteral feeding is to provide nutrition via a functioning gastrointestinal tract for the long term in patients who cannot otherwise eat or eat enough.

Patients in this group often have neurologic disorders, such as stroke or malignancies of the head, neck, or esophagus. Less commonly, enteral access is desired for decompression of the stomach in severe gastroperesis or abdominal carcinomatosis and intestinal obstruction. It may be indicated in severe burns and in patients with Crohn's disease.

10.3   PROPHYLACTIC ANTIBIOTICS
FOR ENTERAL ACCESS PROCEDURES

Several studies have shown that prophylactic antibiotics reduce the incidence of peristomal wound infection after endoscopic enteral access.[3,4] Administering antibiotics at the time of the procedure has been shown to be a cost-effective strategy.[5] There is some suggestion that percutaneous access wound infections with methicillin-resistant *Staphylococcus aureus* (MRSA) are more common in patients receiving the usual prophylactic antibiotics if they happen to have nasopharyngeal colonization with MRSA. MRSA decolonization has been suggested in such individuals, but this issue is still being debated.[6]

10.4   TYPES OF ENDOSCOPIC ENTERAL ACCESS

10.4.1   ENDOSCOPIC NASOENTERIC ACCESS

Enteral nutrition is sometimes delivered by blind placement of a feeding tube, such as a Dobbhoff feeding tube into the stomach, ensuring correct placement with the use of a stethoscope or plain radiograph and will not be discussed any further here. Sometimes it is necessary to deliver feeding into the jejunum in an attempt to prevent aspiration in ill patients or patients who have gastroperesis or gastric outlet obstruction from tumor involvement. Nasojejunal (NJ) feeding tubes are frequently placed with the aid of an endoscope.

Endoscopic passage of an NJ feeding tube generally requires conscious sedation. Some of the more common techniques are described below:

1. *The NJ tube with a suture attached to its tip is passed into the stomach via a nostril.* The patient is then endoscoped and the suture at the tip of the feeding tube is grasped with a forceps and the scope advanced into the distal duodenum where the NJ tube is released. Sometimes the tube is inadvertently pulled back into the stomach when the endoscope is withdrawn. One way to overcome this is to use a double channel scope and through the second channel put down an endoclip to attach the suture to the wall of the intestine before withdrawing the endoscope.
2. *The guide-wire technique.* In this method the endoscope is advanced to the distal duodenum or jejunum and a floppy tip 0.035 guide wire is advanced as far out into the jejunum as possible. The endoscope is then slowly withdrawn as the wire is fed into the biopsy channel. The NJ tube is then pushed over the wire into the distal duodenum or jejunum and the guide wire removed. Sometimes this procedure is easier when done with fluoroscopic guidance. The NJ tube now requires oral-to-nasal transfer. In this final maneuver, a short transfer tube, usually supplied with the NJ tube kit, is passed into a nostril and retrieved from the throat and brought out of the mouth. The feeding tube or guide wire is threaded into this tube and advanced so that it comes out from the nostril. The transfer tube is then slid off the NJ tube or guide wire. Sometimes the guide wire (placed through the nose) to the jejunum has to be held under tension with a biopsy forceps while the tube is fed over the stiffened guide wire.
3. *Nasal endoscopy with ultrathin endoscope for placement of NJ tube.* This technique avoids the need to perform the oral-to-nasal transfer of the feeding tube since the digestive tract is accessed via the nostril. An ultrathin endoscope is passed through a nostril into the duodenum and a guide wire passed through its biopsy channel into the distal duodenum or jejunum. The endoscope is then removed as the wire is carefully fed into the channel to keep the wire in place. Next the NJ tube is pushed blindly over the wire into position in the small bowel.
4. *Nasally inserted NJ tubes guided by conventional endoscopes.* With an endoscope in the midesophagus or stomach, NJ tubes with guide wires in them to stiffen them can be introduced via the nostril and guided by the endoscope keeping the NJ tube tip well ahead of the scope at all times. Once the feeding tube is in place, the scope is carefully withdrawn while the stiffening wires hold the NJ tube in place. Finally the wires are removed from the feeding tubes.
5. *Through the scope jejunal tube placement.* Commercial 9 F and 11 F nasojejunal feeding tubes can be placed through the channel of either a pediatric colonoscope or therapeutic endoscope. This is quick and easy, but an extension tube, such as a snare, sometimes has to be used for very deep jejunal placement because the tube disappears into the channel before the tip of the scope exits the mouth.

10.4.2 Endoscopic Percutaneous Enteral Access

Percutaneous access is usually preferred if enteral nutrition is likely to be required for greater than one month. Percutaneous endoscopic gastrostomy (PEG) is the most commonly performed technique for enteral feeding by the gastroenterologist. In certain situations, such as recurrent aspiration, severe gastroperesis, or previous gastric surgery, it may be preferable to deliver the feed directly into the proximal small intestine. This is achieved either by extending a feeding tube passed through the PEG tube into the jejunum or placing a feeding tube directly into the jejunum percutaneously. These techniques are described below.

10.4.2.1 Percutaneous Endoscopic Gastrostomy (PEG)

Following informed consent, these patients undergo an upper endoscopy generally requiring sedation. Because of the risk of aspiration, the patients head is elevated to 30° during the procedure. Following a brief examination of the pylorus and duodenum, the scope is withdrawn to the upper stomach and the abdominal wall palpated over the potential PEG site area to look for point indentation through the endoscope. Usually at about the same time, transillumination of light from the scope is seen on the abdominal wall further allowing the best site selection for PEG. One should avoid placing a PEG too close to the costal margin or large abdominal scars from previous surgeries because of the risk of the bowel being adherent to these surgery sites. Once a site is selected, the skin is marked either with ink or pressure indentation from a needle cap and the area cleaned with antiseptic. The selected site is anesthetized with lidocaine to raise a wheal. The needle is frequently slowly advanced into the stomach under direct vision. Next a 1-cm incision is made in the skin with a scalpel through which the trocar is pushed into the stomach, again under direct vision. During this time, a snare is introduced through the scope into the stomach. The guide wire supplied in the PEG kit is then introduced through the trocar sheath after the needle has been removed. The guide wire tip is grasped in the snare as it enters the stomach and the endoscope is then pulled out of the patient with the guide wire. Next, depending on whether one uses a pull-type or a push-type PEG tube, one would either push a PEG tube over the guide wire or pull it by tying it to the PEG tube and pulling it into position. Once the PEG tube is in position, an external skin bolster is slid over the PEG tube and brought against the skin to hold the PEG in place. It is important not to tighten the bolster because pressure necrosis or, worse still, necrotizing fasciitis could occur. In fact, it's good practice to leave a loose fit, i.e., 1- to 2-cm slide for the PEG tube. The site is then covered with gauze. PEG feeding can be started three to six hours after PEG placement.[7]

10.4.3 Percutaneous Endoscopic Gastrostomy/Jejunostomy

In this technique, a jejunal feeding tube is placed through an existing PEG tube or as a one-step procedure where a PEG is placed in the usual way and a jejunal tube is placed into position via the PEG. PEG tubes are usually 20F or 24F and most manufacturers now make jejunal feeding tubes that will fit snugly onto these to prevent leakage, which was a problem in the past. Bard Access Systems

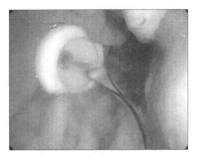

FIGURE 10.1 The jejunal feeding tube is grasped by its string with a biopsy forceps as it emerges through the percutaneous endoscopic gastrostomy (PEG) dome in the stomach.

(Salt Lake City, Utah) makes a one-piece PEG tube that narrows down to a jejunal feeding tube.

Various techniques have been described to pass the jejunal feeding tube through the PEG. It is our preference to use a therapeutic double channel endoscope for this procedure. Then the PEG tube is grasped as it enters the stomach through the PEG dome (Figure 10.1) with a biopsy forceps and taken through the pylorus and as far into the duodenum as possible (Figure 10.2). An endoclip is then introduced through the second channel of the endoscope and the jejunal tube anchored with a clip to the distal duodenal or jejunal wall (Figure 10.3 and Figure 10.4). Placing a flexible 0.035 guide wire inside the jejunal feeding tube makes the process easier both in terms of taking the wire as far as possible into the small bowel, but it also helps hold the clipped tube in place as the endoscope is withdrawn. Once the endoscope is back in the stomach, it is necessary to make sure the feeding tube is not looped in the stomach, but goes directly from the PEG dome to the pylorus (Figure 10.5). If not, the feeding tube needs to be advanced farther into the jejunum.

It is important to make sure that the jejunal tube goes directly from the PEG through the pylorus and into the distal duodenum. Any significant looping of the tube in the stomach will cause it to fall back into the stomach. Some endoscopists prefer to anchor the tip of the jejunal feeding tube in the small bowel before scope withdrawal. This is done by placing a string loop at the tip of the tube and anchoring this to the bowel wall with an endoclip.

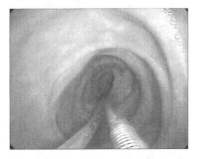

FIGURE 10.2 The endoscope is then advanced through the pylorus and the biopsy forceps advanced farther, taking the feeding tube deeper into the distal duodenum.

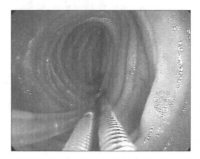

FIGURE 10.3   The feeding tube is now anchored to the jejunal wall with an endoscopically introduced clip through the second channel of the endoscope.

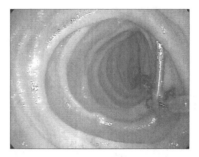

FIGURE 10.4   One or more endoscopically placed clips may be required to secure the feeding tube.

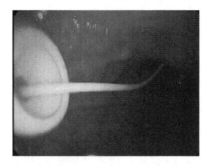

FIGURE 10.5   It is important that the intragastric portion of the jejunal feeding tube does not loop in the stomach but advances directly from the percutaneous endoscopic gastrostomy (PEG) dome to the pylorus, otherwise it may in time fall back into the stomach.

10.4.4   Direct Percutaneous Jejunostomy

A jejunal feeding tube is placed directly into the small bowel just distal to the ligament of Treitz using a pediatric colonoscope or an enteroscope. This procedure is similar to the PEG placement, but is technically more difficult to perform. It is our practice to have two physicians perform this—the endoscopist, and the assistant or the "skin" person.

10.4.4.1 The Technique

Following sedation and 0.5 mg glucagon as an antimotility agent, a pediatric colonoscope or enteroscope is introduced into the patient in the supine or left lateral position. Care is taken to minimize the amount of air put into the stomach to make looping of the scope less likely. Once the scope is advanced in the duodenum, the "skin" doctor looks for transillumination. The endoscope is advanced until the light is seen through the abdominal wall or as far as the endoscope will go. If no transillumination is seen, then the endoscopy is slowly withdrawn while looking for the light. At the same time, poking the left side of the abdomen with the index finger looking for indentation can help localize the potential site for percutaneous endoscopic jejunostomy (PEJ) placement. It is important to see a discreet point indentation at the area of transillumination for site selection and the next step. Once this site is confirmed, it is marked, cleaned with iodine, and draped. The site is then anesthetized with 1% lidocaine to raise a wheal. A 22- or 25-G needle that is at least 1.5 inches is used for this as it is also long enough to enter the jejunum. A 1-cm skin incision is then made with a scalpel. The introducer trocar needle is then placed through this cut into the jejunum and caught by the awaiting snare much like during a PEG placement. The blue loop wire is then inserted through the trocar after the needle in withdrawn, grasped by the snare, and pulled out of the patient's mouth. Then, just like in PEG tube placement, a standard 20F pull-type gastrostomy tube is tied to the wire and pulled back into position. Some prefer to check the position of the PEJ dome before terminating the procedure by repeating the endoscopy. Below are a few "rules of thumb" that we follow:

1. Do not proceed in the absence of good transillumination. This may require moving the scope tip in all four quadrants within the small bowel to look for it.
2. Make sure you get a good point indentation with your index finger before making the final site selection.
3. If you have trouble staying in the jejunum with your needle or trocar, grasp it with a snare quickly to maintain your position.

The success rates for endoscopic PEJ range from 72 to 100%, this is lowest in obese patients and highest in patients who have had previous gastrointestinal surgery, such as Bilroth-II.[8–13] Shetzline et al. demonstrated a high rate of success when using fluoroscopy in oblique views to reach as close to the skin as possible with the enteroscope for site selection. They also used ultrasound to locate solid organs to avoid complications. In seven patients, they had 100% success with no complications.

The major complication rate in the literature is about 2 to 4% and includes colon perforation, significant bleeding and abdominal wall abscess, persistent entrocutaneous fistula, jejuno–colonic fistula, and skin infections. Deaths have occurred from complications.[13]

Direct percutaneous endoscopic jejunostomy (DPEJ) seems to require fewer endoscopic interventions than PEG/J when used long term (greater than six months).[14] These DPEJ tubes may be replaced with replacement J-tubes that have a 3 to 5 mL balloon anchor or internal bolster introduced blindly with a stylet. The DPEJ has to be at least four weeks old for replacement tubes to be placed so that a tract has formed and the bowel doesn't come away from the abdominal wall leading to a "free perforation" and possible peritonitis.

10.5   ENTERAL FEEDING FOLLOWING FEEDING TUBE PLACEMENT

During the past 40 years, there has been a veritable explosion in the field of clinical nutrition, based in large part on studies on hospital malnutrition.[15,16] Subsequently, the concepts of nutrition support and nutrition pharmacology have received widespread attention, spawning the development of (1) evaluative methods for nutrition support, (2) a broad range of both enteral and parenteral formulas and feeding devices, and (3) professional organizations devoted to the science of nutrition support. While early in this growth process, parenteral nutrition was hailed as the innovation that would reverse all hospital-associated malnutrition, limitations of parenteral nutrition (cost, infection risk, negative effects on metabolism, and intestinal epithelial cell structure and function) have relegated it to instances in which enteral nutrition is contraindicated, i.e., with gastrointestinal tract dysfunction. The old adage: "If the gut works, use it" remains the guiding principal and, thus, the focus has been on enteral support via a myriad surgically, endoscopically, or manually placed feeding tubes.

10.5.1   THE DECISION FOR TUBE FEEDING

The decision to provide enteral nutrition is generally based on medical diagnosis, coupled with client history of undernutrition, and/or anticipated or ongoing suboptimal oral nutrition. Major indications are dysphagia and anorexia, either of which may be associated with a variety of primary medical diagnoses. The sole contraindication is mechanical obstruction of the gastrointestinal (GI) tract; in this case, access and feeding may be possible distal to the point of obstruction.

Enteral nutrition support may be initiated either on an out- or inpatient basis, and restricted to inhospital use, or continued in the home setting. Medicare coverage guidelines, frequently followed by third-party carriers, have guidelines for coverage of home enteral nutrition, including a projected minimum duration of 90 days. Although it would appear intuitively obvious, client and/or caregivers should be screened for the ability to transition enteral care into the home (clean and safe home environment, knowledge of tube, care/feeding by tube, and ability to troubleshoot problems). Arrangements with a homecare company with 24-hour availability for troubleshooting, and visits by a homecare nurse will help ensure independence of the client and support system. Additional information and support are available from the Oley Foundation (www.oley.org).

Tube feeding may be delivered into the stomach, duodenum, or jejunum; the site of administration is related to projected duration of tube feeding and site-specific gastrointestinal function. For example, for short term (<1 month) support, nasoenteric tube feeding may be an option. Feedings may then be delivered into the stomach or more distally. To minimize the risk of aspiration or avoid increasing severity of gastroesophageal reflux, placement of the tip past the third portion of the duodenum or the ligament of Treitz is utilized. A prokinetic agent (erythromycin or metoclopramide) may be given prior to tube insertion to facilitate small intestinal tip placement. The primary advantage of nasoenteric tubes is bedside and outpatient placement. Potential complications are many, from nasal discomfort and clogging of small bore tubes to the GI tract, or respiratory trauma and perforations.

For other clients for whom nutrition support will be necessary beyond 30 days, the option of endoscopic, fluoroscopic, or surgical tube placement is considered. Similar placement sites are utilized, again considering diagnosis and functional assessment of the gastrointestinal tract.

10.5.2 NUTRITION ASSESSMENT

Once the decision is made concerning the need for an enteral feeding device, goal nutrients are determined for the individual client. This task is generally accomplished by a registered dietitian, and is based on sex, age, activity, oral nutrient intake, preexisting nutritional status/deprivation, and ongoing medical condition and medications.

Dietary Reference Intakes: Recommended intakes for individuals[17] are generally the starting points for determining nutrient requirements. Baseline energy requirement is calculated using firstly the Harris Benedict Formula, where BEE = basal energy expenditure, and ABW = actual body weight:

Males: 66.5 + (13.8 × ABW in kg) + (5 × height in cm) (6.8 × age in years) = BEE in kcal

Females: 655.1 + (9.6 × ABW in kg) + 1.8 × height in cm) – (4.7 × age in years) = BEE in kcal.

Alternative (and more easily recalled) formula is the Owen formula:

Males: BEE in kcal/day = 879 + 10.2 × weight

Females: BEE in kcal/day = 795 + 7.2 × weight,

Or the Mifflin formula (more accurate than the Owen over wide range of BMI values):

Males: BEE in kcal/day = 5 +10 (weight in kg) + 6.25 (height in cm) – 5 (age in years)

Females: BEE in kcal/day = 161 + 10 (weight in kg) + 6.25 (height in cm) – 5 (age in years)[18]

To the basal energy expenditure, activity and/or injury factors are multipliers to reach total energy expenditure (BEE × AF × IF = TEE):

Activity Factors (AF)
    Bed rest: 1.2
    Ambulatory: 1.3
    Sepsis: 1.6

Injury Factors (IF)
    Minor surgery: 1.2
    Skeletal trauma: 1.35
    Severe burns: 2.1

Baseline protein requirements are based on weight, with modifications for stress. The adult protein requirement is 0.8 – 1 g/kg/d, but increases to 1 to 2 g/kg/d for moderate stress, and 2 to 2.5 g/kg/day with severe stress.

For example, a 65-year-old female, currently at her ideal body weight of 110 pounds (50 kg) for a height of 5'2" (157 cm) is admitted to a hospital from an assisted living center for the problems of Alzheimer's disease and anorexia due to acute cholecystitis. By the Mifflin formula, her BEE = –161 + 10 (50 kg) + 6.25 (157 cm) – 5(65 years), or 995 kcal/day. Currently on bed rest, her activity factor is 1.2, giving her a kcal requirement of 1,194 kcal/d. Estimated protein requirement is 40 to 50 g/day.

Various tools are available for the assessment of nutritional deprivation, including subjective global assessment of malnutrition,[19,20] the Waterlow criteria for malnutrition.[21] Then using a combination of nutrient requirements for age and sex, together with a factor for preexisting malnutrition, macronutrient goals exceeding baseline requirements may be determined.

Despite several available tools for calculation of nutrient repletion, reassessment of the individual client's nutritional progress by anthropometrics is vital to prevention of overnutrition or continuing undernutrition.

10.6 ADMINISTRATION OF ENTERAL FEEDINGS

10.6.1 ADVANCING FEEDINGS

Little data is available on initial rates and volume of feeding. Although initial diluting of formulas has been employed in the past, there is data pointing to greater risk of microbial contamination in diluting formulas, as the lower osmolality and higher pH may contribute to microbial growth.[22]

In medically stable clients, progression of feeding rates and volumes to reach goal nutrients may take place over a 24- to 48-hour time period. Conversely, in cases of medical instability (in particular gastrointestinal instability), or preexisting malnutrition, progression to goal nutrition may require greater than one week. In cases of preexisting malnutrition, care should be taken to avoid refeeding syndrome by careful monitoring and correction of electrolytes and fluid balance.

10.6.2 INTERVAL VERSUS CONTINUOUS FEEDINGS

Regardless of enteral feeding device employed, delivery of nutrients is by interval (bolus) or continuous feedings, or a combination of the two methods. Interval feedings may be provided by gravity drip or enteral feeding pump, while continuous feedings are uniformly delivered via pump. Both interval and continuous feedings have uses and complications, with interval feedings more closely simulating mealtimes.

Interval feedings are generally administered by gravity drip every several hours throughout the day. The client is able to tolerate volumes of 240 to 400 ml delivered over 10 to 20 minutes (in adults), and the frequency of feeding is linked to volume tolerance. This route of administration is easy to teach to caregivers, as there is no need for training on feeding pump use. In addition, the client is free to ambulate and engage in physical activity between feedings. This method is the least costly in terms of dollars and time, as well as least restrictive to the client.

Unfortunately rapid bolus use is associated with significantly lower esophageal sphincter pressure, allowing reflux of gastric contents;[23] this pressure change is not observed in the continuously fed or slower interval fed population. In addition, bloating can be the consequence of delayed gastric emptying or gastroparesis, thus limiting the tolerance for rapid bolus feeding.

Gastric residual volumes are checked as a means to prevent overfilling the stomach, which contributes to gastroesophageal reflux, aspiration, and discomfort due to bloating. At this time, accepting occasional residual volume of 250 ml in an adult has been recommended due to the observation of increased nutrient delivery using this value.[24] A prokinetic agent may be employed to accelerate gastric emptying, with either metoclopramide or erythromycin considered.

Data regarding the relationship between gastric residual volume and aspiration remains insufficiently studied.[24] No research has identified a gastric residual volume associated with either aspiration or gastrointestinal intolerance, and aspiration has been noted in association with zero residual volume. However, incidence of aspiration is greater in association with GRV >250 ml.[25,26] For a more complete discussion of research concerning gastric residual volume, the reader is referred to the recent ASPEN Enteral Nutrition Practice Recommendations.[27]

Interval feedings may also be administered by feeding pump, thus allowing a controlled and slower delivery rate, an alternative useful for patients experiencing nausea, vomiting, bloating, or abdominal pain with gravity interval feedings. Feedings are then delivered via enteral feeding pump, with infusion time determined by tolerance. This method is more restrictive to client movement due to the need for a mechanical device for feeding delivery. The caregiver requires additional training in use of the pump and priming the extension tubing for pump use. Rental or purchase fees for the pump are also considerations, as is the need for an external power source.

Enteral feedings can be delivered via continuous drip to clients intolerant of interval feedings. This method minimizes diarrhea and aspiration events,[28] and the hours of feedings may be linked to sleeping hours, 24 hours continuously, or any duration between.

Due to discomfort (as evidenced by bloating, cramps, diarrhea) with rapid delivery of hyperosmolar solutions into the jejunum, continuous feedings are preferred with intrajejunal feeding devices. Continuous drip feedings are also preferred in the critically ill population as a means to minimize aspiration events.

In instances where intestinal absorptive capacity is compromised, as in the case of the young child with short bowel syndrome, use of both interval feedings during the day and nocturnal continuous feedings may allow for improved volume and calorie tolerance, less diarrhea, and overall improved growth rate without subjecting the child to continuous connection to a pump while awake.

10.6.3 Minimizing Aspiration Risk

Due to the risk of aspiration, gastric feedings should be given in the upright position. For clients restricted to bed, a 30- to 45-degree head of bed elevation is recommended over supine positioning to decrease incidence of aspiration pneumonia. This angle may not avoid aspiration, as studies have documented aspiration even in the semirecumbent position.[29] A recent prospective study of ventilated clients has documented a significant decrease in tracheal secretion pepsin when bed elevation is >30%.[30] Additionally in this study, risk of pneumonia was four times greater among aspirating clients.

In cases where this angle is contraindicated (prone position, unstable spine, hemodynamic instability), use of transpyloric feeding, or use of a prokinetic agent may be considered. Although blue dye (FD&C Blue No. 1 and methylene blue) have traditionally been added to formulas to aid in the diagnosis of aspiration, dye is insufficiently sensitive in detecting pneumonia, and overdosing has been associated with increased risk of mortality.[30] Testing of tracheal secretions by the glucose oxidase method has additionally fallen out of favor given the presence of glucose in the tracheal secretions of unfed clients.[31]

10.6.4 So Now, What Do I Put In This Tube?

Gone are the days when the home blenderized tube feeding diet was the only alternative to the two commercially intact protein formulas for tube feeding. Currently there are many formulas available differing in degree of macronutrient hydrolysis, special additives, and selected indications. Due to cross-manufacturer similarities in products, most healthcare institutions stock a limited formulary of items.

With knowledge of the individual's gastrointestinal anatomy and function, nutrient requirements, and feeding site (gastric versus small intestinal), coupled with any nutrient modifications imposed by disease state, an enteral formula may be selected.

Commercially available formulas, often termed *medical nutritionals*, are preferred to a home-prepared blenderized formula due to concerns of sanitation, nutrient adequacy, and consistency of proximate composition. Many of these products are designed solely for tube feeding, as palatability is poor. Composed of intact protein (casein, soy, whey), glucose polymers and/or lactose, and a mixture of long and medium chain fats, standard formulas are designed to be used as a sole source of nutrition or as a supplement to oral feedings in clients with functional gastrointestinal tract. Hence, these are generally the first formulas utilized. Standard formulas provide 1 to 1.2 kcal/ml and are generally isotonic (approximately 300 mOsm) and low in residue.

Due to the frequency of lactose intolerance in both adults and children, a number of formulas are lactose-free. Some preparations also contain fiber, which may be beneficial in clients with fiber-responsive constipation or diarrhea, or irritable bowel syndrome.

For clients tolerating intact protein, but requiring a more protein-dense formula (specific indications: postsurgical or trauma, sepsis, promotion of wound healing), several formulas provide approximately 30% protein. The protein source is generally casein. These are often suffixed high protein or high nitrogen (HN). Lower osmolality remains a feature.

In clients, volume restricted or intolerant formulas providing 1.5 or 2.0 kcal/ml may be used. With these formulas, though, osmolality is increased. Protein concentration is generally greater to allow protein requirements to be met in less volume. Due to less free water in these formulas, clients should be monitored for hydration status.

10.6.4.1 Protein Modifications

More specialized formulas may contain hydrolyzed protein (to peptides and/or amino acids), facilitating use in protein sensitive or allergic patients. Formula osmolality, as well as cost, increases with protein hydrolysis. Calorie concentration is generally 1 kcal/ml. These products have been marketed for the treatment of gastrointestinal stress, such as in the treatment of active inflammatory bowel disease (IBD).

The most elemental formulas provide free amino acids as well as glucose polymers, and either a combination of medium chain triglycerides and long chain fats or negligible fat. As expected, these are expensive and have limited use due to high osmolality.

Branched chain amino acid fortified formulas are marketed for use in advanced liver disease. In hepatic encephalopathy, decreased serum branched chain amino acids (BCAA) and elevated aromatic amino acids have been noted. Use of specialized BCAA-supplanted formula is based on the ability of BCAA to interfere with aromatic amino acid's ability to cross the blood–brain barrier. Clinical observation has noted no benefit of these formulas when compared to medical treatment of encephalopathy with lactulose or neomycin.[32] Conversely, benefit upon nitrogen balance[33] and survival of a malnourished population[34] has been noted with BCAA supplemented formulas.

10.6.4.2 Immune Enhancing Nutrients

Recently a number of nutrients have been added to enteral formulas based largely on animal studies demonstrating benefit: glutamine, arginine, nucleotides, and omega 3 fatty acids.

The amino acid glutamine, a nucleotide precursor, is essential for rapidly dividing cells. Supplementation has been studied in the following scenarios: trauma/burn, neonatal care, and bone marrow transplantation with varying benefit on infection rates (benefit seen in BMT,[35] trauma/burns;[36] however, not in preterm infants.[37] The so-called "immune-enhancing" mixture includes glutamine, arginine, and omega 3 fatty acids. Several costly formulas, including this cocktail, are commercially available, but data regarding improvement in clinical outcomes remain limited, with meta-analysis suggesting reduction in infection rate, ventilator days, and length of stay, but no change in mortality.[38–39] On the other hand, a large, well implemented study found no effect upon outcomes.[40]

10.6.4.3 Disease Specific Formulas

In diabetic- or glucose-intolerant clients, the option of reduced carbohydrate formula is available. To compensate for the carbohydrate reduction and maintain a kcal concentration of 1 kcal/ml, a greater percentage of kcal are derived from fat. These formulas maintain normal osmolality.

For clients with fat malabsorption from bile salt deficiency or lymphatic disorder, formula containing medium chain triglycerides (MCT) as the predominant fat source is utilized. MCT-predominant formula provides intact carbohydrate and fat, so in cases of compromised gastrointestinal tract function where hydrolysates are preferred, a negligible fat, hydrolyzed protein and carbohydrate formula may be more appropriate.

Pulmonary formulas are polymeric, but supply less carbohydrate as a means to decrease the respiratory quotient. These formulas, like the diabetic formulas are high in fat, and in addition may provide antiinflammatory omega 3 fatty acids and increased kcal density of 1.5 kcal/ml.

10.7 CONCLUSIONS

Nutritional support is important for good outcomes in the critically ill patients and those with chronic disease who cannot ingest an adequate diet or have severe gastroperesis. Early enteral nutrition seems to have better outcomes in all groups where the gut is functional compared to parenteral nutrition. Endoscopic enteral access provides a means of delivering nutrition to these patients without the need for surgery. The techniques for endoscopic enteral access are safe and effective and should be in the armamentarium of every gastroenterologist. The most appropriate nutritional formulas require a knowledge of the particular patient's nutrition and energy requirements.

REFERENCES

1. Daly JM, Lieberman MD, Goldfine J, Shou J, Weintraub F, Rosato EF, Lavin P. Enteral nutrition with supplemental arginine, RNA, and omega-3 fatty acids in patients after operation: immunologic, metabolic, and clinical outcome. *Surgery*. 1992 Jul;112(1):56–67.
2. Kudsk KA, Croce MA, Fabian TC, Minard G, Tolley EA, Poret HA, Kuhl MR, Brown RO. Enteral versus parenteral feeding: effects on septic morbidity after blunt and penetrating abdominal trauma. *Ann Surg*. 1992 May;215(5):503–11; discussion 511–3.
3. Lipp A, Lusardi G. Systemic antimicrobial prophylaxis for percutaneous endoscopic gastrostomy. *Cochrane Database Syst Rev*. 2006 Oct 18;(4):CD005571; review.
4. Ahmad I, Mouncher A, Abdoolah A, Stenson R, Wright J, Daniels A, Tillett J, Hawthorne AB, Thomas G. Antibiotic prophylaxis for percutaneous endoscopic gastrostomy— a prospective, randomised, double-blind trial. *Aliment Pharmacol Ther*. 2003 Jul 15;18(2):209–15.
5. Külling D, Sonnenberg A, Fried M, Bauerfeind P. Cost analysis of antibiotic prophylaxis for PEG. *Gastrointest Endosc*. 2000 Feb;51(2):152–6.
6. Horiuchi A, Nakayama Y, Kajiyama M, Fujii H, Tanaka N. Nasopharyngeal decolonization of methicillin-resistant *Staphylococcus aureus* can reduce PEG peristomal wound infection. *Am J. Gastroenterol*. 2006;101(2):274–7.
7. Choudry U, Barde CJ, Market R, et al. Percutaneous endoscopic gastrostomy: a randomized prospective comparison of early and delayed feeding. *Gastrointest Endosc* 1996;44:164–7.

8. Mellert J, Naruhn MB, Grund KE, Becker HD. Direct endoscopic percutaneous jejunostomy (EPJ): clinical results. *Surg Endosc.* 1994 Aug;8(8):867–9; discussion 869–70.

9. Shike M, Latkany L, Gerdes H, Bloch AS. Direct percutaneous endoscopic jejunostomies for enteral feeding. *Gastrointest Endosc.* 1996 Nov;44(5):536–40.

10. Bueno JT, Schattner MA, Barrera R, Gerdes H, Bains M, Shike M. Endoscopic placement of direct percutaneous jejunostomy tubes in patients with complications after esophagectomy. *Gastrointest Endosc.* 2003 Apr;57(4):536–40.

11. Barrera R, Schattner M, Nygard S, Ahdoot M, Ahdoot A, Adeyeye S, Groeger J, Shike M. Outcome of direct percutaneous endoscopic jejunostomy tube placement for nutritional support in critically ill, mechanically ventilated patients. *J Crit Care.* 2001 Dec;16(4):178–81.

12. Maple JT, Petersen BT, Baron TH, Gostout CJ, Wong Kee Song LM, Buttar NS. Direct percutaneous endoscopic jejunostomy: outcomes in 307 consecutive attempts. *Am J Gastroenterol.* 2005 Dec;100(12):2681–8.

13. Shetzline MA, Suhocki PV, Workman MJ. Direct percutaneous endoscopic jejunostomy with small bowel enteroscopy and fluoroscopy. *Gastrointest Endosc.* 2001 May;53(6):633–8.

14. Fan AC, Baron TH, Rumalla A, Harewood GC. Comparison of direct percutaneous endoscopic jejunostomy and PEG with jejunal extension. *Gastrointest Endosc.* 2002 Dec;56(6):890–4.

15. Dark DS, Pingleton SD. Nutrition and nutrition support in critically ill patients. *J Int Care Med* 1993;8:16.

16. Robinson G, Goldstein M, Levine GM. Impact of nutritional status on DRG length of stay. *JPEN* 1987;11:49.

17. Institute of Medicine. Food and Nutrition Board. Dietary reference intakes: recommended intakes for individuals. *National Academy of Sciences,* 2004.

18. Frankenfield DC, Rowe WA, Smith JS et al. Validation of several established equations for resting metabolic rate in obese and nonobese people. *J Am Diet Assoc* 2003;103:1152.

19. Detsky AS, McLaughlin JR, Baker JP et al. What is subjective global assessment of nutritional status? *JPEN* 1987;11:8.

20. Secker DJ, Jeejeebhoy KN. Subjective global nutritional assessment for children. *Am J Clin Nutr* 2007;85:1083.

21. Waterlow JC. Classification and definition of protein-calorie malnutrition. *Br Med J* 1972;3:566.

22. Campbell SM. *Preventing Microbial Contamination of Enteral Formulas and Delivery Systems.* Columbus OH: Abbott Laboratories, Ross Products Division, 2000.

23. Coben RM, Weintraub A, DiMarino AJ et al. Gastroesophageal reflux during gastrostomy feeding. *Gastroenterol* 1994;106:13.

24. Kattlemann KK, Hise M, Russell M et al. Preliminary evidence for a medical nutrition therapy protocol: enteral nutrition for critically ill patients. *J Am Diet Assoc* 2006;106:1226.

25. Metheny NA, Schallom L, Oliver DA et al. Gastric residual volume and aspiration in critically ill patients receiving gastric feedings. *Am J Crit Care* 2008;17:512.

26. Metheny NA, Dahms TE, Chang YH et al. Detection of pepsin in tracheal secretions after forced small-volume aspiration of gastric juice. *JPEN* 2004;28:79.

27. Bankhead R, Boullata J, Brantley S et al. ASPEN enteral nutrition practice guidelines. *JPEN* 2009;33:122–67.

28. Ciocon JO, Galindo-Ciocon DJ, Tiessen C et al. Continuous compared with intermittent tube feeding in the elderly. *JPEN* 1992;16:525.

29. Torres A, Serra-Batlles J, Ros E et al. Pulmonary aspiration of gastric contents in patients receiving mechanical ventilation: the effect of body position. *Ann Int Med* 1992;116:540.

30. Metheny NA, Clouse RE, Chang YH. Tracheobronchial aspiration of gastric contents in critically ill tube fed patients: frequency, outcomes and risk factors. *Crit Care Med* 2006;34:1.

31. Metheny NA, Dahms TE, Stewart BJ et al. Verification of inefficiency of the glucose method in detecting aspiration associated with tube feeding. *MedSurg Nursing* 2005;14:112.

32. Eriksson LS, Conn HO. Branched chain amino acids in the treatment of encephalopathy: an analysis of variants. *Hepatology* 1989;10:228.

33. Marchesini G, Dioguardi FS, Bianch GP et al. Long-term oral branched chain amino acids treatment in chronic hepatic encephalopathy: a randomized double blind casein-controlled trial. *J Hepatol* 1990;11:92.

34. Cabre E, Gonzalez-Huiz F, Abad-Lacruz A et al. The effect of total enteral nutrition on the short-term outcome of severely malnourished cirrhotics: a randomized controlled study. *Gastro* 1990;98:715.

35. Schloerb PR, Amare M. Total parenteral nutrition with glutamine in bone marrow transplant and other clinical applications. *JPEN* 1993;17:407.

36. Houdijk AP, Rijnsburger ER, Jansen J et al. Randomized trial of glutamine-enriched nutrition on infectious morbidity in patients with multiple trauma. *Lancet* 1998; 352:772.

37. van den Berg A, van Elburg RM, Westerbeek EA et al. Glutamine enriched enteral nutrition in very-low birth weight infants and effects on feeding tolerance and infectious morbidity: a randomized controlled study. *Am J Clin Nutr* 2005;81:1397.

38. Beal RJ, Bryg DJ, Bihari DJ. Immunonutrition in the critically ill: a systemic review. *Crit Care Med* 1999;27:2799.

39. Heyland DK, Novak F, Drover JW et al. Should immunonutrition become routine in critically ill patients? A systemic review of the evidence. *JAMA* 2001;286:944.

40. Kieft H, Roos AN, van Drunen JD et al. Clinical outcomes of immunonutrition in a heterogeneous intensive care population. *Int Care Med* 2005;31:524.

11 Self-Expanding Metallic Stents in the Management of Malignant Esophageal, Gastric Outlet, and Duodenal Obstructions

Francis W. Chan and Priya A. Jamidar

CONTENTS

11.1 OVERVIEW OF ESOPHAGEAL CARCINOMA AND MALIGNANCIES RESPONSIBLE FOR GASTRIC OUTLET OBSTRUCTION

The treatment of upper gastrointestinal tract cancers continues to be a challenge to clinicians. Esophageal carcinoma and malignancies that cause gastric outlet or duodenal obstruction are particularly distressing to both the patient and clinician due to their frequent late stage of presentation as well as their adverse effects on quality of life. The incidence of esophageal adenocarcinoma has been increasing worldwide, while that of esophageal squamous cell carcinoma is decreasing.[1,2] Moreover there has been a significant increase in the proportion of patients presenting with Stage IV adenocarcinoma.[3] Consequently, approximately 50 to 60% of patients have incurable disease at the time of presentation.[4] Based on the histologic organization of the esophagus, squamous cell carcinoma typically occurs in the midesophagus, whereas adenocarcinoma typically occurs in the distal esophagus. Early esophageal carcinomas typically appear as superficial plaques or ulcerations while more advanced lesions can present as strictures or ulcerating and bleeding esophageal masses. Because this malignancy develops as an intraluminal lesion, the advanced stage malignancies most commonly cause symptoms of dysphagia or odynophagia. Other presentations include iron deficiency anemia, overt gastrointestinal bleeding, or tracheoesophageal fistula. In the subset of patients with late stage disease, therefore, palliative therapy is focused on relieving symptoms of dysphagia.

Malignancies are the etiology of up to 39% of cases of gastric outlet obstruction.[5] Malignant gastric outlet and duodenal obstruction can be caused by intrinsic or extrinsic effects of a tumor. Pancreatic adenocarcinoma with extension to the stomach or duodenum can commonly cause extrinsic obstruction, and if invading through the bowel wall, can also cause intrinsic obstruction of the lumen. The incidence of pancreatic adenocarcinoma is 7.1 per 100,000 people.[6] Of affected patients, retrospective reports indicate that gastric outlet obstruction can occur in up to 15 to 25%.[7] Other common malignancies that cause gastric outlet obstruction include distal gastric cancer, small bowel neoplasms, gastric lymphoma, and peritoneal carcinomatosis. Patients with gastric outlet or duodenal obstruction typically present with severe nausea and vomiting, abdominal distension, early satiety, and abdominal pain.

11.2   METHODS OF PALLIATION

11.2.1   ESOPHAGEAL OBSTRUCTION

Because such a large percentage of patients with esophageal cancer present with incurable and unresectable disease, the goals of management for these patients typically focus on palliation of the disease. Modalities that are utilized for palliation include external beam radiation therapy (EBRT), chemoradiotherapy, brachytherapy, endoscopic balloon dilatation, endoscopic laser ablation, and endoscopic stenting with plastic or metal stents.

EBRT and chemoradiotherapy can be successful in 40 to 88% of patients, but improvements in swallowing function can take up to two months.[8,9] For patients with advanced disease and a limited lifespan, the duration of time required to derive benefit from this modality may not be acceptable. Brachytherapy is also an effective palliative modality in greater than 70% of patients. However, similar to EBRT and chemoradiotherapy, the palliative effect is delayed, with some patients deriving peak relief of dysphagia 30 days after therapy.[10] Moreover, up to 30% of patients subsequently develop fibrotic strictures.[11] Although laser therapy also has been used successfully for treatment of malignant dysphagia, patients frequently require multiple treatment sessions at four- to six-week intervals, and some patients require esophageal dilatation prior to laser therapy, which confers a 5 to 9% risk of perforation.[12,13] Conventional plastic endoluminal stents also have been used to treat esophageal malignant obstruction. The benefits of this type of therapy include rapid relief of dysphagia symptoms after stent placement and treatment success with single session therapy. However, plastic stents are often technically challenging to place. Due to the large external diameters of the delivery systems, patients often require prestenting esophageal dilatation to accommodate the stent. This consequently incurs a perforation rate of 5 to 19%.[14] The small internal diameters of the stent lumen also may limit improvement in dysphagia scores. Finally, the procedure-related mortality with plastic endoluminal stents is high, ranging from 2 to 4% up to 16%.[11]

The limitations of these alternative modalities have spurred the development of self-expanding metallic stents (SEMS). The application of SEMS for palliation of gastrointestinal luminal obstruction was pioneered in the early 1990s and has revolutionized the management of malignant luminal obstruction. Overall, SEMS appear to be safer than plastic stents while maintaining equivalent clinical benefits in regards to the relief of dysphagia. Therefore, SEMS have largely surpassed plastic stents for palliation of malignant obstruction. In two randomized controlled trials comparing SEMS and plastic stents, SEMS were found to have lower procedure-related complication rates including perforation, lower procedure-related mortality, and lower rates of stent migration.[9, 15]

11.2.2 GASTRIC OUTLET AND DUODENAL OBSTRUCTION

Malignant gastric outlet and duodenal obstruction are common late complications of pancreatobiliary and gastric cancers. Because of the late presenting symptoms, patients frequently have limited management options. At diagnosis, approximately 85% and 40% of pancreatic and gastric cancers, respectively, are inoperable.[16] The few patients that present with early stage, localized disease may be candidates for curative surgical resection. More commonly, due to its late presentation, this malignancy is amenable only to palliative therapy. If patients are operative candidates, open or laparoscopic gastrojejunostomy is the primary approach for surgical palliation. Open and laparoscopic gastrojejunostomy are associated with morbidity and mortality rates as high as 30% and 15%, respectively.[17] Studies comparing open versus laparoscopic gastrojejunostomy have shown that the laparoscopic approach may have a lower morbidity and mortality as well as a shorter length of hospital stay, and shorter time to oral intake.[18-20] Unfortunately, because most patients present with late stage disease, surgical palliation is frequently not a viable option.

Nonsurgical methods for palliation include radiation therapy, balloon dilatation, laser ablation, and SEMS. In studies comparing SEMS with gastrojejunostomy, SEMS has been found to have lower postprocedure complications, more rapid resumption of normal oral intake, and shorter lengths of hospital stay.[19,21-23]

11.3 STENTS AND CHARACTERISTICS

SEMS are composed of several different types of metals and are designed specifically for use in the biliary tree, esophagus, small bowel, and colon. Each stent has different performance characteristics that are based on the type of metal alloy, delivery system, length and diameter of the closed and open stent, radial force exerted by the open stent, degree of shortening that occurs upon opening of the stent, and the presence or absence of a stent covering.

SEMS are commonly constructed of nitinol, stainless steel, combination alloys, or polyester and silicone. The material from which the stent is constructed and the lattice pattern of the metal contribute to the radial force characteristics of each individual stent. Delivery systems also vary with some stents that are deployed through-the-scope (TTS), while others are non-TTS stents that are placed over-the-wire and deployed via fluoroscopic guidance. The length and diameter (open and closed) vary and can be selected based on the dimensions and characteristics of the obstructing mass. The degree of shortening that may occur with stent expansion should be taken into account when selecting the appropriate stent length. Lastly, the selection of covered versus uncovered stents has important implications in regards to migration risk, tumor overgrowth, and the presence or absence of an enteric fistula.

Currently, in the United States there are three companies who manufacture U.S. Food and Drug Administration (FDA)-approved esophageal stents. Conventionally, FDA-approved esophageal stents also have been used for gastric outlet and duodenal obstruction. Boston Scientific (Natick, Massachusetts) produces the Wallflex® Duodenal and the Wallstent® Colonic and Duodenal Stent (Figure 11.1), the Ultraflex® NG (covered and uncovered), and the Polyflex® Esophageal stents (Figure 11.2). Cook Medical (Bloomington, Indiana) produces the Esophageal Z-Stent® in covered, uncovered, and antireflux versions (Figure 11.3) and the Evolution Controlled Release Stent® (Figure 11.4). Alveolus (Charlotte, North Carolina) produces the Alimaxx-E®. The characteristics and specifications of these stents vary in regards to their deployment diameter, length, flanges, covered versus bare metal construction as well as some additional factors (Table 11.1).

The Wallstent Colonic and Duodenal uncovered stent can be used for lesions in both the upper and lower gastrointestinal tract. It is manufactured from Elgiloy®, which is a cobalt–chromium–nickel-based alloy that is compressed into a 10 French delivery system. The stent is available with fully expanded diameters of 20 and 22 mm. Both of these diameters are available in 60 or 90 mm lengths.

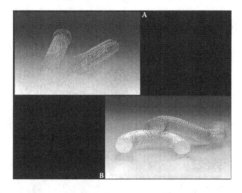

FIGURE 11.1 Boston Scientific Stents. (A) Wallflex Duodenal Stent; (B) Wallstent Colonic and Duodenal covered and Wallflex Duodenal uncovered stent.

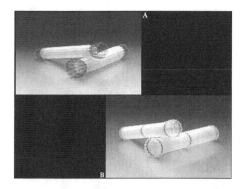

FIGURE 11.2 Boston Scientific Stents. (A) Ultraflex NG covered stent; (B) Polyflex Esophageal stent.

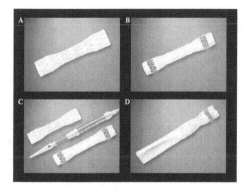

FIGURE 11.3 Cook Medical Stents. (A) Esophageal Z-stent, fully coated; (B) Esophageal Z-stent, uncoated flange; (C) Esophageal Z-stent, fully coated and uncoated flange with delivery device; (D) Esophageal Z-stent with Dua Antireflux Valve.

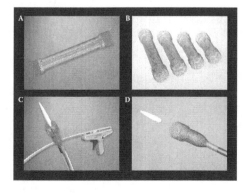

FIGURE 11.4 Cook Medical Stents. (A and B) Evolution Controlled Release Stent; (C and D) Evolution Controlled Release Stent with delivery device.

TABLE 11.1
Esophageal and Duodenal Stents: Specifications and Characteristics

Stent	Composition	Stent Diameter	Stent Length	Additional Characteristics
Boston Scientific				
Wallstent Colonic and Duodenal Stent	Elgiloy	20, 22 mm	60, 90 mm	Through the scope/over the wire deployment, reconstrainable up to 79% deployment
Wallflex Duodenal	Nitinol (nickel-titanium)	22 mm diam/27 mm flare	60, 90, 120 mm	Through the scope/over the wire deployment, flared distal end, reconstrainable up to 70% deployment
Ultraflex NG Stent System, uncovered	Nitinol (nickel-titanium)	18 mm diam/ 23 mm flare	70,100, 150 mm	Large Proximal Flare, available in proximal and distal release system, 48–54% shortening with deployment
Ultraflex NG Stent System, covered	Nitinol (nickel-titanium) w/ polyurethane cover	18 mm diam/ 23 mm flare, 23 mm diam/28 mm flare	100, 120, 150 mm	Large Proximal Flare, available in proximal and distal release system, 48–54% shortening with deployment
Polyflex Esophageal Stent	Polyester w/ Silicone cover	16 mm diam/20 mm flare, 18 mm diam/23 mm flare, 21 mm diam/25 mm flare	90, 120, 150 mm	Proximal flare, designed to be removable, 36–41% shortening with deployment
Cook Medical				
Esophageal Z-Stent Fully Coated	Stainless steel	18 mm/25 mm flared ends	80, 100, 120, 140 mm	Over the wire deployment, flared proximal and distal ends, no shortening with deployment
Esophageal Z-Stent Uncoated Flange	Stainless steel	18 mm/25 mm flared ends	80, 100, 120, 140 mm	Over the wire deployment, uncoated flared proximal and distal ends, no shortening with deployment

TABLE 11.1 (CONTINUED)
Esophageal and Duodenal Stents: Specifications and Characteristics

Stent	Composition	Stent Diameter	Stent Length	Additional Characteristics
Esophageal Z-Stent with Dual Antireflux Valve	Stainless steel	18 mm/25 mm flared ends	80, 100, 120, 140 mm	Over the wire deployment, flared proximal and distal ends, pressure-sensitive "windsock" at distal end to prevent reflux, no shortening with deployment
Evolution Controlled Release Stent	Nitinol (nickel-titanium) w/ silicone internal and external cover	20 mm/25 mm flared ends	80, 100, 125, 150 mm	Flared proximal and distal ends, controlled release with recapture of stent possible up to "point of no return" indicator on deployment device
Alveolus				
Alimaxx-E	Nitinol (nickel-titanium)	18, 22 mm (proximal flare 5 mm greater, distal flare 3 mm greater)	70, 100, 120 mm	Flared proximal and distal ends

The Wallflex Duodenal uncovered stent is composed of Nitinol, which is a nickel–titanium alloy that possess thermal elastic memory. This alloy is constructed with a certain diameter at specific temperatures, then cooled and compressed into a delivery device. When deployed at body temperature, the stent reexpands in an attempt to regain its original size, diameter, and configuration. Because of the characteristics of this alloy, these stents foreshorten when deployed. In addition, they reach their maximal diameter over the course of several days after the stent has been inserted. The Wallflex stent is compressed into a 10 French through-the-scope, over-the-wire delivery catheter. It has a flared distal end with radiopaque markers and clear transition zone and can be recaptured for repositioning of the stent up to approximately 70% deployment. The stent is available in one diameter with an expanded diameter of 22 mm with a 27 mm flare and lengths of 60, 90, and 120 mm.

The Ultraflex NG is manufactured from Nitinol and is available in polyurethane covered and uncovered form. This stent has a proximal flare and, in covered form, the body is covered while the proximal and distal ends remain uncovered. The uncovered stent is available in one diameter with a 18 mm diameter body and 23 mm diameter flare with lengths of 70, 100, and 150 mm.

The covered stent is available in two diameters with an 18 mm diameter body with 23 mm flare, or 23 mm diameter body with 28 mm flare. Length options for the covered stent are 100, 120, and 150 mm.

The Polyflex Esophageal stent is not a self-expanding metallic stent. Rather, it is a new generation of self-expanding plastic stents composed of silicone and polyester. It has a proximal flare, is designed to be removable, and is packaged in a 12, 13, or 14 mm diameter delivery device. The stent is available with a 16 mm body diameter with 20 mm flare, 18 mm body with 23 mm flare, or 21 mm body with 25 mm flare. Each of these sizes is offered in 90, 120, and 150 mm lengths.

The Esophageal Z-stent is composed of stainless steel, flared at the proximal and distal ends, and is available in three forms: fully coated, uncoated flange, and antireflux. This stent features over-the-wire delivery via a 31 French delivery system. It is available with an 18 mm diameter body with 25 mm flared ends and lengths of 80, 100, 120, and 140 mm.

The Evolution Controlled Release uncovered stent is the newest stent and is composed of Nitinol with a silicone internal and external cover. The primary feature of this device is the ability to slowly and incrementally deploy this stent while maintaining the ability to recapture the stent up to a "point of no return" as indicated on the 8 mm diameter delivery device. The stent is flared at the proximal and distal ends and is available in a 20 mm diameter body with 25 mm flared ends in lengths of 80, 100, 125, and 150 mm.

Lastly, the Alimaxx-E is an uncovered Nitinol stent with flared proximal and distal ends. The proximal flare is 5 mm greater and the distal flare is 3 mm greater than the expanded stent body diameter. It is available in 18 and 22 mm body diameters with lengths of 70, 100, and 120 mm.

11.4   TECHNICAL CONSIDERATIONS REGARDING PLACEMENT

Once a thorough evaluation and staging of the primary tumor has been completed and the patient has been deemed a candidate for palliative care, the decision must be made regarding the desired modality. If endoscopic therapy is chosen, SEMS placement is most frequently the treatment of choice. Placement of SEMS typically involves fluoroscopic guidance combined with endoscopic visualization. Before placement of the stent, exact localization and extent of the tumor must be established. In various studies, this initial step has been performed via upper gastrointestinal series with barium contrast or Gastrografin, cross-sectional imaging, or direct visualization by endoscopy.

11.4.1   ESOPHAGEAL OBSTRUCTION

Both the stricture length and lumen diameter must be assessed. An exact measurement of the stricture length determines the length of the stent that will be inserted. The techniques utilized to assess stricture length are determined by the degree of stenosis. If the stenosis is mild to moderate, the length of the stricture can be measured directly during endoscopy as the endoscope traverses the length of the mass and stricture. However, if the stenosis is severe, fluoroscopy with contrast dye injection must often be used to assess the stricture length. A guide wire can be passed through the stenosis followed by a balloon catheter. Contrast dye is then injected through the catheter distal to the stricture and examined under fluoroscopy.

Not only is the lumen diameter important for the measurement of stricture length, but it also determines the feasibility of direct stenting. Each stent is packaged with a unique delivery device. The diameter of the narrowed lumen must be able to accommodate the external diameter of this delivery device in order for the stent to be accurately and securely inserted. If the lumen diameter does not accommodate the diameter of the endoscope, an assessment must be made as to whether the lumen will accommodate the delivery device. In the event that the stenosis does not allow passage of the delivery device, the stricture will then require predilatation with either Savary or balloon dilatation. Just as predilatation increases perforation risk in the placement of plastic endoluminal stents, predilatation for placement of SEMS may also increase perforation risks over no predilatation. However, this concern is theoretical as no controlled trials have compared SEMS placement with and without predilatation. This rate, however, is lower than that of predilatation for plastic stents.[9,15] This difference in perforation risk is likely due to the larger diameter delivery devices of plastic stents.

Because delivery devices are uniquely constructed for each individual stent, they vary by stent type and medical device manufacturer. The early studies with SEMS were conducted in the early 1990s when the majority of stent delivery devices did not utilize through-the-scope delivery systems. Most early stents were developed for fluoroscopic, over-the-wire delivery and insertion. Contrast was typically injected into the lumen to outline the location and length of the stricture. Based on the fluoroscopic images, radiopaque markers were then placed on the skin to mark the upper and lower borders of the tumor. These markers then served to guide placement of the stents. Alternatively, direct fluoroscopy while visualizing the radiopaque borders of the stent itself has been used to guide placement. Although some current stents still utilize fluoroscopic, over-the-wire placement, many of the currently available stents utilize a combination of fluoroscopic, over-the-wire and, through-the-scope delivery techniques. This maximizes the ability of the endoscopist to accurately place the stent on the first attempt while minimizing the risk of migration and misplacement.

When choosing a stent, there are several factors that must be taken into consideration: the stent diameter and length, radial force, degree of shortening upon expansion, and the use of covered versus uncovered stents. Because the stent diameter will determine poststenting lumen diameter, larger stent diameters presumably facilitate resumption of a more normal diet that includes solid foods. Smaller diameter stents may continue to limit patients to liquid or semisolid food intake, have a higher risk of stent migration, tissue overgrowth, and food impaction.[24] Therefore, the stent diameter should be maximized while simultaneously conforming to the limits set by the native diameter of the enteral lumen. However, perforations and fistulas that develop after stent placement can form due to pressure necrosis that may be more likely with larger stents.[24] Particular care should be taken for stents placed in patients who have undergone radiation therapy. In at least one report, patients who have undergone radiation therapy and chemotherapy prior to stent placement have a higher risk of complications, including perforations.[25]

The desired length of the stent will be determined by the extent and length of the esophageal stricture. For mid- to distal-esophageal and gastroesophageal junction disease, the inserted stent should be approximately 4 cm longer than the stricture, such that approximately 2 cm of the stent will extend beyond both the proximal and distal borders of the stricture to maximally reduce tumor overgrowth as well as stent migration. This is particularly important in stents placed across the gastroesophageal junction. In this location, the distal end of the stent will be freely hanging into the gastric lumen and will not be in apposition to a mucosal surface. Therefore, only the proximal end of the stent is in contact with and anchored to normal esophageal mucosa. Because the stent should extend 2 to 3 cm beyond the borders of the stricture, individual stent characteristics must be known prior to stent selection. Because there are a number of stents that foreshorten when fully expanded, the closed length of each individual stent does not necessarily reflect the fully deployed and opened length of the stent. This degree of shortening must be taken into account when selecting the stent length.

Proximal esophageal malignant strictures pose additional challenges. Due to the proximity of these proximal lesions to the upper esophageal sphincter, there have been concerns regarding the risk of proximal stent migration and asphyxiation, tracheal compression, pain, and discomfort. Most studies involving esophageal SEMS for malignant palliation have excluded proximal esophageal lesions. However, there have been several small studies evaluating stenting of proximal lesions.[26,27] In these studies, success rates were high when the proximal end of the stents were positioned within the upper esophageal sphincter.

Lastly, the selection of a covered versus uncovered stent has significant implications. If the primary indication for stent placement is for palliation of a malignant obstruction or stricture, either a covered or uncovered stent can be used. However, if an obstruction/stricture exists concurrently with a tracheoesophageal fistula, only a covered stent can be used.

11.4.2 Gastric Outlet and Duodenal Obstruction

Like esophageal obstructions, assessing the stricture length and lumen diameter in gastric outlet obstruction and duodenal obstruction prior to stent placement is also imperative. The techniques by which this evaluation is performed are similar and consist of either direct endoscopic visualization or fluoroscopic assessment with contrast dye injection. Most lesions causing gastric outlet obstruction will be within reach of a standard upper endoscope. For lesions distal to the second or third portion of the duodenum, a colonoscope or enteroscope may be required to access the stricture.

Depending on the severity of the gastric outlet or duodenal obstruction, predilatation may be required prior to advancing the stent delivery device. Dilatation can be performed with a pneumatic balloon. Because many of the stents that are utilized for esophageal strictures also are used for gastric outlet and duodenal obstruction, the techniques used for stent localization are very similar and are based on the individual stent characteristics and specifications. Localization and insertion is performed either via fluoroscopy and over-the-wire placement or via fluoroscopy and over-the-wire/through-the-scope placement.

The stent chosen should be approximately 4 cm longer than the length of the obstruction to allow an appropriate degree of contact between the stent and the normal mucosa. Oftentimes stents that are placed across the pylorus into the duodenum will traverse the ampulla. In these situations, several case series have described a significant rate of biliary obstruction in up to 50% of patients.[28,29] Therefore, consideration should be given to inserting a biliary stent concurrently with a gastroduodenal stent. If not performed concurrently, biliary obstruction developing after gastroduodenal stent placement may not be able to be managed endoscopically because the stent overlying the ampulla will frequently impair access to the common bile duct. In such cases, percutaneous biliary drainage may be required.

11.5   ESOPHAGEAL OBSTRUCTION OUTCOMES

Stenting of lesions in the esophagus and the gastroesophageal junction (GEJ) with SEMS has a high technical and clinical success rate and an acceptably low rate of complications. The majority of studies with SEMS have been performed in Europe where the stents utilized differ from those that are available and Food and Drug Administration (FDA)-approved in the United States. As such, much of the data regarding success rates are based on stents that are not available in the United States. Moreover, many of the studies that do include FDA-approved stents predate the most recent iteration of stents produced by the medical device companies. Therefore, much of the data must be extrapolated from these studies and applied to stents available in the United States.

In most studies, technical success rates have been defined by the ability to accurately deliver and expand the stent in the desired location on the first procedural attempt. In most studies evaluating placement of SEMS in the esophagus, technical success rates have been reported to be greater than 95%.[9,25,30–33] For stents placed in the distal esophagus and across the GEJ, success rates do not differ significantly from midesophageal stent placement.[34]

Clinical success rates have largely been measured by patient-reported symptoms. Most studies utilize a four-stage dysphagia score. A score of 0 corresponded to the ability to eat a normal diet; 1, the ability to eat some solid foods; 2, the ability to eat semisolids; 3, the ability to drink liquids only; and 4, complete dysphagia. Most studies have shown dramatic reductions in dysphagia scores with the majority of patients improving by 2 grades. Most patients had mean scores of 2 to 3 prior to stenting and scores of 0 to 1 poststenting.[15,31,33,35,36] However, palliation of esophageal stenosis due to extrinsic malignant compression may have less dramatic improvements in dysphagia scores.[34]

The primary procedure related complications that result from SEMS placement include aspiration in 6 to 20% of patients,[30,33,37] pain in up to 25%,[32,33] severe bleeding in up to 10%,[31,32,35,37] and perforation in up to 6%.[31,37] Late complications, such as stent migration, occur in up to 13%[31,35] and recurrent dysphagia or tumor ingrowth/overgrowth occurs in up to 30%.[9,15,31,33,35,37] In addition to these potential complications that may occur with esophageal stenting, there are unique challenges and risks involved when placing stents across the GEJ. Because the distal end of the stent is not in firm apposition with a mucosal surface, but rather projects into the gastric lumen, stent migration is more likely.[11] In addition, increased rates of bleeding complications and reflux have been noted with stents placed at the GEJ.[34]

11.6 GASTRIC OUTLET AND DUODENAL OBSTRUCTION OUTCOMES

Similar to esophageal and GEJ stenting, treatment of gastric outlet and duodenal obstruction with SEMS has a high success rate and low complication rates. The majority of the data originate from Europe, using stents that either are not available in the United States or are outdated by newer stent technology.

Like esophageal stenting, technical success is defined by the ability to accurately deploy the stent in the location of interest on the first attempt. One large systematic review of palliative stenting for gastric outlet obstruction (GOO) included an analysis of 1,046 patients who underwent stent placement. The overall technical success rate was 96%.[6]

Clinical benefit has been defined based on patient symptom scores. The Gastric Outlet Obstruction Scoring System (GOOSS) score has been used for this purpose in most studies. In the GOOSS, a score of 0 denotes no oral intake, 1 represents liquid intake, 2 indicates soft foods, and 3 represents solid food/full diet. Reported clinical success rates have typically been defined by improvement of one stage in the GOOSS. These success rates range from 75 to 92%.[21,23,28,29,38–40] In one large meta-analysis, 11% of patients did not experience a clinical improvement after GOO stenting. The primary causes of this failure included progression of disease (61%), early stent migration (20%), and errors in stent placement and deployment (15%).[42]

The most common complications of GOO stenting include bleeding in 1.5% of patients,[40] common bile duct (CBD) obstruction in 44 to 71%,[21,28] recurrent obstruction in 9 to 22%,[28,29,40–42] perforation in 1 to 6%,[29,39–42] and stent migration in up to 1.5 to 14%.[21,29,39–42] Recurrent obstruction is most commonly caused by tumor overgrowth or ingrowth. This typically can be treated successfully by repeat endoscopic intervention.

11.7 POSTSTENT CARE

Nutritional guidelines have not been studied or established for patients in whom SEMS have been placed. Most patients derive clinical benefit within one to seven days of stent placement. For nitinol stents, in particular, the reduction of dysphagia may not be immediate due to the physical properties of the nitinol. Because these stents possess thermal elastic memory, it may take several days for these stents to reach their maximal diameter. Unlike nitinol, other stents manufactured from other materials typically take on their maximal diameter upon deployment.

In general, for esophageal, gastric outlet, and duodenal stents, patients are typically started on clear liquid diets within one day of the stenting procedure. In some centers, patients undergo an esophagram poststenting to determine the patency of the stent and to rule out perforation prior to resuming oral intake. A clear liquid diet is typically initiated 24 hours poststenting. Once patients have proved their ability to take liquids, they can slowly be advanced to full liquids, puree/semisolid food, and, if tolerated, a full diet. However, patients should avoid high residue foods, such as leafy vegetables. Patients should continue to eat whatever foods they tolerate while avoiding foods that trigger symptoms of dysphagia. As previously mentioned, recurrent obstruction due to tumor ingrowth or overgrowth can be as high as ~25%. These patients who are affected by recurrent dysphagia and obstruction should be evaluated for repeat stenting procedures.

11.8   CONCLUSIONS

Self-expanding metal stents have become the standard of care for the treatment of malignant symptomatic obstructions in the upper gastrointestinal tract for those patients who are not deemed to be operative candidates. Data regarding the usage of SEMS indicate that, when used by experienced clinicians in the appropriate candidates, this technology provides rapid clinical improvement with a low complication rate. The benefits derived from this treatment provide patients comfort and improved quality of life during their finals stages of life.

REFERENCES

1. Blot WJ. Esophageal cancer trends and risk factors. *Semin Oncol.* 1994 Aug;21(4): 403–10.
2. Bollschweiler E, Wolfgarten E, Gutschow C, Holscher AH. Demographic variations in the rising incidence of esophageal adenocarcinoma in white males. *Cancer.* 2001 Aug 1;92(3):549–55.
3. Daly JM, Karnell LH, Menck HR. National Cancer Data Base report on esophageal carcinoma. *Cancer.* 1996 Oct 15;78(8):1820–8.
4. Müller JM, Erasmi H, Stelzner M, Zieren U, Pichlmaier H. Surgical therapy of oesophageal carcinoma. *Br J Surg.* 1990 Aug;77(8):845–57.
5. Awan A, Johnston DE, Jamal MM. Gastric outlet obstruction with benign endoscopic biopsy should be further explored for malignancy. *Gastrointest Endosc.* 1998 Nov;48(5):497–500.
6. Jeurnink SM, van Eijck CH, Steyerberg EW, Kuipers EJ, Siersema PD. Stent versus gastrojejunostomy for the palliation of gastric outlet obstruction: a systematic review. *BMC Gastroenterol.* 2007 Jun 8;7:18.
7. Tendler D. Malignant gastric outlet obstruction; Bridging another divide. *Am J Gastroenterol.* 2002 Jan;97(1):4–6.
8. Coia LR, Soffen EM, Schultheiss TE, Martin EE, Hanks GE. Swallowing function in patients with esophageal cancer treated with concurrent radiation and chemotherapy. *Cancer.* 1993 Jan15;71(2):281–6.
9. Knyrim K, Hans-Joachim W, Bethge N, Keymling M, Vakil N. A controlled trial of expansile metal stent for palliation of esophageal obstruction due to inoperable cancer. *NEJM.* 1993; 329(18);1302–1307.
10. Marjolein YV, Homs MSc, Ewout W, et al. Single-dose brachytherapy versus metal stent placement for the palliation of dysphagia from oesophageal cancer: multicentre randomised trial. *Lancet.* 2004 Oct;364(9444):1497–1504.
11. Shimi SM. SEMS in the management of advanced esophageal cancer: a review. *Semin Laparoscopic Surg*; 2000 Mar;7(1):9–21.

12. Adam A, Ellul J, Watkinson AF, Tan BS, Morgan RA, Saunders MP, Mason RC. Palliation of inoperable esophageal carcinoma: a prospective randomized trial of laser therapy and stent placement. *Radiology.* 1997 Feb;202(2):344–8.

13. Dallal HJ, Smith GD, Grieve DC, Ghosh S, Penman ID, Palmer KR. A randomized trial of thermal ablative therapy versus expandable metal stents in the palliative treatment of patients with esophageal carcinoma. *Gastrointest Endosc.* 2001 Nov;54(5):549–57.

14. Tan BS, Mason R, Adam A. Minimally invasive therapy for advanced oesophageal malignancy (review). *Clin Radiol.* 1996 51:828–826.

15. DePalma GD, diMatteo, E, Romano G, Fimmano A, Rondinone G, Catanzano C. Plastic prosthesis versus expandable metal stents for palliation of inoperable esophageal thoracic carcinoma: a controlled prospective study. *Gastrointest Endosc.* 1996 May;43(5):478–82.

16. Kaw M, Singh S, Gagneja H, Azad P. Role of self-expandable metal stents in the palliation of malignany duodenal obstruction. *Surg Endosc.* 2003;17:646–650.

17. Chopita N, Landoni N, Ross A, Villaverde A. Malignant gastroenteric obstruction; therapeutic options. *Gastroinest Endoscopy Clin N Amer.* 2007 Jul;17(3):533–44.

18. Choi YB. Laparoscopic gatrojejunostomy for palliation of gastric outlet obstruction in unresectable gastric cancer. *Surg Endosc.* 2002 16(11);1620–6.

19. Mittal A, Windsor J, Woodfield J, Casey P, Lane M. Matched study of three methods for palliation of malignant pyloroduodenal obstruction. *Br J Surg.* 2004 Feb;91(2):205–9.

20. Fiori E, Lamazza A, Volpino P, Burza A, Paparelli C, Cavallaro G, Schillaci A, Cangemi V. Palliative management of malignant antro-pyloric strictures. Gastroenterostomy vs. endoscopic stenting. A randomized prospective trial. *Anticancer Res.* 2004 Jan–Feb;24(1):269–71.

21. Jeurnink SM, Steyerberg EW, Hof G, van Eijck CH, Kuipers EJ, Siersema PD. Gastrojejunostomy versus stent placement in patients with malignant gastric outlet obstruction: a comparison in 95 patients. *J Surg Oncol.* 2007 Oct 1;96(5):389–96.

22. Maetani I, Tada T, Ukita T, Inoue H, Sakai Y, Nagao J. Comparison of duodenal stent placement with surgical gastrojejunostomy for palliation in patients with duodenal obstructions caused by pancreaticobiliary malignancies. *Endoscopy.* 2004 Jan;36(1):73–8.

23. Maetani I, Akatsuka S, Ikeda M, Tada T, Ukita T, Nakamura Y, Nagao J, Sakai Y. Self-expandable metallic stent placement for palliation in gastric outlet obstructions caused by gastric cancer: a comparison with surgical gastrojejunostomy. *J Gastroenterol.* 2005 Oct;40(10):932–7.

24. Verschuur EML, Steyerberg EW, Kuipers EJ, Siersema PD. Effect of stent size on complications and recurrent dysphagia in patient with esophageal and gastric cardia cancer. *Gastrointest Endosc.* 2007 Apr;65(4):592–601.

25. Kinsman KJ, DeGregorio BT, Katon RM, Morrison K, Saxon RR, Keller FS, Rosch J. Prior radiation and chemotherapy increase the risk of life threatening complications after insertion of metallic stents for esophagogastric malignancy. *Gastrointest Endosc.* 1996;43(3);258–60.

26. Conio M, Caroli-Bosc F, Demarquay JF, Sorbi D, Maes B, Delmont J, Dumas R. Self-expanding metal stents in the palliation of neoplasms of the cervical esophagus. *Hepatogastroenterology.* 1999 Jan–Feb;46(25):272–7.

27. Bethge N, Sommer A, Vakil N. A prospective trial of self-expanding metal stents in the palliation of malignant esophageal strictures near the upper esophageal sphincter. *Gastrointest Endosc.* 1997 Mar;45(3):300–3.

28. Adler DG, Baron TH. Endoscopic palliation of malignant gastric outlet obstruction using self-expanding metal stents: experience in 36 patients. *Am J Gastroenterol.* 2002 Jan;97(1):72–8.

29. Mosler P, Mergener KD, Brandabur JJ, Schembre DB, Kozarek RA. Palliation of gastric outlet obstruction and proximal small bowel obstruction with self-expandable metal stents: a single center series. *J Clin Gastroenterol.* 2005 Feb;39(2):124–8.

30. Ellul JP, Watkinson A, Khan RJ, Adam A, Mason RC. Self-expanding metal stents for the palliation of dysphagia due to inoperable oesophageal carcinoma. *Br J Surg.* 1995 Dec;82(12):1678–81.

31. Siersema PD, Hop WC, van Blankenstein M, van Tilburg AJ, Bac DJ, Homs MY, Kuipers EJ. A comparison of 3 types of covered metal stents for the palliation of patients with dysphagia caused by esophagogastric carcinoma: a prospective, randomized study. *Gastrointest Endosc.* 2001 Aug;54(2):145–53.

32. Kozarek RA, Raltz S, Brugge WR, et al. Prospective multicenter trial of esophageal Z-stent placement for malignant dysphagia and tracheoesophageal fistula. *Gastrointest Endosc.* 1996 Nov;44(5):562–7.

33. Schmassmann A, Meyenberger C, Knuchel J, Binek J, Lammer F, Kleiner B, Hürlimann S, Inauen W, Hammer B, Scheurer U, Halter F. Self-expanding metal stents in malignant esophageal obstruction: a comparison between two stent types. *Am J Gastroenterol.* 1997 Mar;92(3):400–6.

34. Siersema PD, Marcon N, Vakil N. Metal stents for tumors of the distal esophagus and gastric cardia. *Endoscopy.* 2003 Jan;35(1):79–85.

35. Cowling MG, Hale H, Grundy A. Management of malignancy oesophageal obstruction with self expanding metallic stents. *Br J Surg.* 1998 Feb;85(2):264–6.

36. Sumiyoshi T, Gotoda T, Muro K, Rembacken B, Goto M, Sumiyoshi Y, Ono H, Saito D. Morbidity and mortality after self-expandable metallic stent placement in patients with progressive or recurrent esophageal cancer after chemoradiotherapy. *Gastrointest Endosc.* 2003 Jun;57(7):882–5.

37. Lecleire S, Di Fiore F, Antonietti M, Ben Soussan E, Hellot MF, Grigioni S, Déchelotte P, Lerebours E, Michel P, Ducrotté P. Undernutrition is predictive of early mortality after palliative self-expanding metal stent insertion in patients with inoperable or recurrent esophageal cancer. *Gastrointest Endosc.* 2006 Oct;64(4):479–84.

38. Del Piano M, Ballarè M, Montino F, Todesco A, Orsello M, Magnani C, Garello E. Endoscopy or surgery for malignant GI outlet obstruction? *Gastrointest Endosc.* 2005 Mar;61(3):421–6.

39. van Hooft J, Mutignani M, Repici A, Messmann H, Neuhaus H, Fockens P. First data on the palliative treatment of patients with malignant gastric outlet obstruction using the WallFlex enteral stent: a retrospective multicenter study. *Endoscopy.* 2007 May;39(5):434–9.

40. Phillips MS, Gosain S, Bonatti H, Friel CM, Ellen K, Northup PG, Kahaleh M. Enteral stents for malignancy: a report of 46 consecutive cases over 10 years, with critical review of complications. *J Gastrointest Surg.* 2008 Nov;12(11):2045–50.

41. Dormann A, Meisner S, Verin N, Wenk Lang A. Self-expanding metal stents for gastroduodenal malignancies: systematic review of their clinical effectiveness. *Endoscopy.* 2004 Jun;36(6):543–50.

42. Nassif T, Prat F, Meduri B, Fritsch J, Choury AD, Dumont JL, Auroux J, Desaint B, Boboc B, Ponsot P, Cervoni JP. Endoscopic palliation of malignant gastric outlet obstruction using self-expandable metallic stents: results of a multicenter study. *Endoscopy.* 2003 Jun;35(6):483–9.

12 Management of Chronic Malabsorption

Piyush Tiwari, Manreet Kaur, and Bhaskar Banerjee

CONTENTS

12.1 INTRODUCTION

Malabsorption is a global term that includes a wide variety of impaired digestive and absorptive disorders that are found in diverse gastrointestinal diseases. The severity and breadth of clinical manifestations of malabsorption can differ widely depending on the unabsorbed nutrients. The clinical features are collectively called the *malabsorption syndrome*. This chapter will provide general guidelines to help detect, diagnose, and treat malabsorptive disorders and their symptoms. Before discussing malabsorption, it is important to consider the normal process of digestion and absorption of dietary food as listed below.[1]

- Lubrication of food along with its movement through the alimentary tract.
- Mechanical and enzymatic breakdown of fats, proteins, and carbohydrates.
- Reabsorption of nutrients and water, and transportation of nutrients to the liver via the portal vein and lymphatic system.
- Production of nutrients, such as biotin and vitamin K, by intestinal bacteria.

Any disruption in the above steps can result in malabsorption, which is the impaired ability to digest or absorb nutrients across the intestinal mucosa into the blood stream.[2]

12.2 PHYSIOLOGY OF DIGESTION AND ABSORPTION

The normal physiology of digestion and absorption is outlined below.

12.2.1 FAT

Dietary fat is largely composed of long chain fatty acids (LCFAs), which esterify to form triglycerides. Fat is digested to form free fatty acids and monoglycerides through the process of lipolysis, which is initiated by gastric lipase in an acidic pH of 4.5 to 6. Most of the lipolysis is performed by pancreatic lipase in the alkaline medium of the duodenum and jejunum. In order to traverse through the thin aqueous layer covering intestinal mucous membrane, free fatty acids form hydrophilic *mixed micelles* in combination with conjugated bile acids, phospholipids, and cholesterol. Micelles undergo cellular uptake and disintegrate to individual components, following which free fatty acids resterify to generate triglycerides. Along with B lipoprotein, cholesterol, and cholesterol ester, triglycerides form *chylomicrons* that exit into the lymphatic system to reach the liver. Medium chain fatty acids (present in coconut oil) do not require lipolysis and subsequent reesterification. Upon mucosal absorption, they reach the liver via the portal vein.)[3] Short chain fatty acids are synthesized by colonic bacteria from nonabsorbed carbohydrates reaching the colon, and require absorption through the colonic mucosa with sodium chloride (NaCl) and water.

12.2.2 CARBOHYDRATE

Dietary carbohydrate is found in the form of starch, disaccharides, and glucose. Salivary amylase, pancreatic lipase, and intestinal mucosal brush border cell surface disaccharidase, sequentially digest carbohydrates to form monosaccharides (glucose, galactose, and fructose) that are absorbed in the small intestine through an active sodium (Na)-dependent process with the help of the cell membrane transport carrier protein SGLT (sodium-dependent glucose transporters). Fructose absorption is facilitated by GLUT 5 transport protein.

12.2.3 PROTEIN

Dietary protein is ingested as polypeptides and then converted to tripeptides, dipeptides, and amino acids by gastric pepsin and pancreatic trypsin prior to absorption in the small intestine.

12.2.4 ENTEROHEPATIC CIRCULATION

Approximately 500 mg of primary bile acids (cholic acid and chenodeoxycholic acid) are synthesized in the liver daily from cholesterol. Bile acids are conjugated with glycine and taurine and secreted into the duodenum. In the small intestine, bile acids form micelles with digested dietary fat to aid their absorption. The remaining bile acids are absorbed by the terminal ileum for return to the liver (enterohepatic circulation). A small amount of conjugated bile acid enters the colon and is rapidly deconjugated and converted to secondary bile acids (deoxycholic acid and lithocholic acid) by colonic bacteria, prior to their excretion in stool. The daily fecal loss of bile acid is compensated by hepatic synthesis, which has a limited capacity. The entire bile acid pool is recirculated about six to eight times during a 24-hour period.

12.2.5 MINERALS AND VITAMINS

The absorption of fat-soluble vitamin A, D, E, and K occurs with dietary fat absorption. Fat malabsorption thus disrupts the absorption of fat soluble vitamins. Most vitamins, including water soluble vitamin B and C, are absorbed mainly in the jejunum, but vitamin B_{12} is absorbed in the ileum. Dietary vitamin B_{12} is liberated from diet proteins and binds to R-binder protein (present in salivary and gastric secretion) in the acidic pH of stomach, and later released free again in the alkaline pH of the duodenum secondary to pancreatic enzymes. Vitamin B_{12} further binds to an intrinsic factor (a protein secreted by gastric parietal cells) and reaches the terminal ileum where this complex is attached to the specific mucosal receptors for vitamin B_{12} absorption. An increase in stomach pH[4] and/or decrease in duodenal pH interferes with the release of vitamin B_{12} from dietary and R-binder proteins, respectively, and impair vitamin B_{12}-intrinsic factor complex formation, and, hence, cause vitamin B_{12} malabsorption.

About 25 to 75% of ingested calcium is absorbed actively in the duodenum. Through vitamin D derivatives, Ca^{2+} absorption is adjusted and regulated to body needs. Calcium absorption is inhibited by phosphates and oxalates, which form insoluble salts with Ca^{2+} in the intestine.

Dietary iron is absorbed in the duodenum by a regulated process to maintain body iron homeostasis as iron excretion is not regulated. Dietary iron exists in the forms of heme and nonheme, which are present mainly in red meat and in vegetables, cereals, and white meat, respectively. Nonheme dietary iron is released by acid digestion in the stomach, and before mucosal absorption, reduced to the ferrous (Fe^{2+}) ion by ascorbic acid and an iron-regulated ferric reductase protein (Dcytb, Cybrd1),[5] which is present on the apical membrane of enterocytes.

12.2.6 WATER AND ELECTROLYTE BALANCE

Every day the intestines are exposed to about 2,000 ml of ingested fluid and 7,000 ml of secretions from the gastrointestinal secretory glands. Ninety-eight percent of this fluid is reabsorbed, limiting the daily fluid loss to about 200 ml with stool. Only small amounts of water move across gastric mucosa, but water movement is bidirectional across the mucosa of the small and large intestines in response to osmotic gradients, which influences stool volume and consistency.

12.3 ETIOLOGY OF MALABSORPTION

Malabsorption may be extensive or partial, depending on the number of malabsorbed nutrients. Diffuse mucosal pathology or reduced mucosal absorptive surface, e.g., in celiac disease, may result in extensive malabsorption of almost all nutrients, where symptoms are readily apparent. Partial malabsorption results from the diseases that disrupt the absorption of only specific nutrients, e.g., defective B_{12} absorption in patients with pernicious anemia. The etiology of malabsorption can be classified in three categories (Table 12.1).

12.4 DIAGNOSTIC EVALUATION OF MALABSORPTION

Since malabsorption can be the end result of a variety of disorders, its clinical presentation may vary. Malabsorption can be approached in following manner:[6,7]

1. **Suspicion of Malabsorption**—The classic manifestations of extensive malabsorption are diarrhea with pale, greasy, voluminous, foul-smelling stools; weight loss despite adequate food intake; mild abdominal discomfort; and distention along with flatus. These symptoms can be attributed to the presence of unabsorbed fat and carbohydrate that affects intestinal NaCl and water transport to increase stool volume. Moreover, bacterial fermentation of unabsorbed carbohydrates releases foul-smelling hydrogen and methane gas. Partial forms of malabsorption may present solely with the symptoms that are attributable to the particular nutrient in question. However, many malabsorptive disorders may only have nonspecific clinical presentations, such as loose stools and malaise. The suspicion of malabsorption is generally made based on the patient's history, clinical features, and routine blood investigations, and can sometimes be quite subtle. Details are summarized in Table 12.2.

2. **Confirmation of Malabsorption**—Once suspicion of malabsorption has been raised, the next logical step is to confirm its presence. Measuring low serum level after ingesting a nutrient and/or its decreased urinary excretion can help confirm malabsorption. Similarly, increased excretion of a nutrient in stool supports its malabsorption.[8] List of tests performed to evaluate and confirm presence of malabsorption is mentioned in Table 12.3.

3. **Finding the Cause of Malabsorption**—This often requires more investigations. Several invasive (endoscopy with biopsy, capsule endoscopy, ERCP, or EUS) and noninvasive (abdominal CT scan, MRI, ultrasound, x-rays) tests are used. If history suggests a particular cause, testing can be directed to confirm the diagnosis. The order of testing and choice of a particular test should be individualized and according to available resources. The ultimate goal is to find or to exclude a disease that causes malabsorption. A diagnostic algorithm to evaluate malabsorption is shown in Figure 12.1.[9]

TABLE 12.1

Etiological Classification of Malabsorption Based on Pathophysiology

Site of Malabsorption	Pathophysiology	Example of Disease	Causative Mechanism
Luminal Phase (Carbohydrates, proteins, and fats are hydrolyzed and solubilized in the lumen by intestinal mucosal, pancreatic, and biliary secretions)	1. Impaired nutrient hydrolysis	Chronic pancreatitis, pancreatic resection, cystic fibrosis pancreatic cancer, congenital pancreatic enzyme deficiencies	Absent or decreased level of pancreatic enzyme
		Zollinger–Ellison syndrome	Inactivation of pancreatic enzyme from gastric acid hypersecretion
		Short bowel syndrome	Inadequate mixing of nutrients, bile, and enzymes
		Enterokinase deficiency	Inability of pancreatic proenzymes to convert to active enzymes
	2. Impaired micelle formation	Cirrhosis, Parenchymal liver diseases	Decrease hepatic synthesis of bile acid
		Primary biliary cirrhosis, chronic cholestasis, Primary sclerosing cholangitis	Decrease bile secretion in duodenum
		Anatomical abnormality (*small bowel diverticulosis, blind loop, stricture*)	Bacterial overgrowth causes deconjugation of bile and subsequently diminishes micelle formation
		Impaired motor abnormality (*scleroderma, diabetic neuropathy*), enterocolic fistula	
		Terminal ileitis, e.g., Crohn's disease, ileal resection	Impaired bile absorption second to ileal mucosal disease
	3. Impaired nutrient processing and availability for absorption	Pernicious anemia, gastric resection	Lack of intrinsic factor causes vitamin B_{12} deficiency
		Atrophic gastritis	Diminished gastric acid secretion causes vitamin B_{12} deficiency secondary to impaired cleavage of vitamin B_{12} and R-binding protein
		Postbillroth II procedure	Inadequate mixing and disorganized enzyme release

(continued)

TABLE 12.1 (CONTINUED)
Etiological Classification of Malabsorption Based on Pathophysiology

Site of Malabsorption	Pathophysiology	Example of Disease	Causative Mechanism
Mucosal Phase (Carbohydrates, peptides, and fats are further hydrolyzed and packaged for absorption)	1. Impaired brush border hydrolysis	Lactase deficiency	Acquired disaccharidase defect; most common cause of intestinal brush border enzyme deficiency
		Sucrase-isomaltase enzyme deficiency	Congenital disaccharidase defect
		Acrodermatitis enteropathica	Autosomal recessive metabolic disorder affecting the zinc uptake
	2. Impaired mucosal nutrient absorption	Crohn's disease, celiac/collagenous/tropical sprue, AIDS enteropathy, chemotherapy and radiation enteritis, nongranulomatous ulcerative jejunoileitis, eosinophilic gastroenteritis	Damaged mucosal surface secondary to inflammation
		Intestinal lymphoma and amyloidosis, systemic mastocytosis, immunoproliferative small intestinal disease (IPSID)	Mucosal and submucosal infiltration affecting absorption
		Bacterial overgrowth, Giardiasis, Whipple's disease, cryptosporidiosis, microsporidiosis, and other parasitic diseases, mycobacterium avium-intracellulare, AIDS enteropathy	Mucosal and submucosal infestation by microorganism impairs absorption
		Cystinuria	Defect in dibasic amino acid transport
		Hartnup disease	Defect in neutral amino acid transport

TABLE 12.1 (CONTINUED)
Etiological Classification of Malabsorption Based on Pathophysiology

Site of Malabsorption	Pathophysiology	Example of Disease	Causative Mechanism
Postabsorptive Phase (Absorbed nutrients are packaged and exported to vein and lymphatic system to reach liver)	1. Impaired lymphatic flow	Intestinal lymphangiectasia, Milroy disease	Congenital abnormality, affecting lymphatic flow
		Whipple disease, intestinal neoplasm, tuberculosis	Acquired abnormality, causing disruption in lymphatic flow
	2. Impaired chylomicron absorption	Abetalipoproteinemia	Absent beta lipoprotein causing defect in chylomicron transport to lymphatic system

12.5 MANAGEMENT OF MALABSORPTION

The primary goals of managing patients with malabsorption should include:

- Control of diarrhea
- Correction of nutritional deficiencies and maintaining an optimal nutritional status
- Correcting the cause

Because the underlying etiology of malabsorption varies in patients, the following section details certain general principals of management.

12.5.1 CONTROL OF DIARRHEA

Diarrhea is usually the most common and troublesome manifestation of malabsorption. The cause of diarrhea has an impact on its treatment. For example, in steatorrhea secondary to pancreatic insufficiency, enzyme supplementation with 25,000 to 40,000 units of porcine lipase per meal using pH-sensitive pancreatin microspheres is recommended (Table 12.4). In case of treatment failure, the dose should be increased, compliance checked, and alternative causes of malabsorption excluded. Addition of PPI/H2 blocker therapy may help to increase the efficacy of pancreatic enzyme supplement.[10] Still, in most patients, fat digestion cannot be completely normalized by standard therapy and the diarrhea may not resolve entirely.

Bile salt malabsorption from terminal ileal disease or resection can result in a secretory choleretic diarrhea that responds to treatment with bile salt-binding resins (cholestyramine, colestipol).[11] These resins can cause flatulence and bloating that may interfere with compliance and absorption of other oral medications. In patients that have undergone extensive resection of terminal ileum (usually >100

TABLE 12.2
Clinical Features and Routine Laboratory Tests Suggesting Nutrient Deficiency

Clinical Features	Nutrient Deficiency
Bleeding	Vitamin K, protein malnutrition
Night blindness, xerophthalmia, follicular hyperkeratosis	Vitamin A
Peripheral neuropathy, ataxia	Vitamin B_{12} and thiamine
Dermatitis	Vitamin A, zinc, and essential fatty acid deficiency
Anemia	Iron, folate, vitamin B_{12}
Tetany, paresthesia, pathologic fracture, positive Chvostek and Trousseau sign	Calcium, vitamin D, and magnesium malabsorption
Glossitis, cheilosis, stomatitis, acrodermatitis	Iron, vitamin B_{12}, folate, and vitamin A malabsorption
Amenorrhea and decrease libido	Protein/calorie malabsorption, second hypopituitarism
Azotemia and hypotension	Fluid and electrolyte depletion
Weakness, muscle wasting, weight loss	Protein/calorie malabsorption, anemia, electrolyte depletion
Steatorrhea	Fat malabsorption
Seizure	Biotin deficiency
Edema, ascites	Protein deficiency

Laboratory Tests	Nutrient Deficiency
Microcytic anemia, low serum iron and ferritin level, thrombocytosis	Iron
Macrocytic anemia, low vitamin B_{12} and folate level, increase serum methylmalonic acid, and homocysteine level	Vitamin B_{12} or folate
Hypokalemia	Potassium and magnesium malabsorption
Low blood urea nitrogen, creatinine and albumin	Protein malnutrition
Low serum calcium and vitamin D level, high serum alkaline phosphatase	Calcium, vitamin D, fat, and magnesium
Elevated INR	Vitamin K and fat malabsorption
Low carotene level	Vitamin A

cm), the loss of bile salt may exceed the liver's ability to compensate with increased synthesis, and, hence, treatment with bile salt-binding resins often worsens diarrhea[12] (in this case, steatorrhea). Definitive treatment comprises the administering of exogenous bile acids. Synthetic preparations are preferred as they are resistant to bacterial deconjugation by colonic flora that can contribute to secretory diarrhea.

In the absence of fat or bile acid malabsorption, diarrhea may be secondary to rapid transit of contents through the intestine. Nonspecific antidiarrheal medications help prolong the intestinal transit time and increase rectal sphincter tone (Table 12.4). Dosages of these medications may need to be titrated with careful

TABLE 12.3
List of Tests to Confirm Malabsorption of Specific Substrate

Test	Result
Protein malabsorption	Generally not performed due to technical difficulties
Alpha-antitrypsin fecal clearance	Suggest protein-losing enteropathy as a cause for protein malabsorption
Carbohydrate malabsorption	After 25 g of D-xylose ingestion, failure of blood
D-xylose absorption test	D-xylose levels to rise above 20 mg/100 ml at 1 hour and above 22.5 mg/100 ml at 3 hours, or failure of urinary output to exceed 4.5 g in 5 hours suggests carbohydrate malabsorption secondary to proximal intestinal dysfunction;[17] falsely positives in diabetes mellitus, renal insufficiency; false negative in small bowel bacterial overgrowth
Oral glucose, sucrose, lactose tolerance test	Similar to D-xylose test
Breath hydrogen tests	Greater than 10–20 ppm breathe hydrogen after ingestion of specific carbohydrate substrate is consistent with malabsorption;[18] false positive in bacterial overgrowth; false negative in hydrogen nonexcretors (18% of population)
Fat malabsorption	It is very simple to perform, but commonly the result of
Qualitative fecal fat excretion	this test is equivocal, and can have false positive secondary to medication usage (orlistat, mineral oil, etc.)
Quantitative fecal fat excretion (48–72 hour stool collection)	Test is more accurate for fecal fat analysis, but difficult to perform; mainly used for fat malabsorption follow-up study; adherence to an 80- to 100-g/daily fat diet is required
Near infrared reflectance analysis of fecal fat[19]	Not used commonly, but may be the test of choice in future
Vitamin B$_{12}$ malabsorption	It is mainly used to evaluate function of ileum in patients
Schilling test	with diarrhea or malabsorption
Bile acid malabsorption	
Quantitative fecal bile acid excretion	"Gold standard," but difficult to perform
SeHCAT (selenium-75-labeled taurohomocholic acid) test	Sensitive indicators of ileal bile acid malabsorption, but difficult to perform;[20] false positive in diarrhea
Bacterial overgrowth test	These tests are performed more commonly. Every test
14C-glycocholic acid breath test	performed in this category works on the principle that
14C-xylose breath test	bacterial overgrowth will metabolize nutrients more
Glucose (lactose) breath hydrogen test	rapidly, and would release substrates, which would be absorbed and expired, but these tests have low sensitivity and specificity
Quantitative culture of jejunal aspirate (>105 CFU/ml)	"Gold standard" test for this diagnosis

(continued)

TABLE 12.3 (CONTINUED)
List of Tests to Confirm Malabsorption of Specific Substrate

Test	Result
Tests for exocrine pancreatic insufficiency	Low concentration in presence of steatorrhea is
Stool chymotrypsin concentration	suggestive of pancreatic insufficiency
Fecal elastase test	Low level of stool elastase is sensitive only for advance state pancreatic insufficiency
Serum trypsinogen level	Although not specific, but very low level <20 ng/ml is sensitive for pancreatic insufficiency
Secretin/CCK tests (direct pancreatic stimulation)	Complex analysis, but more accurate test; performed only at a few centers

attention to potential adverse effects, such as dry mouth, urinary retention, dizziness, and drowsiness.

12.5.2 CORRECTION OF NUTRITIONAL DEFICIENCIES

An important goal of managing patients with malabsorption is detecting the early and often subtle signs of nutrient malabsorption. The individual with malabsorption also must be monitored for signs of dehydration and loss of calories. Malabsorption of dietary fat can lead to deficiency of fat soluble vitamins (A, D, E, and K), which often occur in a cluster. Diffuse ileal disease can lead to deficiency of one or more water soluble vitamins. Iron and folic acid supplementation are usually required in celiac disease.[13] Calcium and magnesium supplementation are required after extensive small intestinal resection or in any setting where there is severe fat malabsorption.

The daily requirement of vitamins and nutrients, along with common manifestations of deficient states are given in Table 12.5. Patients with ongoing malabsorption and deficient states may require nutrient supplementation with several times the daily requirement to replete body stores. For example, patients with gastric resection and Whipple's procedure are at increased risk for iron, vitamin D, and calcium deficiency, which can lead to metabolic bone disease. Weekly doses of 50,000 IU of vitamin D administered for four to six weeks is required to replete levels and attenuate cortical bone loss. Serum levels of 25(OH) vitamin D, calcium, and parathyroid hormone levels should be checked following the initial supplementation and annually thereafter along with bone mineral density of the hip and lumbar spine.[14]

12.5.3 TREATMENT OF UNDERLYING DISEASE AND DIET MODIFICATION

Dietary restrictions can prove beneficial in alleviating diarrhea in patients with malabsorption. Specific dietary restriction varies with the underlying conditions as follows.

- Gluten-free diet in celiac sprue.
- Fat restriction in exocrine pancreatic insufficiency.

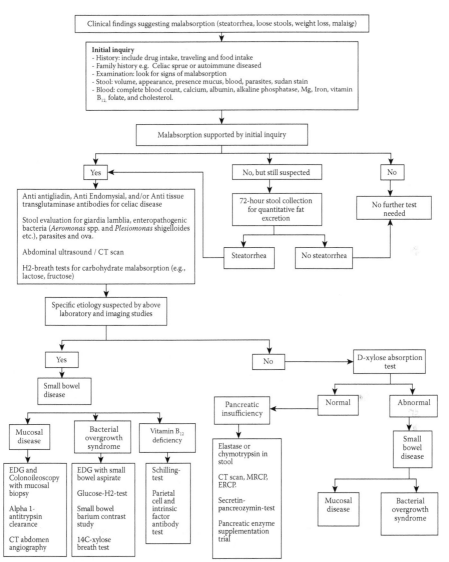

FIGURE 12.1   Diagnostic algorithm for evaluation of malabsorption. (From Porter, R. (Ed.). *Merck Manual of Diagnosis and Therapy*, 18th ed. Hoboken, NJ: John Wiley & Sons, 2008. With permission.)

- Removal of a particular carbohydrate from the diet in patients with isolated disaaccharidase deficiencies (lactose intolerance, fructose intolerance).
- Consumption of daily calories in six small meals in patients with rapid intestinal transit.
- Patients with steatorrhea, who have an intact colon, benefit from a diet restricted in long chain triglycerides (e.g., most of the dietary fat). Medium chain triglycerides (in coconut oil) do not require bile salts for absorption and are a useful caloric supplement in these patient populations.

TABLE 12.4

List of Medicines Commonly Used for Treatment of Diarrhea

Medications and Dosages

Antidiarrheals

Diphenoxylate/ Atropine (*Lomotil*) 2.5 mg/.025 mg tab PRN, maximum daily dose 8 tabs

Loperamide (*Imodium*) 2 mg capsule, maximum daily dose 16 mg

Deodorized Tincture of Opium: 0.6 ml Q4H PRN

Pancreatic enzyme supplements

Viokase, Creon, Pancrease, etc.:25,000–40,000 units of lipase with meals; titrate as needed

Bile salt-binding resins

Cholestyramine: 4 to 8 gm in divided doses; max daily dose 24 gm

Colestid (*Colestipol*) 2 to 16 gm per day in divided doses

Bile salt supplements

Cholyl sarcosine (synthetic preparation): 2 to 4 gm with meals

Dessicated ox bile (available without prescription)

Similarly, resolution of symptoms can be achieved by treating specific disease processes causing malabsorption:

- Antibiotics, such as rifaximin, a poorly absorbed antibiotic to treat bacterial overgrowth.[15]
- Oral 5-ASA, corticosteroids, anti-TNF (tumor necrosis factor) to treat Crohn's disease.
- Long-term antibiotics (tetracycline) and folic acid for six months to treat tropical sprue Supplements, such as B_{12}, iron, and other vitamins may also be needed.[16]
- Protease and lipase supplements are helpful in pancreatic insufficiency.
- Proton pump inhibitor (PPI) therapy and surgical resection of sporadic gastrinoma in Zollinger–Ellison syndrome.
- Long-term antibiotics (e.g., trimethoprim-sulphamethoxazole for one year) to treat Whipple's disease.

The goal of management is maintaining adequate nutritional status with oral intake while avoiding parenteral nutrition. Some patients may require nutritional supplements if they are unable to maintain ideal body weight. Management of chronic malabsorption can be challenging and requires multiple attempts at dose adjustments of medications and dietary modifications before arriving at a successful regimen.

TABLE 12.5
Daily Recommended Dose Supplement of Nutritional Substrates

Nutrient	RDA /AI	Manifestations of Deficiency State
Vitamin A	900 μg/d	Night blindness
		Follicular hyperkeratosis
Vitamin D		
20–49 yrs	5 μg/d (200 IU)	Osteomalacia /osteoporosis
50–69 yrs	10 μg/d (400 IU)	(Monitor serum 25(OH) vitamin D levels
> 70 yrs	15 μg/d (600 IU)	during replacement)
Vitamin E	15 mg/d	Spinocerebellar ataxia
		Myopathies
Vitamin K	120 μg/d	Petechiae ecchymosis
Vitamin B_{12}	2.4 μg/d	Anemia (megaloblastic)
		Peripheral neuropathy
Folate	400 μg/d	Anemia (megaloblastic)
Vitamin B_6	1.3–1.7 mg/d	Seborrhoeic dermatitis
		Atrophic glossitis
		Angular cheilitis
Niacin	14–16 mg/d	Dermatitis
		Pellagra (diarrhea, dermatitis, and dementia) in severe cases
Thiamine	1.1–1.2 mg/d	Peripheral neuropathy
		Encephalopathy
Riboflavin	1.1–1.3 mg/d	Angular cheilitis
		Scaly dermatitis
Iron		
Females 18–50 yrs	18 mg/d	Anemia
> 51 yrs	8 mg/d	Koilonychia ("spoon nails")
Males	8 mg/d	
Calcium		Tetany
Males and females	1000 mg/d	Muscle weakness
20–50 yrs	1200 mg/d	Fractures
> 51 yrs		Osteoporosis
Magnesium	300–400 mg/d	Required for normal calcium levels
Zinc	8–11 μg/d	Acrodermatitis
Selenium	55 μg/d	Osteoarthropathy
		Mental retardation (deficiency extremely rare in United States)
Copper	900 μg/d	Anemia
		Pancytopenia
		Peripheral neuropathy
		Ataxia

REFERENCES

1. Phillips, SF. The growth of knowledge in human digestion and absorption. *Gastroenterology* 1997;112:1404.
2. Riley, SA, Marsh, MN. Maldigestion and malabsorption. In *Gastrointestinal and Liver Disease*. Feldman, M, Scharschmidt, BF, Sleisenger, MV (Eds), WB Saunders, Philadelphia 1998, p. 1501.
3. Jeppesen, PB, Mortensen, PB. The influence of a preserved colon on the absorption of medium chain fat in patients with small bowel resection. *Gut* 1998;43:478–83.
4. Marcuard, SP, Albernaz, L, Khazanie, PG. Omeprazole therapy causes malabsorption of cyanocobalamin (vitamin B_{12}), *Ann of Int Med*. 1 Feb 1994;120;3:211–15.
5. McKie AT, Barrow D, Latunde-Dada GO, Rolfs A, Sager G, Mudaly E, Mudaly M, Richardson C, Barlow D, Bomford A, Peters TJ, Raja KB, Shirali S, Hediger MA, Farzaneh F, Simpson RJ. An iron-regulated ferric reductase associated with the absorption of dietary iron. *Science*. 2001 Mar 2;291(5509):1755–59. Epub 2001 Feb 1.
6. Romano TJ, Dobbins JW. Evaluation of the patient with suspected malabsorption. *Gastroenterol Clin North Am* 1989;18:467.
7. Harewood GC, Murray JA: Approaching the patient with chronic malabsorption syndrome. *Semin Gastrointest Dis* 1999;10:138.
8. Abdelshaheed NN, Goldberg DM. Biochemical tests in diseases of the intestinal tract: their contribution to diagnosis, management, and understanding the pathophysiology of specific disease states. *Crit Rev Clin Lab Sci*. 1997;34:141. (PMID: 9143817)
9. Beers MH Berkow, R. *The Merck Manual of Diagnosis and Therapy*, 18th ed., Robert Porter (Ed). Hoboken, NJ: John Wiley & Sons, 2008. Available at: http://www.merck.com/mmpe (accessed on October 1, 2009).
10. Bruno MJ;,Haverkort EB;,Tytgat GN;,van Leeuwen DJ. Maldigestion associated with exocrine pancreatic insufficiency: implications of gastrointestinal physiology and properties of enzyme preparations for a cause-related and patient-tailored treatment. *Am J Gastroenterol* 1995 Sep; 90(9):1383–93.
11. Schiller LR. Management of diarrhea in clinical practice. *Rev Gastroenterol Disorders* 2007;(suppl 3):S27–38.
12. Hofman AF, Poley JR. Role of bile acid malabsorption in pathogenesis of diarrhea and steatorrhea in patients with ileal resection. *Gastroenterology* 1972;62:918.
13. Johnston SD, Watson RG, McMillan SA, McMaster D, Evans A. Preliminary results from follow-up of a large-scale population survey of antibodies to gliadin, reticulin and endomysium. *Acta Paediatr Suppl* 1996 May;412:61–64.
14. Basha B, Rao S, Han ZH, Parfitt M. Osteomalacia due to vitamin D depletion: a neglected consequence of intestinal malabsorption. *American Journal of Med*. 2000 Mar;108:296–300.
15. Quigley EM, Quera R. Small intestinal bacterial overgrowth: roles of antibiotics, prebiotics, and probiotics. *Gastroenterology*. 2006;130:S78–90. (PMID: 16473077)
16. Nath SK. Tropical sprue. *Curr Gastroenterol Rep*. 2005;7:343–49. (PMID: 16168231)
17. Casellas F, Malagelada JR. Clinical applicability of shortened D-xylose breath test for diagnosis of intestinal malabsorption. *Dig Dis Sci* 1994;39:2320.
18. Simren M, Stotzer PO: Use and abuse of hydrogen breath tests. *Gut* 2006;55:297–303.
19. Stein, J, Purschian, B, Bieniek, U, et al. Near-infrared reflectance analysis: a new dimension in the investigation of malabsorption syndromes. *Eur J Gastroenterol Hepatol* 1994;6:889.
20. Merrick, MV. Gallbladder and colonic retention of SeHCAT: A re-evaluation. *Eur J Nucl Med* 1994;21:988.

13 Total Parenteral Nutrition
Theory and Application in Hospitalized Patients

Dominic Reeds

CONTENTS

13.1 INTRODUCTION

Most hospitalized patients are able to meet their nutritional needs through voluntary consumption of a regular diet. Determining which hospitalized patients may benefit from nutrition support (NS) is challenging. This chapter will provide guidance in the assessment of nutritional status, macronutrient requirements, the use of total parenteral nutrition (TPN), and clinical cases. Where possible, these suggestions have been made using evidence-based medicine; however, for many issues in nutrition support, there are no prospective clinical trials to provide guidance and, thus, conclusions have to be drawn from a synthesis of the literature.

13.2 NUTRITIONAL ASSESSMENT

There are no simple, clinically available methods for accurately determining nutritional status in hospitalized patients. Practitioners are forced to rely on surrogate measures, many of which lack objective data to support their use.

13.2.1 PLASMA PROTEINS

Plasma protein markers have been purported to reflect nutritional state since the 1950s.[1] The value of these measurements may be as prognostic factors rather than measures of nutritional status.[2,3] Plasma albumin and prealbumin concentration are affected by many clinical factors including inflammation, hepatic and renal function, clinical acuity, and fluid shifts[4] making interpretation impossible. Further, calorie or protein restriction in healthy patients does not appear to affect the plasma concentration of albumin and prealbumin. Patients who undergo bariatric surgery maintain normal plasma albumin concentration despite up to 35% weight loss[5] and patients with anorexia nervosa typically have normal concentrations of plasma proteins despite very low body mass index (BMI). At this time, the plasma concentration of albumin and prealbumin concentration should not be used to determine "nutritional status" or to guide changes in protein or calorie delivery in patients receiving NS.

13.2.2 BODY WEIGHT

Body weight is also often used as a surrogate measure of nutritional status. It is often assumed that patients who have a low BMI (<18.5 kg/m^2) are underweight and are at greater risk for development of complications related to malnutrition. Similarly, patients who are overweight or obese are often felt to be at low risk for developing malnutrition due to large energy stores in adipose tissue. It is clear that obese people are normally able to tolerate starvation for longer periods of time than leaner patients. A 70 kg (154.3 lb) man provided fluids and electrolytes has sufficient fat stores to tolerate ~60 days of fasting before death, whereas the longest documented case of a supervised fast is that of an obese patient who fasted for 382 days without complications.[6] BMI is not always accurate in identifying patients with malnutrition. Extremely obese patients with excessively rapid weight loss (for example, through gastric bypass with complications) may have signs and symptoms consistent with severe malnutrition despite being obese. While measurement of body weight would seem to be a simple measurement, it is often unreliable in a hospital setting due to rapid changes in body fluid status and methods of weighing (bed weight versus bedside weight).

Weight change may be the most helpful clinical measure. Clinical data indicates that an unintentional weight loss of >10% in the six months prior to hospitalization is associated with worse clinical outcomes.[7] It is not clear, however, whether this is because of malnutrition itself or whether weight loss is a surrogate marker of more severe or chronic underlying illness. Nevertheless, it is reasonable to regard patients with an unintentional weight loss of more than 10% in the six months prior to hospitalization as at increased risk of complications and to consider earlier use of NS in this setting.

13.2.3 SUBJECTIVE GLOBAL ASSESSMENT

This process involves the combination of a focused history and physical exam to assess recent macronutrient intake and the impact that macronutrient deficiency has had on body composition and function.[8] The findings from this assessment rank patients as well nourished, moderately malnourished, or severely malnourished. These criteria may predict the likelihood of developing postoperative complications.[8] Again, it should be noted that these medical complications may not be due directly to malnutrition or modified by institution of TPN, but rather identify patients at greater risk of morbidity and mortality.

13.3 MACRONUTRIENT NEEDS

Prior to considering the use of any form of nutrition support, it is critical to understand caloric requirements and macronutrient needs. In adults, caloric needs are determined primarily by basal metabolic rate, which represents the number of calories that are required to meet the energetic needs of maintaining homeostasis (e.g., brain activity, heart contraction). In most people, activity makes only a minor contribution (~20%) to daily energy expenditure. Daily resting energy expenditure may be estimated by a predictive equations, the most widely used of which is the Harris–Benedict (HB) equation:[9]

Men: 66 + (13.7 × weight in kg) + (5 × height in cm) – (6.8 × age in years)

Women: 665 + (9.6 × weight) + (1.8 × height) – (4.7 × age)

The energy expenditure of a noncritically ill adult with a BMI of 20 to 25 kg/m^2 may be estimated by adding 10 to 20% to the HB equation to account for activity, and results in an energy requirement of 25 to 30 kcal/kg/day. Providing excessive amounts of calories increases the risk of metabolic abnormalities including hyperglycemia, hyperlipidemia, and acidosis, and the risk of infectious complications. In critically ill adults, it is especially important to minimize the risk of overfeeding and TPN should provide calories equal to, or perhaps less than that predicted by HB. Government guidelines suggest that energy expenditure be increased by 300 kcal/day during pregnancy.[10]

13.3.1 EFFECT OF CHANGES IN BODY WEIGHT

As patients become progressively more obese, most of the weight gain (75%) is adipose tissue and only a minor component is skeletal muscle. Both adipose tissue and skeletal muscle have relatively low energy requirements compared to visceral tissues. While resting, energy expenditure increases with increasing adiposity, the number of calories per kg body weight per day actually *declines*. Therefore, in obese patients, an adjusted body weight should be used to prevent overfeeding:

Adjusted body weight = ideal body weight + (actual ideal body weight × 0.25)

In patients who are underweight, the majority of body weight is made up of lean, metabolically active tissue, so while their absolute daily energy expenditure is lower than that of a larger person, the relative number of calories per kg body weight per day *increases* as BMI becomes smaller. A patient with a BMI <15 kg/m^2 may have energy requirements of 35 to 45 kcal/kg/day or 300 to 500 kcal greater than that predicted by HB. Energy needs supplied by TPN may be determined using BMI-based regimens.[11]

13.3.2 PROTEIN REQUIREMENTS

Critically ill patients may lose up to 1% of their lean body mass per day[12] and the primary goal of NS is to attenuate these losses. The amount of protein that is required by a patient is dependent upon endogenous needs (determined by the amount of lean body mass), exogenous protein losses (e.g., chylothorax, nephrotic syndrome), and clinical status. Protein requirements should be calculated on the basis of ideal body weight (IBW), even in obese patients. In healthy patients, 0.8 g/kgIBW/day of protein will meet estimated protein needs for ~98% of the population. Most hospitalized patients should receive protein intake of 0.8 to 1.5 g/kgIBW/day; however, several common clinical conditions increase protein requirements including hemodialysis (1.2 to 1.4 g/kg IBW/day) and peritoneal dialysis (1.3 to 1.5 g/kgIBW/day). The number of nonprotein calories supplied also affects protein needs. As caloric intake declines (such as in hypocaloric feeding), protein needs increase, and it is critical to remember that if the decision is made to feed a patient hypocalorically that protein intake should be liberalized (up to 2 g/kg IBW/day). Providing more than 1.5 g/kgIBW/day of protein per day does not appear to attenuate negative nitrogen balance in most hospitalized patients who are being fed eucalorically.[12] Protein intake may need to be restricted in patients with chronic renal failure who are not being dialyzed, acute renal failure (0.8 to 1.0 g/kg IBW/day) and in patients with hepatic encephalopathy.[11] Patients who have exogenous protein losses (e.g., chylothorax , surgical drains) should have the daily volume and the concentration of protein in fluid losses measured to estimate additional protein needs.

13.3.3 FAT

Adipose tissue is the largest energy storage depot in adults and during illness these lipids are mobilized to supply fuel to vital organs. It is recommended that patients receive more than 5% of total daily calories from fat to prevent deficiency of the essential fatty acids linoleic and linolenic acid.[13] At a minimum, 2% of total energy should be obtained from linoleic acid and 0.5% from linolenic acid.[11]

13.3.4 CARBOHYDRATE

There is no absolute requirement for carbohydrate because glucose can be synthesized from precursors including glycerol and gluconeogenic amino acids. Most body tissues rely on fatty acid oxidation during starvation; however, several body tissues including bone marrow, white and red blood cells are dependent on glucose. Glycogen stores are exhausted in ~24 hours of starvation and, subsequently, hepatic gluconeogenesis is increased and insulin sensitivity is reduced to promote sparing of glucose for glucose-requiring tissues. Insulin resistance promotes release of gluconeogenic amino acids from skeletal muscle and hydrolysis of triglycerides to release fatty acids and glycerol. During prolonged periods of starvation, the kidneys and liver are the major sources of glucose and patients with renal or hepatic dysfunction are at increased risk of life-threatening hypoglycemia.

13.4 PARENTERAL NUTRITION

In patients who are unable to receive enteral feeding, parenteral nutrition may be a life-saving intervention. It is often not clear when TPN should be initiated because it is not known when negative caloric balance becomes clinically harmful. While cross-sectional studies suggest that failure to meet caloric needs is associated with worse outcomes,[14] it is not clear whether the caloric deficit itself contributes to morbidity or more likely whether failure to tolerate feeding is a predictor of poorer outcomes. Conversely, some data suggests that in obese patients, caloric restriction (permissive underfeeding) during critical illness may be beneficial, causing shorter ICU stays and reduced antibiotic use.[15] The period of time that each patient will tolerate starvation is highly variable and depends on body fat reserves, muscle mass, weight history, and clinical scenario. Parenteral nutrition is generally initiated when a patient with normal body weight has been, or it is anticipated will be, unable to meet 25% of their energy intake for 10 to 14 days; however, there is no prospective data to support this cutoff.

13.4.1   TPN Solutions

TPN solutions provide macro- and micronutrients, trace elements, and vitamins to meet the estimated needs of each patient. In general, these solutions are provided as a single bag that contains all of these substrates.

13.4.1.1   Amino Acid Formulation

Most standard TPN solutions contain amino acids at a concentration between 3 and 15%, at a ratio of ~50:50 between "essential" and "nonessential" amino acids. Most commercially available formulas lack the nonessential amino acids glutamine, glutamate, aspartate, asparagine, tyrosine, and cysteine. It is not known whether this deficiency affects the efficacy of TPN. Modified formulations of TPN have been marketed for use in patients with specific disease states, such as solutions with greater amounts of branched-chain amino acids for patients with hepatic encephalopathy or greater amounts of essential amino acids for patients with renal dysfunction. These formulations allow for provision of greater amounts of protein without development of encephalopathy in patients with severe underlying liver disease.[16] The benefit of TPN supplemented with essential amino acids in patients with renal failure may not necessarily provide clinical benefit.[17]

13.4.1.2   Carbohydrate

Most TPN formulations provide carbohydrate in the form of 5 to 30% dextrose. As the dextrose is provided as dextrose monohydrate, it provides 3.4 kcal/gram. Infusion of dextrose stimulates insulin release, inhibits lipolysis, suppresses the release of amino acids from skeletal muscle, and may be "protein-sparing," reducing amino acid oxidation.

13.4.1.3   Fat

TPN provides lipid as a fat emulsion with the lipids from soy or safflower oil. These lipids provide sufficient linoleic and linolenic acid to prevent fatty acid deficiency. These fatty acids form lipid micelles that are similar in size to chylomicrons. Recent focus[18] has been placed on the importance of large particle sizes in these emulsions as particles greater than 1 μm are associated with poorer clearance, and greater uptake by the reticuloendothelial system, possibly promoting fat buildup in end organs and immune dysfunction.[19] Lipid infusion allows minimization of calories provided as carbohydrate, which may help prevent development of hyperglycemia and lower the risk of respiratory acidosis.

Lipid infusion is associated with a number of medical complications including pulmonary syndromes,[20] impaired immune function,[21] and hypersensitivity reactions which may be fatal[22] and should not be infused at a rate of greater than 1 kcal/kg/hour to lessen the chances of complications. Lipid infusion may aggravate hypertriglyceridemia, especially in patients with preexisting hyperlipidemia and a plasma lipid profile should be measured during TPN infusion. If plasma triglycerides are >400 mg/dl before institution of TPN, interventions should be taken to treat this condition prior to institution of lipid-containing TPN.

13.4.2 TPN Use

Prior to providing TPN, a full clinical and biochemical assessment of the patient should be made including current nutritional status and medical co-morbidities. Close attention should be paid to conditions that affect glucose and lipid metabolism. Biochemical measurement should include a basic metabolic profile, calcium, glucose, phosphorous, and plasma triglyceride concentration. Body weight and fluid balance should be monitored daily.

13.4.2.1 TPN Regimens

It is impossible to provide a uniform prescription for TPN that is suitable for all patients. In general, the first step is to estimate the number of calories that the patient will require. Sufficient lipid (9 kcal/g) is provided to meet approximately 30% of total daily calories. Amino acid (4 kcal/g) needs are calculated based on ideal body weight and co-morbidities. The remaining calories are then provided as carbohydrate (3.4 kcal/g).

In patients who are believed to be at low risk of refeeding syndrome (normal body weight without a recent history of significant weight loss or calorie restriction) and are at low risk for development of volume overload, TPN may generally be initiated at goal calories infused over a 24-hour period. The duration of infusion of TPN may be tapered to infuse over a 12-hour period in most patients, with close attention to hyperglycemia, hyperlipidemia, and observation for development of heart failure. Blood sugars should be monitored before and at regular intervals during infusion of TPN, with a goal of <150 mg/dl. If during titration of TPN, the blood glucose (BG) is consistently >200 mg/dl, then the rate of TPN infusion should not be increased until glycemic control has been achieved. In patients with type 1 diabetes, insulin may be added to the TPN fluid at a ratio of 1 unit/15 g of carbohydrate. Higher doses may be necessary in patients with type 2 diabetes, critical illness, or receiving medications that lower insulin sensitivity. If patients require an additional corrective dose of insulin during TPN, half of this amount of insulin should be added to the following days TPN. A plasma triglyceride concentration greater than 400 mg/dl during TPN infusion requires either reduction in the rate of lipid infusion or removal of lipid altogether.

13.4.2.2 Catheter Care

Careful attention should be paid to the central catheter, with dressing changes every 24 to 48 hours. A 0.22 μm filter should be used in line with lipid-free TPN, and a 1.2 μm filter should be used with lipid-containing TPN. These filters should be changed whenever the TPN is changed. (*Note*: **TPN should not be disconnected and then restarted for any reason.**) TPN should not be infused through central lines placed in the groin because of the high risk of infection. Patients receiving TPN should be monitored by a nutrition support team as this reduces complications.[23]

13.4.2.3 Complications

TPN is not a risk-free intervention. It carries a clear risk of infection and should be used cautiously in immunocompromised patients (e.g., chemotherapy, neutropenia, renal failure). Long-term TPN is associated with development of many complications including liver failure. The risk of TPN-associated liver disease is greatest in patients with (1) short residual intestinal length, (2) excess caloric delivery, (3) patients receiving continuous (noncycled) TPN, and (4) inability to consume any oral feeding. TPN is also associated with a number of metabolic abnormalities including osteoporosis, hyperglycemia, hyperlipidemia, and fluid and salt overload.[24,25]

13.5   CASE STUDIES

13.5.1   Case 1

A 72-year-old woman is admitted to the general hospital ward with a week-long history of abdominal pain. She lives with her husband who says she has had a good appetite. Her past medical history is significant for type 2 diabetes, hypertension, coronary artery disease, dyslipidemia, and obesity. On admission, she is receiving lisinopril, hydrochlorthiazide, glipizide, simvastatin, and aspirin. She smokes 1 pack per day and drinks socially. On exam, she is obese, 5 feet, weight 100 kg (220 lb), blood pressure (BP) 140/100, pulse (P) 110, respiratory rate (RR) 22, temperature (T) 38.9° C (102° F). Her jugular venous pressure is elevated. Her abdomen is diffusely tender. A CT scan demonstrates a colonic mass with complete obstruction. She undergoes a colectomy with ileostomy placement. After 24 hours, she is still unable to eat because of persistent nausea and vomiting. A nasogastric tube is placed with improvement in symptoms. A request is made by the surgical service for NS evaluation and consideration of TPN.

13.5.1.1   Management Plan

The initial question is whether TPN will benefit the patient. TPN is not risk free in this clinical setting as diabetics have a significantly greater risk of central line associated gram-negative infections than nondiabetics.[26] A record of the patients weight history would be helpful, as while she is obese, it is possible that she had lost greater than 10% of her body weight. A clinical assessment should be made to determine volume status, and to assess for any other potential sources of protein loss, such as nephrotic syndrome, given her diabetes. If surgical drains are present, then the daily volume and protein content of the drainage should be measured.

It is commonly believed that (1) metabolic rate is dramatically increased by critical illness or trauma and (2) routine use of perioperative NS in patients who are unable to eat after surgery improves outcomes. Several studies suggests that in the absence of burn injury, head trauma, or the use of sympathomimetic medications, energy expenditure is not significantly increased in critical illness or with infection.[27,28] It has yet to be proved that patients who undergo surgical procedures, who had good preoperative nutritional status benefit from routine use of TPN, and data suggests that conservative care with intravenous (IV) fluids alone may be the best treatment. One prospective study randomized 300 patients undergoing major elective surgery to either TPN beginning within 24 hours of surgery or intravenous fluids containing ~500 kcal/day as dextrose.[29] Each regimen was continued until patients were either able to voluntarily meet their caloric needs or until day

15. There was no difference in clinical outcomes between the two groups. When patients who received TPN were grouped with those who were randomized to TPN, but were unable to tolerate goal feeding rates, mortality appears to have been greater in the TPN group. These data suggest that in patients in whom it is predicted will not be able to eat for up to 15 days, routine use of TPN is of no benefit. Furthermore, patients who are unable to tolerate goal TPN rates are at increased risk of poor outcomes.

On the basis of the Case 1 patient's obesity, stable preoperative weight history, and lack of significant protein losses, TPN is not recommended at this time and enteral feeding should be initiated when able.

13.5.1.2 Follow-Up Evaluation

The patient undergoes diuresis and conservative management. Evaluation reveals only trace proteinuria. After receiving maintenance intravenous fluid and electrolytes for a further 10 days, the patient continues to have a postoperative ileus and fails to tolerate attempts at enteral feeding. The surgical team requests "aggressive" TPN because the patient has been in negative caloric balance and there is concern that this increases the risk of poor outcome.

13.5.1.3 Management Plan

It is not unreasonable to consider TPN in a patient who has been unable to eat for 10 days; however, again it is unlikely that even a further delay in feeding will result in poorer outcomes. Negative caloric balance has been shown in some studies to be predictive of poorer clinical outcomes in hospitalized patients, with the greatest impact in the first week after the insult,[14] this may be an associative rather than a causative relationship.

The goal of TPN in this patient should be to minimize negative nitrogen balance. Providing calories in excess needs increases the risks of hyperglycemia, hyperlipidemia, hepatic steatosis, metabolic acidosis, and a greater risk of infectious complications. Hypocaloric feeding(i.e., permissive underfeeding) could permit mobilization of the patient's endogenous lipid stores, improve insulin sensitivity, and lower the risk of metabolic complications.[27] Cross-sectional studies indicate that providing between 33 and 67% of predicted energy expenditure is associated with improved clinical outcomes in critically ill patients.[30] Prospective studies have shown that hypocaloric feeding in obese, critically ill patients does not result in worse clinical outcomes and may reduce antibiotic usage, probably by lowering hyperglycemia and infection risk.[15] Providing additional amounts of protein to patients receiving hypocaloric diets appears to minimize loss of lean body mass. Providing ~10 to 12 kcal/kg adjusted body weight per day as TPN with 1.5 to 2 g of protein per kg ideal body weight and 30% of calories from fat would be a reasonable initial TPN regimen. Prolonged periods (>two to three weeks) of hypocaloric feeding should be used cautiously in critically ill patients as this intervention has not been shown to be beneficial for extended periods of time. Blood sugars should be optimized prior to initiating TPN to prevent severe hyperglycemia. Given preexisting type 2 diabetes, providing at a ratio of 1 unit of insulin for every 10 grams of carbohydrate in the TPN will lower the risk of hyperglycemia.

13.5.2 CASE 2

An 82-year-old man is transferred to your hospital from a local nursing home after suffering a stroke. He was found in bed that morning with new onset dysarthria and confusion. According to the nursing home records, the patient had stable body weight prior to transfer. His past medical history is remarkable only for hypertension and Alzheimer's disease. He takes hydrochlorthiazide and aspirin. He never smoked or drank alcohol. On exam, he is 5 feet 6 inches tall and weighs 70 kg (154 lb); BP 150/94, P 80, RR 12, T 37° C (98.6° F). He is dysarthric, but in no apparent distress. He has poor dentition. His neck veins are flat. Lungs are clear. He is normally ambulatory, but is currently confined to bed. His basic metabolic profile and CBC are unremarkable. His son, who is an internist, requests that his father receive early nutrition because he believes that this improves outcomes in hospitalized patients who are unable to eat.

While early nutrition support is probably indicated in patients with low body weight, it is not clear that early nutrition support itself improves outcomes in hospitalized patients. Recent studies have shown that early protocols to raise the awareness of the role of early nutrition in ICUs have indeed shortened the time span between admission and initiation of NS, but no benefit in outcomes occurred.[31] The FOOD trial randomized patients, who suffered a stroke causing dysphagia, to early enteral nutrition using a nasogastric (NG) tube or late placement (~seven days after admission).[32] As anticipated, the early NG tube placement group received enteral feeding earlier than the late group and had slightly improved mortality rates. Unfortunately, the degree of severe morbidity (requiring 24-hour care) was greater in the early group, corresponding to almost exactly the number of people who may have benefited from early feeding. On the balance of the data, it is unlikely that early enteral nutrition will improve the outcome in this patient, and could increase the risk of complications including GI bleeding or aspiration. It is unlikely that TPN will provide clinical benefit and may increase the risk of infectious complications. The preferred treatment may be to provide supportive care including intravenous fluids, but not feeding enterally until the prognosis is more clear.

13.5.3 CASE 3

You are asked to provide care to a 22-year-old white female who is admitted for anorexia nervosa. She reports that she consumes 600 kcal per day and exercises on a treadmill for one hour per day. She uses alprazolam and caffeine to suppress her hunger. She denies shortness of breath or swelling, but does feel cold. She has no significant past medical history other than prior admissions for anorexia. On exam she appears cachectic; she is 5 feet 2 inches, weighs 34 kg (75 lb), BMI 14.1, P 40, RR 12, T 35° C (95° F). Her jugular venous distention (JVD) is not elevated, heart sounds are distant, point of maximal impulse (PMI) is the fifth intercostal space at the anterior axillary line. Laboratory studies are remarkable for a sodium of 132 mEq/L, potassium of 3.2 mEq/L, glucose of 42 mg/dl, albumin of 4.3 g/dl, hematocrit of 28% with a mean corpuscular volume of 72 uL. You are consulted for management.

13.5.3.1 Management

In order to understand management, an understanding of the changes in body composition, organ function, and substrate metabolism is necessary. This patient is at high risk of refeeding syndrome given her low body weight and chronic starvation.[33] This syndrome, which was initially reported in concentration camp victims, has been reported in patients with starvation who receive aggressive refeeding. This is manifested with a lowering of serum potassium and magnesium when carbohydrate is provided, due to an influx of these salts from the plasma into the intracellular compartment, and is exacerbated by increases in plasma insulin concentration. Ventricular tachyarrhythmias and sudden death are common in patients with extremely low BMI and may be preceded by QT prolongation.[34] The patient should receive an EKG and be monitored on telemetry. Also plasma phosphate concentration often declines dramatically following refeeding in malnutrition due to use in the synthesis of ATP. This may be manifested with EKG abnormalities, muscle weakness including heart failure, and diaphragmatic weakness precipitating respiratory failure.[35-37] Glucose intolerance is common in patients who are suffering from starvation. Prolonged starvation results in hypoglycemia, promotes lipid mobilization with increased dependence on fatty acids, and preservation of glucose for use by glucose-requiring organs. Carbohydrate should be used as necessary to prevent hypoglycemia, but patients should be closely monitored for subsequent hyperglycemia.[38] Fluid management may be challenging in starving patients. Prolonged caloric restriction may be accompanied by a dilated cardiomyopathy with low cardiac mass, low stroke volume, and bradycardia. This may be confounded by a reduction in renal mass inhibiting the ability to excrete a free water load. Further, hyperinsulinemia during refeeding promotes sodium resorption and places these patients at high risk for developing volume overload and pulmonary congestion.[39] Loss of subcutaneous adipose tissue places patients at risk of hypothermia and bedsores from loss of cushioning over bony prominences. All patients should receive intravenous thiamine prior to refeeding to prevent development of Wernicke's encephalopathy.[40]

13.5.3.2 Management Plan

Initial treatment should focus on cautious replacement of necessary fluid and electrolytes with close attention to the prevention of development of volume overload. Patients should receive multivitamins through the intravenous route to ensure adequate absorption. All patients should receive 100 mg of thiamine to prevent the development of Wernicke's encephalopathy after carbohydrate administration.

If the patient is willing, enteral nutrition (EN) should be provided as this allows for more gradual absorption of electrolytes. TPN may be provided if the patient is unwilling or unable to tolerate EN. Patients should receive intermittent, isotonic feeds to prevent fasting hypoglycemia and also overwhelming the ability of the body to metabolize the caloric load. Repletion of potassium and phosphorous should also be made, preferably through the enteral route. Clinicians should be cautious in repletion of these electrolytes because while total body stores are depleted, as these nutrients are buffered in lean body mass, rapid infusions may cause dangerous increases in serum levels of these electrolytes.

The precise formulation of EN or TPN is widely variable from patient to patient so that a universally applicable prescription is not possible, but several key features should be noted. After ensuring that patients are euvolemic, fluid should be restricted to ~800 ml above insensible losses to prevent heart failure. Unless sodium losses are high (e.g., diuretic abuse), sodium should be restricted to ~88 meq (2 g) per day. Body weight should be measured daily as weight gain of greater than 0.25 kg/day or ~1.25 kg/week is suggestive of fluid overload. Caloric delivery should initially be ~15 to 20 kcal/kg/day containing 100 g of carbohydrate to meet the needs of glucose-requiring tissues. Magnesium, phosphorous, and potassium should also be repleted in patients with normal renal function. Close attention should also be made to ensure that patients do not suffer from hypo/hyperthermia and to prevent development of bedsores. Calories may be advanced at up to 200 kcal/day if electrolyte and volume status remain acceptable.

13.5.4   CASE 4

You are asked to provide recommendations for nutritional management of a 62-year-old man with HIV who is admitted with community-acquired pneumonia. The patient had a week-long history of malaise, fever, cough, and shortness of breath. His symptoms persisted despite prescription of oral antibiotics. He has responded slowly to antibiotics over the last 10 days, but subsequently developed *clostridium difficile* colitis. He has been treated with metronidazole orally; however, he has had profound nausea accompanying this therapy. He is now unable to eat due to persistent nausea and has refused nasogastric tube placement. Due to his prolonged period of inanition, the admitting team has requested use of TPN. The patient denies recent weight loss. His past medical history is remarkable for HIV for 15 years, hypertension, and hypertriglyceridemia. He has gained approximately 120 lb after beginning HAART (antiretroviral drug therapy) eight years ago. He reports loss of limb and facial fat, but gain in trunk fat over the last five years. His hypertriglyceridemia has been severe with triglyceride concentrations of 500 to 1000 mg/dl despite fibrate therapy. He does not smoke or use alcohol and denies recreational drug use. On exam, he appears comfortable. He is 5 feet 8 inches, weighs 90 kg (198 lb), BP 130/74, RR 20, T 36.7⁰ C (98° F). He has facial lipoatrophy and prominent veins on his arms and legs. He has darkly pigmented axillary skin. He has diffuse rhonchi with apical wheezes. He has abdominal obesity, but no striae, with a liver edge 4 cm below the right costal margin. His laboratory studies reveal a blood sugar of 250 mg/dl, a white blood cell count of 17,000. His lipid profile reveals a plasma triglyceride concentration of 750 mg/dl, HDL 24 mg/dl, LDL 100 mg/dl.

13.5.4.1   Management

In order to determine how this patient should be managed, it is important to understand the metabolic changes that are seen in patients with HIV. Prior to the availability of HAART, patients with HIV had a progressive course of weight loss with elevated metabolic rate and lipolytic rate, and hypertriglyceridemia, the "HIV wasting syndrome."[41] While use of HAART has improved mortality due to infectious complications, more than 50% of patients develop metabolic abnormalities including loss of adipose tissue on the limbs and/or face (lipoatrophy), gain in trunk fat (lipohypertrophy), hypertriglyceridemia, low plasma HDL, lipid accumulation in the liver (hepatic steatosis), insulin resistance, and skeletal muscle loss.[42–45] This patient has many features of this HIV metabolic syndrome and, as such, is at risk for hyperglycemia and hypertriglyceridemia. Prior to considering TPN in this patient, blood glucose and triglycerides should be brought into control to lower the risk of pancreatitis. Use of an infusion of glucose and insulin to achieve euglycemia will suppress fat release and may rapidly improve hypertriglyceridemia. Discussions should be made with the patient regarding the risks of TPN, in particular the risk of infection given the insulin resistance and hyperglycemia. While the patient is not at immediate risk of development of complications due directly to insufficient calorie intake, it is not unreasonable to consider the use of TPN. If TPN is initiated, he should initially be fed hypocalorically given his obesity and hyperglycemia. Patients with HIV-metabolic syndrome have a reduced capacity to suppress proteolysis during hyperinsulinemia, and are probably at increased risk of loss of lean body mass with hypocaloric feeding,[46] so protein intake should be 2 g/kgIBW/d. Insulin should be added to the TPN regimen at a ratio of 1 unit for every 10 g of carbohydrate. He should initially receive continuous TPN, as infusing the TPN over a shorter period of time may overwhelm the ability of the body to dispose of glucose. Plasma triglyceride concentration should be measured while receiving TPN.

13.5.5 CASE 5

A 45-year-old man with no significant past medical history undergoes endoscopic retrograde pancreatography to evaluate for episodic abdominal pain. Soon after the procedure he develops epigastric abdominal pain. A serum lipase level is elevated and CT reveals pancreatitis. You are consulted by the primary team to provide management recommendations, specifically whether TPN is necessary. On exam, he is afebrile and in moderate distress. His BMI is 27 kg/m2, pulse 110, afebrile, RR 12. On exam, his abdomen is moderately tender.

13.5.5.1 Management

Most patients with mild or moderate acute pancreatitis using Ranson's criteria do not require NS and merely require analgesia and intravenous fluids. Clinical care generally involves preventing oral feeding to minimize pancreatic stimulation. Occasionally, small bowel feeding tubes are placed beyond the ligament of treitz to provide enteral feeding into the jejunum. Several studies have shown that jejunal feeding can be safely given to select patients with pancreatitis, even those with severe disease.[47–49] TPN does not appear to confer clinical benefit in patients with mild or moderate pancreatitis and may increase the risk of bacteremia.[47,49,50] Several trials have compared jejunal tube feeding to TPN.[47–49] In patients with mild or moderate pancreatitis, clinical outcomes showed no difference between jejunal feeding and TPN.[47] Indeed, some data suggest that outcomes may actually be better with jejunal feeding than TPN.[48] While providing ~30% of calories as lipid to patients with pancreatitis appears to be safe and may cause less hyperglycemia, exacerbation of pancreatitis with lipid infusion has been reported.[51] Hypertriglyceridemia is common in patients with pancreatitis, and should be controlled prior to initiation of

TPN. It is likely that this patient will have only mild pancreatitis and he should be managed conservatively. If his symptoms persist and his pancreatitis remains mild or moderate, jejunal feeding should be considered to reduce his risk of complications from TPN.

REFERENCES

1. Rhoads, J. and C.E. Alexander, *Nutritional problems of surgical patients.* Annals NY Acad Sci, 1955. **63**: p. 268–275.
2. Ferguson, R.P., et al., *Serum albumin and prealbumin as predictors of clinical outcomes of hospitalized elderly nursing home residents.* J Am Geriatr Soc, 1993. **41**(5): p. 545–9.
3. Kaysen, G.A., et al., *Trends and outcomes associated with serum albumin concentration among incident dialysis patients in the United States.* J Ren Nutr, 2008. **18**(4): p. 323–31.
4. Klein, S., *The myth of serum albumin as a measure of nutritional status.* Gastroenterology, 1990. **99**(6): p. 1845–6.
5. Seres, D.S., *Surrogate nutrition markers, malnutrition, and adequacy of nutrition support.* Nutr Clin Pract, 2005. **20**(3): p. 308–13.
6. Stewart, W.K. and L.W. Fleming, *Features of a successful therapeutic fast of 382 days' duration.* Postgrad Med J, 1973. **49**(569): p. 203–9.
7. Dewys, W.D., et al., *Prognostic effect of weight loss prior to chemotherapy in cancer patients. Eastern Cooperative Oncology Group.* Am J Med, 1980. **69**(4): p. 491–7.
8. Detsky, A.S., et al., *Evaluating the accuracy of nutritional assessment techniques applied to hospitalized patients: methodology and comparisons.* JPEN J Parenter Enteral Nutr, 1984. **8**(2): p. 153–9.
9. Harris, J.A. and F.G. Benedict, *Standard basal metabolism constants for physiologists and clinicians*, in *The Carnegie Institute of Washington. A biometric study of basal metabolism in man.* 1919, Lippincott: Philadelphia.
10. Gibney, M., H. Vorster, and F. Kok (Eds.) *Introduction to Human Nurition.* 2002, Oxford, U.K.: Blackwell, p. 333.
11. Klein, S. , *A primer of nutritional support for gastroenterologists.* Gastroenterology, 2002. **122**(6): p. 1677–87.
12. Griffiths, R.D., *Muscle mass, survival, and the elderly ICU patient.* Nutrition, 1996. **12**(6): p. 456–8.
13. Barr, L.H., G.D. Dunn, and M.F. Brennan, *Essential fatty acid deficiency during total parenteral nutrition.* Ann Surg, 1981. **193**(3): p. 304–11.
14. Villet, S., et al., *Negative impact of hypocaloric feeding and energy balance on clinical outcome in ICU patients.* Clin Nutri, 2005. **24**(4): p. 502–9.
15. Dickerson, R.N., et al., *Hypocaloric enteral tube feeding in critically ill obese patients.* Nutrition, 2002. **18**(3): p. 241–6.
16. Naylor, C.D., et al., *Parenteral nutrition with branched-chain amino acids in hepatic encephalopathy. A meta-analysis.* Gastroenterology, 1989. **97**(4): p. 1033–42.
17. Kopple, J.D., *The nutrition management of the patient with acute renal failure.* JPEN J Parenter Enteral Nutr, 1996. **20**(1): p. 3–12.
18. Driscoll, D.F., *The pharmacopeial evolution of intralipid injectable emulsion in plastic containers: From a coarse to a fine dispersion.* Int J Pharm, 2008. **368**(1–2):193–8.
19. Olivecrona, G. and T. Olivecrona, *Clearance of artificial triacylglycerol particles.* Curr Opin Clin Nutr Metab Care, 1998. **1**(2): p. 143–51.
20. Skeie, B., et al., *Intravenous fat emulsions and lung function: a review.* Crit Care Med, 1988. **16**(2): p. 183–94.

21. Seidner, D.L., et al., *Effects of long-chain triglyceride emulsions on reticuloendothelial system function in humans*. JPEN J Parenter Enteral Nutr, 1989. **13**(6): p. 614–9.
22. Hiyama, D.T., et al., *Hypersensitivity following lipid emulsion infusion in an adult patient*. JPEN J Parenter Enteral Nutr, 1989. **13**(3): p. 318–20.
23. Nehme, A.E., *Nutritional support of the hospitalized patient. The team concept*. JAMA, 1980. **243**(19): p. 1906–8.
24. Daly, J.M. and J.M. Long, III, *Intravenous hyperalimentation: techniques and potential complications*. Surg Clin North Am, 1981. **61**(3): p. 583–92.
25. Klein, G.L. and J.W. Coburn, *Parenteral nutrition: effect on bone and mineral homeostasis*. Annu Rev Nutr, 1991. **11**: p. 93–119.
26. Sreeramoju, P.V., et al., *Predictive factors for the development of central line-associated bloodstream infection due to gram-negative bacteria in intensive care unit patients after surgery*. Infect Control Hosp Epidemiol, 2008. **29**(1): p. 51–6.
27. Jeejeebhoy, K.N., *Permissive underfeeding of the critically ill patient*. Nutr Clin Pract, 2004. **19**(5): p. 477–80.
28. Raurich, J.M., et al., *Resting energy expenditure during mechanical ventilation and its relationship with the type of lesion*. JPEN J Parenter Enteral Nutr, 2007. **31**(1): p. 58–62.
29. Sandstrom, R., et al., *The effect of postoperative intravenous feeding (TPN) on outcome following major surgery evaluated in a randomized study*. Ann Surg, 1993. **217**(2): p. 185–95.
30. Krishnan, J.A., et al., *Caloric intake in medical ICU patients: consistency of care with guidelines and relationship to clinical outcomes*. Chest, 2003. **124**(1): p. 297–305.
31. Doig, G.S., et al., *Effect of evidence-based feeding guidelines on mortality of critically ill adults: a cluster randomized controlled trial*. JAMA, 2008. **300**(23): p. 2731–41.
32. Dennis, M.S., S.C. Lewis, and C. Warlow, *Effect of timing and method of enteral tube feeding for dysphagic stroke patients (FOOD): a multicentre randomised controlled trial*. Lancet, 2005. **365**(9461): p. 764–72.
33. Solomon, S.M. and D.F. Kirby, *The refeeding syndrome: a review*. JPEN J Parenter Enteral Nutr, 1990. **14**(1): p. 90–7.
34. Isner, J.M., et al., *Anorexia nervosa and sudden death*. Ann Intern Med, 1985. **102**(1): p. 49–52.
35. Silvis, S.E. and P.D. Paragas, Jr., *Paresthesias, weakness, seizures, and hypophosphatemia in patients receiving hyperalimentation*. Gastroenterology, 1972. **62**(4): p. 513–20.
36. Weinsier, R.L. and C.L. Krumdieck, *Death resulting from overzealous total parenteral nutrition: the refeeding syndrome revisited*. Am J Clin Nutr, 1981. **34**(3): p. 393–9.
37. Hayek, M.E. and P.G. Eisenberg, *Severe hypophosphatemia following the institution of enteral feedings*. Arch Surg, 1989. **124**(11): p. 1325–8.
38. Wyrick, W.J., Jr., W.J. Rea, and R.N. McClelland, *Rare complications with intravenous hyperosmotic alimentation*. JAMA, 1970. **211**(10): p. 1697–8.
39. DeFronzo, R.A., et al., *The effect of insulin on renal handling of sodium, potassium, calcium, and phosphate in man*. J Clin Invest, 1975. **55**(4): p. 845–55.
40. Mattioli, S., et al., *Wernicke's encephalopathy during total parenteral nutrition: observation in one case*. JPEN J Parenter Enteral Nutr, 1988. **12**(6): p. 626–7.
41. Nahlen, B.L., et al., *HIV wasting syndrome in the United States*. Aids, 1993. **7**(2): p. 183–8.
42. Reeds, D.N., et al., *Alterations in lipid kinetics in men with HIV-dyslipidemia*. Am. J. Physiol Endocrinol.Metab, 2003. **285**: p. E490–E497.
43. Reeds, D.N., et al., *Alterations in liver, muscle, and adipose tissue insulin sensitivity in men with HIV infection and dyslipidemia*. Am J Physiol Endocrinol Metab, 2006. **290**(1): p. E47–E53.

44. Yarasheski, K.E., et al., *Insulin resistance in HIV protease inhibitor-associated diabetes.* J Acquir. Immune. Defic. Syndr., 1999. **21**(3): p. 209–16.

45. Carr, A., et al., *A syndrome of peripheral lipodystrophy, hyperlipidaemia and insulin resistance in patients receiving HIV protease inhibitors.* Aids, 1998. **12**(7): p. F51–8.

46. Reeds, D.N., et al., *Whole-body proteolysis rate is elevated in HIV-associated insulin resistance.* Diabetes, 2006. **55**(10): p. 2849–55.

47. McClave, S.A., et al., *Comparison of the safety of early enteral vs. parenteral nutrition in mild acute pancreatitis.* JPEN J Parenter Enteral Nutr, 1997. **21**(1): p. 14–20.

48. Windsor, A.C., et al., *Compared with parenteral nutrition, enteral feeding attenuates the acute phase response and improves disease severity in acute pancreatitis.* Gut, 1998. **42**(3): p. 431–5.

49. Kalfarentzos, F., et al., *Enteral nutrition is superior to parenteral nutrition in severe acute pancreatitis: results of a randomized prospective trial.* Br J Surg, 1997. **84**(12): p. 1665–9.

50. Sax, H.C., et al., *Early total parenteral nutrition in acute pancreatitis: lack of beneficial effects.* Am J Surg, 1987. **153**(1): p. 117–24.

51. Lashner, B.A., J.B. Kirsner, and S.B. Hanauer, *Acute pancreatitis associated with high-concentration lipid emulsion during total parenteral nutrition therapy for Crohn's disease.* Gastroenterology, 1986. **90**(4): p. 1039–41.

14 Home Nutrition Support

Carol Ireton-Jones and David S. Seres

CONTENTS

14.1 INTRODUCTION

Enteral and parenteral nutrition are utilized in the hospital when patients cannot take adequate nutrients orally, but require nutrition to support or improve their nutritional status. With hospital stays decreasing in length or patients actually initiating nutrition support therapy without hospitalization, provision of enteral nutrition (EN) and parenteral nutrition (PN) in the home is a very real and viable option for completing a course of nutrition support or as lifetime therapy. The American Society for Parenteral and Enteral Nutrition (ASPEN) has developed guidelines that specifically address the application of home specialized nutrition support (HSNS), stating that HSNS should be used in patients who cannot meet nutrient needs orally and who are able to receive therapy outside of an acute care facility.[1] Additionally, these guidelines state that if HSNS is required, home EN is the preferred route when feasible. However, home PN should be used when the gastrointestinal (GI) tract is not functional or EN/oral intake insufficient to meet nutritional needs. It is also feasible to provide dual therapies, EN and PN in tandem, to achieve nutrient goals.

There is very little randomized controlled data to draw upon to develop specific HSNS recommendations and guidelines. Therefore, much of this chapter is based on the extensive experience of the authors caring for this population and can be considered Level V data—case series, uncontrolled studies, and expert opinion—as used in the newest combined Society of Critical Care Medicine (SCCM) and ASPEN guidelines.[2] The reader should understand that, in the absence of referenced randomized controlled studies, the contents are meant as suggestions. While this chapter focuses primarily on adult care, references are provided for pediatric practitioners as well.

Prior to initiating home PN or EN, there are some key components to assess. These include the patient's and caregiver's ability to manage these therapies at home, the reimbursement options for the patient, and the safety of the home environment. While the technology is certainly available for providing these therapies at home, complications are frequent in the period just after discharge and may be due to the disease process more so than the nutrition therapy.[3] Care must be taken to assure appropriate patient selection and ensure that the selected patient and their caregivers are aware of the responsibilities that are part and parcel of home EN or PN.

HSNS can be initiated at home, bypassing the hospital. Patients who may be candidates include those with oncologic diagnoses, certain GI conditions, or hyperemesis gravidarum. A careful evaluation of the patient's clinical status, biochemical status, and potential response to therapy are particularly important in these patients.[4] When HSNS is started at home, calories should be kept at a minimum for the first several days and increased to goal once tolerance is established. HSNS patients started at home on PN should initially receive a formula containing a low concentration of dextrose, which is increased slowly over the ensuing days for up to one week.

14.2   HOME ENTERAL NUTRITION

Indications for home EN are the same as those applied to hospitalized patients: inability to meet nutritional needs by mouth for an extended period and without contraindication. Typical diagnoses include head and neck cancer, stroke or other neurological disease associated with dysphagia, and gastrointestinal diseases, such as Crohn's disease, short bowel syndrome, or pancreatitis. The presence of significant gut dysfunction does not necessarily rule out the use of the intestine for home EN if proper access is obtained and symptoms and absorption problems are aggressively and successfully managed. This may provide a greater challenge when initiating EN in the outpatient setting. Many more people than previously thought may be managed with home EN, especially in partnership with an experienced home nursing service. It is unusual, however, that home nursing services related to home EN are covered by insurance. This continues to present a challenge in managing complex patients.

It is important to carefully evaluate for a treatable cause for deficient intake prior to considering home EN. A careful review of systems might elicit treatable symptoms. Nausea should be distinguished from symptoms of gastroparesis. In the latter, patients often report vomiting without much warning as well as postprandial bloating or pain. Antinauseants frequently do not help patients with gastroparesis, and prokinetic agents are very poor at treating nausea.[5] Although, if a patient is on maximal antinauseants without resolution of vomiting, a prokinetic agent may be considered. Similarly, constipation and diarrhea can both add to eating difficulties. It is also important to ask the patient whether their sense of taste and smell are intact. For example, the loss of the sense of taste may suggest zinc deficiency.[6] The quality of the food available may make a large difference in intake. Many medications can decrease appetite and affect gastric emptying as well.

Elderly patients are frequently considered for home EN. It is often the case that intake may be optimized with hand feeding. Aspiration is rarely an indication for tube feeding in this population unless the patient is frankly choking. Because disallowing oral intake and initiating EN in patients with aspiration is not believed to decrease the incidence of aspiration pneumonia, the proper indication for home EN is that these patients are not meeting their nutritional needs. Attention to feeding techniques is extremely important in all home EN situations, but especially with fragile patients at risk for aspiration. Patients demonstrated to have swallowing dysfunction should receive a thorough evaluation by a qualified speech pathologist with a request to provide advice on the safest feeding methods as well as evaluation by an otolaryngologist.

14.2.1 ENTERAL ACCESS

Access for home EN is best achieved using a permanent or semipermanent device, such as a gastrostomy or jejunostomy. It is frequent that a home nursing agency, or skilled nursing home for that matter, will reject patients with a temporary nasogastric or nasoenteric tube. If the patient is ambulatory, a gastrostomy is usually preferred so that nourishment may be given in discrete boluses, allowing the patient a maximum of independence and time off the feeding. Some patients with jejunostomies are able to tolerate slow bolus feeds, but these are generally thought to be easier with gastrostomies. Gastrostomies and jejunostomies are both acceptable for infusion feeding (i.e., feeding via a pump), but patients with jejunostomies tend to be less tolerant of concentrated feeding products. Diarrhea may occur as well, particularly if a concentrated feed is used (see below).

14.2.2 FORMULAS

Standard feeding formulas are generally adequate for most patients. Disease-specific feeding products have very limited usefulness and can increase the cost for the feeding product as much as 15-fold. Unless fluid or electrolyte restriction is needed, concentrated and/or renal formulas are not necessary. A moderately concentrated (1.5 kcal/ml) feed may help shorten the delivery time in bolus feeding. As mentioned, concentrated feeds are hypertonic and may be less well tolerated as boluses or when fed into the small bowel. Dialyzed patients are unlikely to benefit and may be harmed by protein restriction. When potassium and phosphorus levels are difficult to control, an electrolyte-restricted formula may be helpful. Hepatic and pulmonary formulas have not proved to improve outcomes.

14.2.3 Initiation of Home EN

Patients tolerating in-hospital EN should be carefully assessed for their ability to manage the feeding process independently at home. If they are unable, or are likely to be too ill, a family member must be available to administer the feeds. Outpatient placement of feeding devices is acceptable, but confirmation by x-ray is strongly recommended before feeding is initiated.

Bolus or nocturnal infusions are the most commonly used feeding schedules for home EN. Gastric access is most appropriate for bolus feeding, but slow bolus feeds have been tolerated in the small bowel. The total daily feeding volume is divided into two to five sessions. Bolus feeds may be administered by gravity or by pump, and may be the initial feeding method when gastric emptying dysfunction is not suspected. One method for bolus feeds utilizes a 60 ml catheter-style syringe, with the piston removed, as a funnel. The syringe is connected to the end of the enterostomy tube and formula and water are poured into the syringe in aliquots. A feeding session using this method should take 15 to 30 minutes. Most patients will tolerate approximately 750 ml at each session (500 ml of feeding product and 250 ml of water). When overfullness and intolerance to volume is encountered, a prokinetic agent should be considered. Gravity bolus feeds may be administered by attaching a feeding bag to the enterostomy and allowing the feed to run in by gravity as well. This usually takes longer, but has the advantage of being relatively hands-free.

Pump infusions may be necessary in patients with jejunostomies and/or marginal gastric emptying. Scheduling the feeding is flexible and should be individualized. Infusions may be given over a range of approximately 8 to 24 hours depending on tolerance and convenience. It is commonly thought that an overnight feed yields maximal daytime freedom. But nocturnal feeds may disrupt sleep when the infusion needs attention (feeding bags do not usually exceed one liter) or when nocturia is induced. With the availability of portable infusion pumps, a daytime-only schedule, in fact, may be preferable. Further, a daytime schedule may make glycemic regulation easier.

Initiating EN for the first time in the home setting should not be done in the absence of a responsible observer because vomiting and aspiration may occur. In the authors' experience, it is more often the case that patients are admitted for nutrition- or hydration-related problems and feeds are initiated during the hospitalization. Feeding goals should be discussed with a nutrition practitioner and there is generally no hurry achieving the goal rate. There are many approaches to assessing tolerance and increasing rates. It is recommended that rates and incremental increases be more conservative in the home setting if the patient is bedbound or gastric dysfunction suspected. A reasonable approach might include starting feeding at 30 to 50% of goal and then increasing by 30 to 50% every day or two. Technical aspects of home EN should be explained well, such as assuring the head of the bed is elevated to 30 degrees and that the proper care and administration techniques are adhered to by the patient or caregiver.

Severely malnourished patients are at risk for refeeding syndrome characterized by hypokalemia, hypophosphatemia, and hypomagnesemia.[7] For these patients, initial feeding goals should be very conservative, for example, 15 to

20 kcal/kg of current weight, until electrolyte stability and tolerance are established. It is suggested that laboratory testing be performed after one to two days, and as often as daily if needed until stable. If there is concern, hospital EN initiation may be preferable. The lack of coverage for home nursing for EN makes home initiation all the more challenging for complex patients. Refeeding syndrome is even more critical in the home PN patient and will be discussed later in this chapter.

14.2.4   Role of the Hospital and Home Clinicians

Proper in-hospital preparation and training of the patient and/or caregivers prior to discharge is crucial. A multidisciplinary assessment should include analysis of the home situation, insurance coverage for feeding product, and the ability for the patient or family to administer EN. Discharge planners should ensure that provisions for continuity of care are in place and communicated to the outpatient provider, particularly when the patient is being discharged from a teaching or hospitalist service that does not provide postdischarge care. Referral to an academic center and/or nutrition support specialist, such as a registered dietitian, should be considered when the home EN issues are complex.

14.2.5   Monitoring of Home EN

Patients receiving home EN should be monitored for tolerance of the feeding, bowel function, weight, and hydration. Monitoring frequency should be individualized, should be more frequent in the initiation period, may be decreased over time given stability, and may be accomplished by phone if there is a reliable patient or caregiver in the home. If the potential for refeeding syndrome is suspected, laboratory testing will be important during the initiation of EN, and longer term for fluid balance and electrolyte disturbances. The monitoring that the patient will receive is often dependent on the home provider of the EN supplies and formula. If a durable medical equipment (DME) company (also called a home medical equipment [HME] company) is providing these, monitoring may consist of assuring that adequate supplies are ordered and delivered because a nutrition support clinician is usually not involved. A home infusion agency that also provides home PN will more likely provide closer clinical monitoring. Therefore, when choosing a provider, it is important to determine who will monitor these patients at home and what type of monitoring will be provided.[8]

14.2.6   Complications of Home EN

As discussed above in Section 14.2.5, life-threatening electrolyte disturbances may occur with the initiation of feeding (by any modality) in severely malnourished patients and, in particular, those with preexisting electrolyte deficiencies.[4,7] In-hospital initiation may be a safer approach for these patients.

Because normal thirst is often bypassed or depressed, dehydration is a serious concern in home EN patients. Standard feeding products are maximally 85% water.

Water supplementation during tube feeding serves two purposes: (1) in addition to hydration, frequent flushing of the feeding tube decreases the risk for clogging, and (2) adequate hydration further prevents constipation. Acidic fluids, such as soda and cranberry juice, should be avoided as routine flushing with these may increase the risk for clogging.

Intolerance to bolus feeding in patients with gastrostomies is quite frequent. Symptoms of overfullness and bloating are most common. The stomach is pulled anteriorly and tacked to the abdominal wall when the tube is placed. This may cause gastric emptying dysfunction. Clinicians caring for a patient on gastric home EN should be careful to screen for these symptoms. Prokinetic agents, such as metoclopramide, are very helpful in treating these symptoms.[5]

Diarrhea is a frequent accompaniment to tube feeding. Often multiple feeding products are tried without benefit. The most frequent cause is either medications or the concentration of the feeding product.[9] Patients receiving home EN are often receiving antibiotics and prokinetics, both known to cause diarrhea. Medications, such as H2 blockers and proton pump inhibitors given to decrease acid secretion, are notorious for causing diarrhea and often overlooked as causative in these patients. Feeds that are hypertonic (greater than 380 mOsm/l) are more likely to cause diarrhea, especially when infused into the small bowel. Finally, the vehicle for any medication given in a liquid form is often 70% sorbitol. Sorbitol is a nonabsorbable sugar that acts as an osmotic agent to increase the water content of the stool. It is very useful in treating constipation in these patients, but can also cause diarrhea if enough is consumed.

14.2.7 LONG-TERM COMPLICATIONS

Despite placement of feeding devices, patients receiving home EN will frequently lose significant amounts of weight due to recurrent mild intolerance causing feeding interruptions. Care must be taken to palliate all gastrointestinal symptoms. Many of the long-term complications of home EN result from problems with the feeding device. When patients gain weight, the abdominal wall thickens. If the bolster holding the enterostomy tube in place is not loosened, tissue around the device will die and the ostomy will enlarge. This causes leakage and is difficult to manage. Alternatively, the bolster may become embedded in the skin, a so-called "buried bumper."[10] An enlargement of the ostomy also may occur in patients if the enterostomy tube is pressed to the side, especially in slender patients.

14.3 HOME PARENTERAL NUTRITION

Parenteral nutrition is indicated for patients who are unable to intake or absorb adequate nutrients enterally. Common diagnoses associated with home PN include short bowel syndrome, bowel obstruction, enterocutaneous fistula, radiation enteritis, and intractable nausea or vomiting.

For hospitalized patients, PN may be used for a relatively short period of time to accommodate a nonfunctioning small bowel due to an acute injury or episode with recovery of bowel function and return to an oral diet prior to discharge. However, in many cases, the recovery of bowel function is impeded or extended and, therefore, the acute episode may be complete and the patient ready for discharge, yet requiring PN for adequate nutrient intake. Patients who require a continuation of their PN therapy or will require long-term or lifetime support, such as patients with short bowel syndrome, are candidates for home PN therapy. As mentioned previously, a multidisciplinary assessment of each patient's clinical status, home environment, and insurance coverage is essential in the discharge process for home PN. A caregiver must be present especially in the early stages of home PN management to assist with all of the logistics of managing the PN therapy and supplies at home.

In preparation for home PN, appropriate access must be obtained. Central parenteral nutrition (CPN), that is PN infused into a large vein, usually the superior vena cava, is most commonly used for patients both in the hospital and at home. Peripheral parenteral nutrition (PPN) is available for both care settings, but is not readily applicable to the home care setting in that it is a short-term therapy (usually less than two weeks) and infused through a midline catheter with limitations on fluids and solution osmolality. Options for intravenous access for home PN are listed in Table 14.1.

14.3.1 TRANSITIONING TO HOME

Patients receiving PN in the hospital are ready to transition to the home care setting when they are clinically and medically stable. Typically, a home infusion provider will organize the home infusion needs for the patient and meet the patient at home with supplies for the infusion therapy on the day of discharge. Patient education regarding administration of the therapy at home should begin in the hospital and culminate on

TABLE 14.1
Venous Access Devices

Device	Location	Needle Skin Puncture Required for Access	Usual Durability	Benefits
Hickman (Tunneled cuffed catheter)	Under skin and exit site	No	Months to years	Infections can often be treated without removing device
Port	Under skin	Yes	Months to years	No exit site
PICC	Under skin and exit site	No	Weeks to months	Inexpensive safe bedside placement possible

Source: Reprinted with permission from Coram, Inc., *Celebrate Life* newsletter.
Note: The table summarizes the characteristics, benefits, and disadvantages of each of these three types of venous access devices.

the first day home with a delivery of required supplies and the first visit by the home infusion nurse. The hospital clinicians managing the patient should provide a final discharge PN order coordinated with the home care/home infusion provider. A home infusion company may provide infusion therapies only with nursing supplied by a home health agency or may provide their own nursing. Experienced home infusion nurses are critical to the success of the home PN therapy as the education received in the hospital is put into action in the home care setting. Appropriate and thorough patient education on home PN therapy, administration of the therapy, and complication prevention (specifically excellent catheter care maintenance) is crucial.

A thorough nutrition assessment should be performed in the home setting as requirements in the hospital are different from those in the home setting. Nutrient needs may change at home as the patient may be more active and return to normal activities while being more sedentary in the hospital or may change as healing occurs. Baseline labs should be established when home PN is started and observed for trends over time. Hypoalbuminemia more often reflects the inflammatory process and is not a good indicator of nutritional status in acute care; however, trends of albumin over time may aid in the overall evaluation of response to therapy.[11]

Determining the home PN formula should take into account the goals of nutrition support (repletion versus maintenance), any preexisting disease process, and nutritional status. Further, it should take into account the patient's lifestyle at home with the goal to infuse less than 24 hours per day, usually 10 to 14 hours per day. For pediatric home PN patients, needs for both growth and development should be considered.

14.3.2 COMPONENTS OF HOME PN

Protein in the form of amino acids, fat as lipid emulsion, and carbohydrate provided as dextrose make up the macronutrients in a home PN formula. Protein requirements may be calculated on a gram per kilogram basis and usually fall into the range of 1.0 to 1.5 gram/kg of body weight (if normal weight). For extremely overweight individuals or those who are underweight, protein needs should be adjusted accordingly. An optimal ratio of protein to carbohydrate and lipid can be achieved by including 15 to 20% of total kcals as protein. Fat is provided as 25 to 30% of total kcals/day. Lipid emulsions should not exceed the 2.5 g of lipid/kg body weight/day or 60% of total kcals. Currently available commercial lipids in the United States are aqueous emulsions of soybean or safflower oil with egg phospholipid as the emulsifier. Patients with egg allergies may not tolerate lipids and should be tested prior to infusion. Lipid emulsions also contain phosphorus that may be important for patients with renal disease as well as a small amount of vitamin K. Carbohydrate serves as the primary energy source and will make up the balance of kcals after accounting for protein and fat. Dextrose in sterile water is used in PN solutions and provides 3.4 kcal/gm. When kcal requirements are balanced (15 to 20 % from protein, 25 to 30% from fat, and the balance of kcals are from dextrose), then the maximum 24-hour glucose infusion rates will be less than 7 mg/kg/minute, which is appropriate for patients with a normal glycemic response.[12] The use of glucose infusion rates to estimate optimal dextrose infusion in home infusion patients is questionable because the majority of home PN patients will receive a cyclic infusion of PN for 10 to 12 hours.

Home PN may be in the form of a Total Nutrient Admixture (TNA), which is a mixture of dextrose, amino acids, and lipids, or a "standard" solution containing amino acids and dextrose only with lipids provided by a separate pump or "piggy-backed" into the central line. Two pumps will be needed if the lipid is not mixed into the home PN and, therefore, this is an added expense and inconvenience in the home situation. Pediatric patients often require two pumps due to compatibility issues when adding lipids to the types of dextrose and amino acid solutions required for the infant or young child.[13]

Multivitamins are added by the patient or caregiver prior to infusion of home PN. The multivitamin content has been developed from standards determined by the Nutrition Advisory Group of the Department of Foods and Nutrition of the American Medical Association (NAG-AMA, 1975, revised 1985, mandated by 2004). If a patient has a documented vitamin or mineral deficiency due to disease state, previous malnutrition, or higher than normal requirements, additional supplementation of individual nutrients should be provided. It is important to monitor for adequacy to assure that the normal dosage is used after supplementation is completed. Long-term home PN patients may need specific, individual trace-element supplements due to potential elevations of copper, manganese, and chromium.[14]

14.3.3 INITIATION OF HOME PN

A majority of patients will be receiving PN in the hospital and will be transitioned from the hospital to the home. Refeeding syndrome has been addressed in this chapter, but should again be discussed in relation to the initiation of home PN. Refeeding syndrome has been defined as the "over-vigorous feeding of the severely malnourished patient." This overfeeding is not helpful and, in fact, is harmful, causing hypophosphatemia, hypokalemia, and hypomagnesemia, which if left untreated can result in serious complications including death. The optimal treatment for refeeding syndrome is prevention. If a patient has been without nutrition for some time and is malnourished, the first level of care should be replenishment of fluids and electrolytes. Then, repletion of nutritional status can occur with a low level of dextrose (100 to 150 g of dextrose) and advanced as tolerated over several days. This rehydration and repletion does not have to happen in the hospital and can be accomplished in the home with a capable home infusion provider.[4]

14.3.4 MONITORING

Home monitoring includes evaluation of laboratory data, physical assessment, as well as self-monitoring that is completed by the patient.[15,16] The frequency of monitoring should decrease as the patient is stable on home PN. A baseline complete metabolic panel, phosphorous, magnesium, and complete blood count (CBC) with differential is obtained initially as a baseline. A basic metabolic profile is needed on an ongoing basis along with specific labs as needed based on clinical status and symptoms. Individual micronutrients may be assessed if deficiency is suspected; however, interpretation of the results and development of a repletion regimen remains a challenge.[14–17] Patients also will need to self-monitor by checking their weight daily or every other day initially, then weekly checking their temperature daily initially and adhering to a glucose monitoring schedule if ordered by their physician. Catheter maintenance is of utmost importance. The physician will order the catheter-care maintenance, with the home-care nurse providing the catheter-care education to the patient. The home nursing provider should provide the catheter care until the patient or caregiver is independent and can successfully manage the care on his/her own. This can be a limiting factor to home PN because, if the patient or caregiver cannot manage the catheter care, alternatives to placement at home should be considered.

Goals of therapy should be established early in the nutrition therapy program and may need to be revised as the patient progresses. Along with observing for tolerance of the home PN regimen is the monitoring of the adequacy of home PN intake. This is particularly important as the patient is transitioning from one nutrition support modality to another (PN to EN or oral). Additionally, when home EN alone is inadequate to support nutrient needs, home PN may be used as well. This is a common occurrence with pediatric patients.[13] The challenge of dual therapies is not in the efficacy of the therapies, but in the need for two to three pumps (one to two for home PN and one for home EN) and insurance coverage for multiple therapies to accomplish the same goal. If transition back to an oral diet or to an enteral feeding is the goal, attention to adequacy of the macro and micronutrient intake during this transition is key. A registered dietitian is well qualified to manage this transition

14.3.5   Home PN Reimbursement

Most commercial payers include coverage of PN at home as a contracted benefit. Governmental payers—Medicare and Medicaid—do reimburse for home PN under specific circumstances. Medicaid reimbursement for home PN varies from state to state and benefits must be verified individually. Medicare reimbursement for home PN is complex and requires that two basic criteria be met initially and then further criteria is evaluated to assure that the therapy will be reimbursed based on clinical criteria.[18] Medicare requires the determination of permanence, which they define as the need for home PN for a long and indefinite duration, 90 days or a lifetime, *and* the presence of malabsorption of nutrients due to small intestinal malabsorption. Further criteria are used to justify the need for home PN, such as recent massive small bowel resection, short bowel syndrome, and failure of EN. One of the first steps in the referral process for home nutrition support for home PN or EN is the verification of the patient's benefits whether from commercial or a governmental payer. The hospital case manager can initiate this or the home care provider can as well upon referral. These individuals are usually highly qualified to assist the referral clinician and patient in understanding their reimbursement for therapies at home.

14.3.6   Complications

Complications of home PN can be divided into metabolic, mechanical, infectious, and psychosocial categories. Metabolic complications include hyper- or hypoglycemia, electrolyte disturbances, and fluid imbalance. Working with qualified clinicians in the home care setting can attenuate these challenges and has proved to be effective in minimizing complications.[19] When a patient is clinically at risk for electrolyte or fluid imbalance, such as a patient with a high output fistula, close clinical monitoring is essential. This includes assessment of labs and careful management of the PN formulation. If a patient is requiring daily changes to their home PN formulation, clinical stability is in question and this patient may be best managed in the hospital or an extended care facility.

Mechanical complications and venous access complications are primarily related to the home PN catheter. Vascular access device complications can be minimized by optimal choice in the venous access device to be used related to the patient's needs as well as fastidious care of the catheter.[20,21] Patients who are receiving home PN (or home EN) also may be receiving other infusion therapies, such as antiinfectives, infusion pain management, subcutaneous medications, or supplemental fluids. Initiation of an antiinfective at home to treat a suspected catheter-related infection can obviate the need for a hospitalization.[19] Assuring that the home infusion provider is well skilled in teaching catheter care techniques and monitoring for complications is of utmost importance in successful home PN therapy. One study has shown that not only does close clinical monitoring by a home nutrition support team consisting of a dietitian, nurse, and pharmacist working with the patient's physician improve clinical outcomes, but it also decreases cost.[19] Details of catheter placement and care require significant attention and are out of the scope of this chapter; however, many excellent resources are available through the American Society for Parenteral and Enteral nutrition (ASPEN: www.nutritioncare.org) and the National Home Infusion Association (NHIA: wwww.nhia.org) as well as The Oley Foundation (800-776-OLEY; www.oley.org).

Along with clinical management, psychosocial support is also essential, especially if this will be a lifetime therapy. A support group (The Oley Foundation) is available specifically for patients receiving home EN or PN and their friends and family. The Oley Foundation provides telephonic support, a newsletter, resources for individuals and families, and a network of people across the country who are also on home EN and PN. Clinicians working with patients on home EN or PN should be aware of The Oley Foundation and provide the contact information to their patients; it is a wonderful resource.

Being outside of the hospital and at home can certainly improve the quality of life of individuals who need continued nutrition therapy. Expert management at home is required and, therefore, the agency that will be providing the home EN or PN should have clinical support and expertise in home nutrition support management.

REFERENCES

1. ASPEN Board of Directors and The Clinical Guidelines Task Force. Guidelines for the use of parenteral and enteral nutrition in adult and pediatric patients. *J Parenter Enteral Nutr* 2002;26S:1SA–8SA.

2. Martindale, RD, McClave SA, Vanek VV, et al. Guidelines for the provision and assessment of nutirtion support therapy in the adult critically ill patient: Society of Critical Care Medicine and American Society for Parenteral and Enteral Nutrition: Executive Summary. *Crit Care Med* 2009;37(5):1757–1761.
3. de Burgoa LJ, Seidner D, Hamilton C, at al. Examination of factors that lead to complications for new home parenteral nutrition patients. *J Infus Nurs*, 2006:29:74–80.
4. Newton AF, DeLegge MH. Home initiation of parenteral nutrition. *Nutr Clin Pract* 2007;22:57–64.
5. Reddymasu SC, McCallum RW. Pharmacotherapy of gastroparesis. *Expert Opin Pharmacotherapy* 2009;10:469–84.
6. Heyneman, CA. Zinc deficiency and taste disorders. *Ann Pharmacother* 1996;30: 186–7.
7. Tresley J, Sheean PM. Refeeding syndrome: recognition is the key to prevention and management. *J Am Diet Assoc.* 2008;108(12):2105–8.
8. Ireton-Jones C. Home enteral nutrition from the provider's perspective *J Parenter Enteral Nutr* (Suppl.) 2002;26(5):S8–9.
9. Eisenberg P. An overview of diarrhea in the patient receiving enteral nutrition. *Gastroenterol Nurs* 2002;25:95–104.
10. McClave S, Neff R. Care and long-term maintenance of percutaneous endoscopic gastrostomy tubes. *J Parenter Enteral Nutr* 2006;30(1): S27–40.
11. Fuhrman P, Charney P, Mueller C. Hepatic proteins and nutrition assessment. *J Am Diet Assoc.* 2004;104(8):1258–64.
12. Wolfe RR, O'Donnell TF, Stone MD, et al. Investigation of factors determining the optimal infusion rate in total parenteral nutrition. *Metabolism* 1980;29(9):892–900.
13. Nguyen PC, Kerner J. Home parenteral nutrition support in pediatrics, In *Handbook of Home Nutrition Support*, Ireton-Jones C and DeLegge M (eds.). Jones and Bartlett: Sudbury, MA, 2007; 223–251.
14. Howard L, Ashley C, Lyon D, Shenkin A. Autopsy tissue trace elements in 8 long-term parenteral nutrition patients who received the current U.S. Food and Drug Administration formulation. *J Parenter Enteral Nutr* 2007;31(1):388–396.
15. Ireton-Jones C, DeLegge M, Epperson LA, et al. Management of the home parenteral nutrition patient. *Nutr Clin Prac* 2003;18:310–317.
16. Siepler J. Principles and strategies for monitoring home parenteral nutrition. *Nutr Clin Prac* 2007;22:340–350.
17. Kelly D. Guidelines and available products for parenteral vitamins and trace elements. *J Parenter Enteral Nutr* 2002;26(5):S34–36.
18. Wojtylak F, Hamilton K. Reimbursement for home nutrition support, In *Handbook of Home Nutrition Support*, Ireton-Jones C and DeLegge M (eds.). Jones and Bartlett: Sudbury, MA, 2007; 389–412.
19. Ireton-Jones C, Hamilton K, DeLegge M. Improving clinical and financial outcomes with parenteral nutrition therapy. *Support Line* 2009;31(1):23–25.
20. Sands MJ. Vascular access in the adult home infusion patient, *J Parenter Enteral Nutr* 2006;30(1):S57–64.
21. Ryder M. Evidence based practice in the management of vascular access devices for home parenteral nutrition therapy. *J Parenter Enteral Nutr* 2006;30(1):S82–93.

15 Intestinal Failure and Liver Disease Related to Parenteral Nutrition and Intestinal Transplantation

Khalid Khan

CONTENTS

15.1   INTRODUCTION

Intestinal failure refers to a patient's inability to maintain life with enteral intake. Short bowel syndrome (SBS), often used synonymously, refers to a malabsorptive state that results from functional and/or anatomic deficiencies of the small intestine. SBS is broadly dichotomous: Congenital anatomic disorders predominate in infancy, whereas intestinal disease and mechanical loss are the major causes of SBS in adults. During intestinal rehabilitation, parenteral fluid, electrolytes, and nutrients are required to sustain life. In the case of anatomic SBS, the small intestine has the ability to morphologically change (i.e., undergo adaptation) to improve function; in addition, surgical options exist for lengthening the intestine in infants.

Ultimately, some patients have no alternative but long-term parenteral nutrition (PN). Although PN is a lifesaving therapy, liver disease may develop, particularly in infants with SBS when the remaining small intestine is extremely short, if no enteral intake is possible and as their time on PN increases. Control of systemic sepsis, scrutiny of the PN content, and progress with enteral feeding may halt or even reverse liver disease, especially if the patient is able to wean off PN. Despite advances in the care of this population, the eventual outcome is poor on long-term PN, especially in infants. Transplantation of abdominal viscera, including the small intestine, makes it possible to prolong life with good quality.

15.2   INTESTINAL FAILURE AND SHORT BOWEL SYNDROME

15.2.1   Etiology

Intestinal failure is most frequently due to anatomic SBS. The most common underlying cause of SBS in adults is small intestinal Crohn's disease.[1] Other causes include a mesenteric vascular event; an infarction from arterial and venous thrombosis, from an arterial embolism, from midgut volvulus, or from complications of surgery; extensive resection after trauma or for tumor removal; and radiation injury. Complications of surgery for obesity are an increasing cause.[2]

Advances in the care of sick newborns have led to the survival of almost all infants who undergo extensive resection of the small intestine. The congenital abnormalities that give rise to most cases of anatomic SBS in infants are gastroschisis, intestinal atresia, and malrotation.[3,4] Sophisticated care of severely premature infants has increased the number of survivors, resulting in an increased proportion of infants with SBS caused by surgery for necrotizing enterocolitis. Other than SBS, intestinal failure is also caused by diffuse neuromuscular dysfunction, such as the total aganglionic form of Hirschsprung disease. Much less common causes are hollow visceral myopathy and neuropathy (e.g., pseudo-obstruction), which can affect adults or children. Diffuse mucosal disease (e.g., microvillus inclusion disease) is fatal in infancy without treatment; malabsorption can occur with polyposis.[5]

15.2.2 PREVALENCE

There is no data on prevalence of intestinal failure in the United States. Widely quoted home PN Registry data from 1992 showed that about 40,000 patients required PN each year during that era in the United States.[6] About 26% of the patients had SBS, although some with malignancy or enteritis from radiation may also have had SBS. For infants, the incidence of SBS was reported as 1,200 of 100,000 live births between 2002 and 2005.[7] Survival rates in children with SBS range from 73 to 89%, making it one of the most lethal conditions in early childhood.[3]

15.2.3 PATHOPHYSIOLOGY

In most patients with SBS, the duodenum is intact, although it may be dysfunctional in those with total aganglionosis or pseudo-obstruction. The jejunum is the site of fluid, electrolyte, and nutrient movement between the gut lumen and the vasculature. To achieve such movement, the mucosa comprises long villi and deep crypts for maximal surface area, the greatest amount of brush border enzyme activity, and large intraepithelial gap junctions. The jejunum is the major site of carrier-mediated absorption of nutrients after digestion of food and its conversion into monosaccharides, amino acids, and peptides. The ileum has relatively shorter villi and tighter gap junctions, resulting in less fluid movement, thereby allowing for better (albeit slower) nutrient absorption. Vitamin B_{12} and bile salts are absorbed through specific receptors in the ileum. Ileal absorption is enhanced by the ileocecal valve, which slows small intestinal transit and increases time spent by nutrients within the ileum. The valve prevents reflux of bacteria from the colon into the ileum. The colon has the ability to reclaim sodium, water, amino acids, and energy from bacterial fermentation of carbohydrates into short-chain fatty acids, which provide colonic mucosal cells with energy.[8,9]

Hormones that regulate secretion and motility are released from the proximal small intestine, most notably, gastrin, gastric inhibitory polypeptide, cholecystokinin, secretin, and motilin. Because the loss of intestine is distal in patients with SBS, secretion of these hormones is usually preserved. Hypergastrinemia occurs in patients with SBS from the loss of negative feedback on gastrin secretion after ileal resection.[10] Gastric acid hypersecretion may lead to peptic ulcers and esophagitis, and may impair absorption by inactivating pancreatic lipase and deconjugating bile salts. Gastric acid suppression may improve water absorption in patients with SBS.[11] The ability to secrete ileal hormones (e.g., enteroglucagon, glucagon-like peptides [GLPs] 1 and 2, peptide YY, and neurotensin) may be lost in patients with SBS.[12] In particular, peptide YY and neurotensin are responsible for the ileal "brake" effect of delaying gastric emptying and slowing intestinal transit time, especially in response to lipids in the ileum.[12,13]

15.2.4 PATHOLOGY AND CLINICAL SPECTRUM

The loss of the small intestine in patients with SBS can be primary or resection-related. Primary loss is common in infants with intestinal atresia or gastroschisis.

Functioning small intestine can be lost as a result of severe small intestinal Crohn's disease in adults, but the more likely culprit is repeated surgical resection. Small intestinal volvulus results in the removal of a variable length of jejunum and ileum. Ileocolic disease may involve removal of ileum, the ileocecal valve, and a proportion of proximal colon. The major cause of ileocolic disease in infants is necrotizing enterocolitis; in older children and adults, Crohn's disease. Most macronutrients are absorbed within the first 100 to 150 cm of jejunum in adults; marked fluid secretion in the jejunum in response to hypertonic feeding is reabsorbed, primarily in the ileum.[6,14,15] Major jejunal resection with a stoma, therefore, will result in nutrient and fluid loss—a loss further complicated by secretion of salt and fluid, which is stimulated by oral intake.[16] A shortened gastric emptying time and rapid transit in the proximal small intestine unchecked by the lack of ileal hormones results in a net secretory response to food.[17] In adults, removal of 60 cm or more of ileum may cause vitamin B_{12} deficiency; removal of 100 cm gives rise to bile salt deficiency and to fat malabsorption from loss of enterohepatic circulation.[18] At least 100 cm of small intestine is necessary in the absence of the colon to prevent intestinal failure, but 35 to 60 cm may suffice when the colon is intact.[19–21] In a pediatric study of mainly small children, patients with >15 cm of small intestine without an ileocecal valve and patients with <15 cm of small intestine with an ileocecal valve had most success at nutritional rehabilitation.[22] The plasma citrulline level is a measure of mucosal mass, therefore the length and adequacy of the remaining small intestine.[2]

Adaptation is the process of expansion of the luminal surface cell mass by which the small intestinal absorptive area increases in response to the patient's nutritional needs. Data from patients who underwent jejunoileal bypass and from animal studies indicate that the intestine lengthens and that its diameter and the height of villi increase, resulting in a larger absorptive surface[23]—a process that continues for two years or more.[24] Some aspects of adaptation occur without such morphologic changes as increased absorption of carbohydrates.[25] In animal studies, small intestinal adaptation is heralded by epithelial hyperplasia within 24 to 48 hours after intestinal resection.[26,27] Although the absorptive area increases, functional immaturity occurs, but gradually improves.[25,26,28] Some nutrients are absorbed much more quickly than others.[29] Gross morphologic change is evident by two to three weeks after intestinal resection.[30] A number of genes whose expression is altered after intestinal resection may play a role in adaptation.[31] Jejunal adaptation is limited to function while the ileum adapts anatomically and functionally resembles the jejunum.[32] The jejunum cannot adapt to absorb vitamin B_{12} after ileal loss. In general, patients with an extremely short small intestinal remnant or with a high jejunal stoma lack sufficient length for adaptation, although there are exceptions.

Data from animal studies indicate that intestinal hormones, in particular, GLP-2, contribute to adaptation.[33,34] GLP-2 is secreted from the ileum and pancreas; postprandial levels are reduced after ileal resection.[35] Animals administered GLP-2 after ileal resection have shown marked villus hyperplasia, enhanced glucose absorption, reduced intestinal permeability, and morphologic adaptive changes in jejunal remnants.[36] Subcutaneous GLP-2 or synthetic variants increase nutrient and fluid absorption.[33] The effect of hormones may be related to an effect on polyamine metabolism. Polyamines, (e.g., spermine) are produced by proliferating tissues, particularly in small intestinal epithelium.[37] Prostaglandin analogues have been shown to be trophic to cells, capable of increasing mucosal mass, and of stimulating adaptation after intestinal resection.[38] Inhibition of prostaglandin synthesis, particularly of the cyclooxygenase pathway, impedes adaptation.[39] Specific hormones may also inhibit adaptation; octreotide, a somatostatin analogue, reduces cell proliferation after intestinal resection; transforming growth factor-beta 1 reportedly inhibits intestinal cellular growth; ghrelin is reduced in patients with SBS, but leptin has been shown to increase carbohydrate absorption.[40–42]

Enteral nutrition is imperative for mucosal health and adaptation. Animal data show that, after small intestinal resection, PN gives rise to atrophy, whereas enteral intake stimulates hyperplasia.[43] The proposed mechanisms include direct stimulation through stimulated secretion of gut hormones and release of trophic secretions from the upper intestinal tract. Direct stimulation is more effective when the workload is increased, such as when the animal's body is dealing with complex (versus simple) carbohydrates.[44] The role of stimulated hormones and secretions has been elegantly described in animal models.[45,46] In animals, intravenous arginine and glutamine have been shown to reduce intestinal permeability.[47,48] Intravenous glutamine supplementation reportedly has a trophic effect on gut hypoplasia and on lamina propria plasma cells that produce immunoglobulin A; it also improves overall gut immunity.[49–51] However, enteral glutamine supplementation appears not to affect intestinal adaptation in animals.[52]

In humans, enteral glutamine improves body weight as well as fluid and electrolyte absorption when growth hormone is added.[53] Long-chain triglycerides, especially arachidonic acid, stimulate intestinal adaptation, an effect related, in part, to stimulation of ileal hormone release.[54]

15.2.5 ENTERAL NUTRITION

The care of patients with SBS includes providing adequate fluid, along with macro- and micronutrients, to prevent malnutrition and deficiency states and to circumvent dehydration and acid-base disturbances. In children and adults, an initial period of PN is warranted immediately after intestinal resection. Adults need about 25 to 35 kcal/kg/day and 1.0 to 1.5 kg/day of protein.[6] Enteral nutrition should be started as soon as possible, and then advanced, as tolerated, to a regular diet. In children with SBS, continuous, steady administration of enteral nutrition is more likely to be tolerated than bolus feeding.[55] In adults with a stoma, eating an increased amount may help maintain an adequate nutritional balance.[56] In adults, protein absorption has been shown to improve with a peptide-based diet, but no consensus exists on the benefit of using elemental supplements.[6] In infants, initial enteral feeds consist of diluted elemental formula. The normal caloric density in infants is 0.67 kcal/ml, in older children, 1 kcal/ml. Feed volume is increased as tolerated. Elemental formulas are not necessary unless formula intolerance or allergy is evident. Semielemental peptide-based formulas with a mixture of long-chain and short-chain fatty acids can be used. Long-chain fatty acids (in particular, highly unsaturated fatty acids) have a stimulatory effect on adaptation.[54] Age-appropriate solid food should be the eventual goal.

Diarrhea is often due to the osmotic load generated by malabsorbed simple carbohydrates. A further osmotic load is created by bacterial action in the colon. Continuous or small bolus feedings, therefore, enhance absorption. Replacing some carbohydrate calories with medium-chain triglycerides may help patients with SBS, especially infants. Small bowel bacterial overgrowth results from abnormal motility and anatomic changes due to intestinal resection, loss of immune tissue, and loss of the ileocecal valve. The consequences include deconjugation of bile acids, which results in increased proximal absorption and in the lack of bile salts for micelle formation and, therefore, leads to diarrhea, colitis and arthritis, D-lactic acidosis, and competitive deficiency of B_{12}, and other nutrients.[57] The usual symptoms are bloating, cramping, diarrhea, and blood loss. The diagnosis is made through a culture of duodenal fluid or a hydrogen breath test. Facultative and anaerobic bacteria are typical. The usual treatment includes broad-spectrum antibiotics. Hypergastrinemia-related fluid secretions may be reduced by histamine$_2$ antagonists. Cholestyramine for binding bile acids may be useful for diarrhea after ileal resection; however, after major resection of the small intestine, it may cause further depletion of bile acids. Other agents that can be of benefit include octreotide,[58] and loperamide or diphenoxylate (which may reduce transit time, but, at the same time, may potentiate bacterial overgrowth). Even when adequate macronutrient intake is maintained, micronutrient deficiencies can develop with either enteral nutrition or PN in patients with SBS.[6] Iron deficiency is common, although both macro- and microcytic anemia may occur. Fat-soluble vitamin deficiency is a concern in patients who have steatorrhea and problems with bile circulation. Jejunal stomas result in loss of electrolytes, particularly sodium and magnesium. Sodium replenishment is likely to be inadequate with hypotonic electrolyte solutions.[59] Patients with diarrhea are at risk for zinc and selenium deficiency, in particular.[60] Even with stomas for decompression, patients with diffuse neuromuscular disease are repeatedly disabled by massive intestinal dilatation and consequent fluid shifts. Dietary supplementation with soluble fiber (in particular, pectin) could have an effect on gut adaptation, but the major benefit of soluble fiber is increasing calories by conversion to short-chain fatty acids in the colon.[61] Careful monitoring, along with dietary restriction of oxalate, may be necessary in symptomatic patients who have lost the ileum.

15.3　LIVER DISEASE RELATED TO PN

PN, a lifesaving treatment for patients with nutritional failure, was introduced into clinical practice almost five decades ago.[62] Short-term PN has few negative consequences, but long-term PN is associated with liver and biliary tract disease, nutritional deficiency, and central venous line complications. Liver disease develops in 40 to 60% of infants with intestinal failure on long-term PN and in 15 to 40% of adults on home PN.[9] The spectrum of disease ranges from gallbladder and biliary disorders to cholestasis, hepatic steatosis and fibrosis, and end-stage liver disease. Once end-stage liver disease is established, survival at one year is only 20 to 30%.[63] Infants typically develop cholestasis, steatosis is usual for adults. Cholelithiasis and biliary sludging occur in both adults and children.[9]

15.3.1 Cholestasis

Cholestasis is the major effect of PN in infants; however, jaundice and hyperbilirubinemia are features of end-stage liver disease in adults and children on PN. Recent data have confirmed that liver disease in patients on PN is strongly associated with poor long-term survival; in a cohort study of 78 children with SBS, the survival rate of patients with cholestasis (direct bilirubin concentration >2 mg/dL) was close to 20%, as compared with 80% in those without cholestasis.[22] The mortality rate is related to the inability to wean off PN.[64] In premature infants (as compared with full-term infants and adults), the bile salt pool is small, hepatic uptake and synthesis of bile salts are poor, and ileal absorption is reduced.[65] Not surprisingly, therefore, cholestasis is associated with prematurity and low birth weight.[66] A factor in the development of cholestasis is conjugation of bile salts, which involves taurine in premature infants; sulfation is a more efficient way of solubilizing toxic bile salts, such as lithocholic acid.[67] Lithocholic acid, produced by intraluminal bacterial deconjugation of bile acids, is toxic, causing reduced bile flow with subsequent cholestasis, gallstones, and bile duct proliferation.[68] Recurrent sepsis is associated with cholestasis; in fact, a bout of sepsis is often the initial event.[69] This is compounded by bacterial overgrowth and bacterial translocation.[70] Also associated with the development of cholestasis are a higher number of laparotomies, lipid emulsions, and the lack of, or delayed, enteral feeding.[9] The relationship between cholestasis and lipid emulsions has been described in both adults and children.[71,72] A lipid infusion rate of >1 g/day has also been reported in adults on home TPN.[72] The mechanism may include macrophage activation caused by excess w-6 polyunsaturated fatty acids in commonly used solutions, leading to an accumulation of hepatic phospholipids and/or phytosterols.[72,73]

15.3.2 Hepatic Steatosis

Hepatic steatosis, the accumulation of lipids, may occur for a number of reasons: an excess of carbohydrate calories (> 8 to 12 mg/kg/d of glucose);[74] excess lipid infusions;[75] deficiencies of essential fatty acids; deficiencies of choline, taurine, or glutathione;[76,77] or the creation of toxic hydroperoxidases from ultraviolet light.[78] Steatosis is reversible with appropriate reduction of calories.[79]

15.3.3 Risk Factors: Enteral Intake, Sepsis, and Constituents of PN

A total lack of enteral feeding is a risk factor for the development of cholestasis; data indicate a reduction in gastrointestinal hormones in patients on PN who are not able to feed enterally,[80] resulting in intestinal and biliary dysfunction.[81] Sepsis also plays a significant role in such patients.[81] Intestinal stasis associated with bacterial overgrowth and bacterial translocation may exacerbate cholestasis especially in infants[82] as well as increase the production of lithocholic acid. Recurrent bacterial sepsis, regardless of the cause, contributes to liver disease related to PN in patients with intestinal failure, especially SBS,[83] and may lead to progressive liver failure.[84] Lack of stimulated cholecystokinin release can cause biliary sludging.[85] Fasting possibly reduces the size of the bile salt pool and decreases bile formation, compounding the difficulties with gallbladder contractility and sludge formation. Taurine or cysteine levels may be reduced by enzymatic immaturity, especially in premature infants;[86] however, adding taurine does not affect PN-related liver disease.[87] Alternatively, in adults with a choline deficiency state, choline supplementation does result in reduced steatosis.[88] Both aluminum toxicity and chromium toxicity are well recognized in patients on PN, but no evidence points to a causal effect in PN-related liver disease.[89,90] The toxic effect of manganese, which is excreted in bile, may be exacerbated in patients with cholestasis. In a study by Fell et al.,[91] high whole-blood manganese concentrations correlated with liver enzyme levels and with the deaths of 4 of 11 children with hypermanganesemia and cholestasis. Stopping or reducing manganese resulted in improvement in nervous system findings and liver function.[92] An excess in lipid emulsions can be expected to lead to hepatic steatosis, hyperlipidemia, and thrombocytopenia.[93] Removing lipid entirely from PN can have a very brief effect in reducing bilirubin.[94] Similarly, data in adults indicate that use of >1 g/kg/d of lipid results in cholestasis.[72] Mechanisms of injury include toxicity from the lipid itself, from accumulation of phospholipids or phytosterols, and from inflammatory cytokines.[72,74,95]

15.3.4 BILIARY SLUDGE AND GALLSTONES

Biliary sludge, gallbladder distention, and gallstones and acalculous cholecystitis are well known in adults and children on long-term PN.[9] Biliary sludge increases with the duration of PN to 100% at 6 to 13 weeks,[96] as does the incidence of gallstone formation.[86] Reduction in cholecystokinin stimulation may be contributory, although other hormone abnormalities may also be significant.[86,97] Endogenous release of cholecystokinin through pulsed infusions of amino acids or by any rate of enteral nutrition, helps to reduce cholestasis.[98] Infusing cholecystokinin has a limited benefit, and side effects may be bothersome.[99]

15.3.5 CLINICAL FEATURES

Liver enzyme elevation may be episodic and related to sepsis, but it eventually becomes persistent and progressively elevated.[70] In 22 children evaluated for combined liver and small intestinal transplantation, bilirubin concentration >12 mg/dL predicted death from end-stage liver disease within six months in 11 of the children.[100] Similarly, 6 of 42 patients on home PN developed end-stage liver disease and died within 10 months of the first bilirubin elevation.[101] Overall, a poor prognosis is associated with cholestatic liver disease in patients on PN.[102] Isolated hepatic fibrosis is also reported with PN, although portal hypertensive features are not prominent.[103] In contrast to children, adults typically do not develop cholestasis early, unless they have biliary or small intestinal obstruction.

15.3.6 Histology

Histopathologic changes in the liver include hepatic steatosis without additional liver injury. Centrilobular cholestasis may be associated with portal inflammation, necrosis, and fatty infiltration that progresses to periportal fibrosis, bile ductular proliferation, and, eventually, bridging fibrosis. Biliary cirrhosis is a late development that may be associated with death within six months.[103]

15.3.7 Clinical Management

Patients with intestinal failure on long-term PN need a dedicated team approach to their care. In the absence of severe fibrosis, cessation of PN may resolve the liver disease.[104] Even a minimal amount of enteral feeding will improve liver and biliary function.[105] Controlling intake of macromolecules and micronutrients is clearly important. If cholestasis is severe, restriction of lipid intake and a strategy to alter omega-3 fatty acid levels can be considered, especially in infants with severe cholestasis.[106] Aggressively managing intravenous line sepsis[107] and controlling bacterial overgrowth, thereby reducing bacterial translocation, are perhaps the most vital components in preventing advancing disease.[108] Adding glutamine has a number of potential benefits (discussed above in Section 15.2.4). In rats, it reverses the depression of hepatocyte mitochondrial metabolism seen with endotoxemia, thereby curing sepsis.[109] In premature infants, supplementation of PN with glutamine has improved the time to full enteral feeding[110] and reduced the incidence of infection.[111] Enteral administration of the yeast *Saccharomyces boulardii* has been proposed to reduce bacterial translocation.[112] Cycling PN may be helpful in reducing its impact on liver disease.[113] While the evidence is mixed on oral ursodeoxycholic acid, it was associated with improved liver function tests in patients on long-term PN.[3]

15.3.8 Nontransplant Outcome

In a 1975 to 2000 review from a North American academic center of the outcome of children on PN for longer than three months, adaptation occurred in the first three years in 77% of survivors.[22] The long-term survival rate at five years on PN approximates 60%.[2]

15.3.9 Nontransplant Surgery for SBS

The most common surgical therapy for intestinal failure is the placement of feeding devices. Some patients with SBS have a proximal small intestinal stoma even when the distal small intestine or the colon is present, but not in continuity. Taking down the stoma allows the intestinal contents to have maximal contact time with the small and large intestine, improving nutrient, fluid, and electrolyte absorption. Removing strictures and tapering dilated areas of intestine improve the function of the small intestine by reducing dysmotility and the potential for bacterial overgrowth. Intestinal lengthening procedures take advantage of the intestinal dilation that often occurs in the foreshortened remaining small intestine. Longitudinal intestinal lengthening was described in 1980 by Bianchi et al. and has now been used widely.[114] The dilated segment of small intestine is symmetrically divided in half longitudinally along the antimesenteric border. The blood flow is preserved by separating the leaves of mesentery with either limb. The lumen is recreated by the formation of two narrower channels, which are then reapproximated to each other in a serial fashion. Results have been favorable.[115] The serial transverse entero-plasty procedure (STEP) was more recently described by Kim et al.[116] It can also be applied to a symmetrically dilated piece of small intestine. It requires no entero-tomies and preserves intestinal vasculature. The procedure consists of applying a surgical stapler along the intestine at a 90-degree angle to the mesentery, alternating sides so as to create a zigzag-shaped channel that is longer and narrower. The recently created STEP registry reported an increase of 116% in enteral tolerance in 38 patients; nearly half were weaned off PN after a median follow-up time of about a year.[117]

15.3.10 ISOLATED LIVER TRANSPLANTS FOR INTESTINAL FAILURE

An isolated liver transplant in children with SBS has enabled some of them to wean off PN.[118] This result suggests a suppressive effect of liver disease on the process of adaptation. Alternatively, an isolated liver transplant may facilitate adaptation by increasing the time available and negative effect of chronic liver disease on growth in patients who would otherwise die of intestinal failure.

15.4 INTESTINAL TRANSPLANTATION

An intestinal transplant (ITx) is a definitive treatment for patients with intestinal failure. Recognized indications for an ITx in the United States include complications of PN, particularly those related to central intravenous line infections and sepsis.[119] Adults on PN can survive for prolonged periods if such complications are contained. An ITx also may be considered for indications not related to intestinal failure, such as a desmoid tumor. The overall mortality rate on the waiting list for intestinal transplant candidates continues to be the highest of all abdominal organs: 25% for adults, 60% for children.[120] Waiting time averages 7.7 months.[2]

15.4.1 TYPES OF GRAFTS

The graft in any particular case can be adapted according to the indication for the ITx, the recipient's anatomy, and the function of the other abdominal organs. The small intestine can be combined with the liver or with any of the abdominal viscera, including the abdominal wall if necessary (according to the "cluster" concept originally proposed by Starzl et al.).[121–122] An isolated ITx has two main variants: (1) if the recipient's abdominal cavity is normal in size (e.g., in case of intestinal pseudo-obstruction), the superior mesenteric artery (SMA) and vein are used for grafting; (2) if the recipient's abdominal cavity is small (e.g., in SBS), the aorta and the vena cava are used for grafting.[123] For a combined liver and intestinal transplant (LITx), separate organs are used for adult recipients, and a composite graft is typical for small children.[124,125] The multiviseral transplant (MVT) has two main variants: (1) the "classic" procedure includes the liver, the stomach with duodenum, the pancreas, and the small intestine; (2) the modified version excludes the liver, but includes the stomach with duodenum, the pancreas, and the small intestine.[126] If the MVT recipient's abdominal domain is limited, the donor needs to be 50 to 75% of the recipient's size.[127] Given the large number of small children who are prospective recipients, size-matched organ availability is a problem.[128] Using a larger donor is the clearest option. Under these circumstances, alternatives for abdominal closure include reducing the recipient's abdominal contents using nonbiologic or biologic mesh, acellular dermal matrix, human skin, a rotational flap, and/or a donor abdominal wall graft implanted into the recipient's iliac or epigastric vessels.[129–132] In some MVT recipients, the donor's colon and spleen have been included with reasonable results. The spleen has been included for technical considerations, the potential of splenic function, and better tolerance.[133] Inclusion of the spleen has been shown to reduce intestinal rejection and to increase response to the pneumococcal vaccine without an increase in the incidence of posttransplant lymphoproliferative disease (PTLD) or graft-versus-host disease.[134] The previous standard of using organs from deceased but heart-beating donors has been expanded by successfully using deceased donors who underwent prior resuscitation, whose blood group did not match the recipient's, who had a positive T-cell cross-match, and who were positive for cytomegalovirus (CMV) even if their recipient was negative.[135]

Living donors have also been used successfully for ITx recipients. The technique, now standard, as described by Gruessner et al.,[136] entails using 120 to 150 cm of the distal jejunum and ileum. The ileocecal valve and a segment of 20 cm of the distal ileum are preserved in the donor to assure normal intestinal sufficiency after donation.[137] Hence, the arterial supply chosen for the graft is the terminal segment of the SMA distal to the takeoff of the ileocecal branch. Computed tomography scans with three-dimensional reconstruction and/or angiography are necessary to accurately evaluate the vasculature and, in particular, the size of the artery. The first living donor LITx involved a sensitized two-year-old recipient. A sequential transplant first used the left lateral segment of the liver from the mother and then the ileal graft, also from the mother, a week later. The outcome was described as good for both the child and the mother.[138] Few such cases have been done overall. The advantage of this technique is that it allows time for desensitization.

15.4.2 Patient and Graft Outcome

The most recent estimates suggest a survival rate of 90% in ITx recipients in centers with the greatest experience.[2] The long-term graft survival rate has remained about 60%; the graft survival rate abruptly worsens in pediatric patients after three years posttransplant.[139] Early deaths are mainly from sepsis (40 to 50%) and rejection (10%).[140] Later deaths are also frequently caused by sepsis and rejection, along with PTLD (6 to 8%, with a peak incidence at two years posttransplant).[141] The outcome of PTLD has improved with rituximab.[142]

15.4.3 NUTRITION

Most patients (>90%) wean off PN after their ITx.[143] Patients are started on PN, then gradually transitioned to enteral feedings. Lymphatic interruption is the rule in ITx recipients; however, chylous ascites is rare. Lipids are gradually initiated four to six weeks after the introduction of a diet. Steatorrhea is usually not a problem. PN is discontinued once 50% of the caloric intake is enteral. Some prefer to use an elemental diet for the first few weeks posttransplant, others have used more liberal protocol without problems.[144] Stoma fluid output is slowed with medication when necessary.

15.4.4 MAINTENANCE IMMUNOSUPPRESSION AND REJECTION

Induction therapy (with IL-2 receptor blockade and/or antilymphocyte or antithymocyte globulin) has resulted in improved graft and patient survival rates in the first year posttransplant; induction agents are now included in some combination in most regimens, along with steroids.[2,145] Tacrolimus is standard for maintenance immunosuppression, allowing many recipients to wean off steroids; sirolimus has been used in combination with tacrolimus to prevent severe rejection.[146] Notably, alemtuzumab has been reduced to only very limited use in children because of a high rate of side effects.[147] In ITx recipients, small intestinal graft acute cellular rejection (ACR) occurs more frequently and is more severe, as compared with any other abdominal organ probably related to the amount of transplanted lymphoid tissue.[147] Historically, a third of ITx recipients did not experience acute rejection; MVT recipients, particularly children.[148] With newer regimens, ACR is now reported to affect only a third of ITx and MVT recipients.[2] Graft loss occurs from severe intractable ACR; chronic allograft dysfunction can occur with repeated episodes of less severe rejection. Subclinical rejection (SCR) has been described; predominantly reported in adults, SCR significantly affects graft and patient survival rates at five years.[149] Graft survival is reduced in recipients showing early vascular lesions. Although acute vascular rejection (AVR) is not well defined, it is related to panel-reactive antibodies (PRAs) and to positive T-cell and B-cell cross-matches.[150] Antirejection therapy for refractory AVR includes OKT3 or thymoglobulin. Antiinflammatory monoclonal antibodies (mAbs) against tumor necrosis factor (TNF)-α have been shown to be effective for acute rejection and may be useful for chronic enteropathy,[151] similar to the results with alemtuzumab.[152] Ultimately, chronic graft loss due to vascular changes cannot be adequately treated and is responsible for the poor long-term outcome in most ITx recipients. A recent finding is that mutations in the gene coding for nucleotide-binding oligomerization domain containing two (NOD2) mutations that are typically associated with Crohn's disease, may have a role in rejection.[153]

15.4.5 COST AND QUALITY OF LIFE

A poor quality of life (QoL) with associated neuropsychological complications is typical of patients with intestinal failure on PN. QoL is improved in transplant patients.[2] A recent review concluded that, because of the limited number of studies and the preliminary nature of findings, strong conclusions cannot yet be drawn regarding QoL in ITx recipients; however, the available limited data were judged as encouraging.[154] The cost of a transplant involving the small intestine has been examined in North America and Europe and is roughly similar.[2] An ITx is cost-effective as early as two years posttransplant, as compared with continued PN.[155]

REFERENCES

1. Raman M, Gramlich L, Whittaker S, Allard JP. Canadian home total parenteral nutrition registry: preliminary data on the patient population. *Can J Gastroenterol.* 2007;21(10):643–8.
2. Fishbein TM. Intestinal transplantation. *N Engl J Med.* 2009;361:998–1008.
3. Duro D, Kamin D, Duggan C. Overview of pediatric short bowel syndrome. *J Pediatr Gastroenterol Nutr.* 2008;47 (Suppl 1):S33–6.
4. Spencer AU, Neaga A,West B, et al. Pediatric short bowel syndrome: redefining predictors of success. *Ann Surg.* 2005;242:403–408.
5. Grant D, Abu-Elmagd K, Reyes J, et al.Intestine Transplant Registry. 2003 report of the intestine transplant registry: a new era has dawned. *Ann Surg.* 2005;241(4):607–13.
6. Buchman AL. Etiology and initial management of short bowel syndrome. *Gastroenterology.* 2006;130(2 Suppl 1):S5–S15.
7. Cole C, Hansen N, Ziegler T, et al. Outcomes of low-birth-weight infants with surgical short bowel syndrome. *J Pediatr Gastroenterol Nutr* 2005;41:507.
8. Btaiche F, Khalidi N. Parenteral nutrition-associated liver complications in children. *Pharmacotherarpy.* 2002;22:188–211.
9. Kelly DA. Intestinal failure-associated liver disease: what do we know today? *Gastroenterology.* 2006;130(2 Suppl 1):S70–7.
10. Williams NS, Evans P, King RF. Gastric acid secretion and gastrin production in the short bowel syndrome. *Gut.* 1985;26:914.
11. Jeppesen, PB, Staun, M, Tjellesen, L, Mortensen PB. Effect of intravenous ranitidine and omeprazole on intestinal absorption of water, sodium, and macronutrients in patients with intestinal resection. *Gut.* 1998;43:763.
12. Nightingale JMD, Kamm MA, van der Sijp JR. Gastrointestinal hormones in SBS. Peptide YY may be the colonic brake to gastric emptying. *Gut.* 1996;39:267.
13. de Miguel, E, Gomez de, Segura IA, et al. Trophic effects of neurotensin in massive bowel resection in the rat. *Dig Dis Sci.* 1994;39:59.
14. Fordtran, JS, Rector, JR Jr, Carter, NW. The mechanisms of sodium absorption in the human small intestine. *J Clin Invest.* 1968;47:884.
15. Glynn CC, Greene GW, Winkler MF, Albina JE. Predictive versus measured energy expenditure using limits-of-agreement analysis in hospitalized, obese patients. *J Parenter Enteral Nutr.* 1999;23:47–154.
16. Nightingale JM, Lennard-Jones JE, Walker ER, Farthing MJ: Jejunal efflux in SBS. *Lancet.* 1990;336:765.
17. Nightingale JMD, Kamm MA, van der Sijp JR, et al. Disturbed gastric emptying in the SBS: evidence for a "colonic brake." *Gut.* 1993; 34:1171.
18. Hofmann AF, Poley JR. Role of bile acid malabsorption in pathogenesis of diarrhea and steatorrhea in patients with ileal resection: response to cholestyramine or replacement of dietary long chain triglyceride by medium chain triglyceride. *Gastroenterology.* 1972;62:918.
19. Nightingale JMD, Bartram CI, Lennard-Jones JE. Length of residual small bowel after partial resection: correlation between radiographic and surgical measurements. *Gastrointestinal Radiol.* 1991;16:305.

20. Jeppesen PB, Mortensen PB. Intestinal failure determined by measurements of intestinal energy and wet weight absorption. *Gut.* 2000;46:701–707.

21. Carbonnel F, Cosnes J, Chevret S, et al. The role of anatomic factors in nutritional autonomy after extensive small bowel resection. *J Parenter Enteral Nutr.* 1996;20:275–280.

22. Quiros-Tejeira RE, Ament ME, Reyen L, et al. Long-term parenteral nutritional support and intestinal adaptation in children with short bowel syndrome: a 25-year experience. *J Pediatr.* 2004;145:157–163.

23. Weinstein LD, Shoemaker CP, Hersh T, Wright HK. Enhanced intestinal absorption after small bowel resection in man. *Arch Surg.* 1969;560–561.

24. Kurkchubasche AG, Rowe MI, Smith SD. Adaptation in short-bowel syndrome: reassessing old limits. *J Pediatr Surg.*1993;28:1069–1071.

25. Urban E, Michel AM. Separation of adaptive mucosal growth and transport after small bowel resection. *Am J Physiol.* 1983;244(3):G295–300.

26. Hanson, WR, Osborne, JW, Sharp, JG. Compensation by the residual intestine after intestinal resection in the rat. 1. Influence of amount of tissue removed. *Gastroenterology.* 1977;73:692.

27. Hanson, WR, Osborne, JW, Sharp, JG. Compensation by the residual intestine after intestinal resection in the rat. II. Influence of postoperative time interval. *Gastroenterology.* 1977;73:701.

28. Bury KD.Carbohydrate digestion and absorption after massive resection of the small intestine. *Surg Gynecol Obstet.* 1972;135(2):177–87.

29. Gouttebel MC, Saint Aubert B, Colette C, Astre C, Monnier LH, Joyeux H. Intestinal adaptation in patients with short bowel syndrome: measurement by calcium absorption. *Dig Dis Sci.* 1989;34(5):709–15.

30. Vanderhoof JA, Burkley KT, Antonson DL. Potential for mucosal adaptation following massive small bowel resection in 3-week-old versus 8-week-old rats. *J Pediatr Gastroenterol Nutr.* 1983;2(4):672–6.

31. Erwin, CR, Jarboe, MD, Sartor, MA, et al. Developmental characteristics of adapting mouse small intestine crypt cells. *Gastroenterology.* 2006;130:1324.

32. Thompson, Effect of the distal remnant in ileal adaptation. *J Gastrointest Surg* 2000; 4:430.

33. Cisler JJ, Buchman AL. Intestinal adaptation in short bowel syndrome, *J Investig Med.* 2005;53:402–413.

34. Jeppesen PB, Hartmann B, Thulesen J, et al. Glucagon-like peptide 2 improves nutrient absorption and nutritional status in short-bowel patients with no colon. *Gastroenterology.* 2001;120:806.

35. Jeppesen PB, Hartmann B, Hansen BS, et al. Impaired meal stimulated glucagon-like peptide 2 response in ileal resected short bowel patients with intestinal failure. *Gut;*1999:559–563.

36. Sigalet DL, Bawazir O, Martin GR, et al. Glucagon-like peptide-2 induces a specific pattern of adaptation in remnant jejunum. *Dig Dis Sci.* 2006;51:1557.

37. Dowling RH. Polyamines in intestinal adaptation and disease. *Digestion.* 1990; 46 (Suppl 2):331.

38. Vanderhoof JA, Grandjean CJ, Baylor JM, Baily J, Euler AR. Morphological and functional effects of 16,16-dimethyl-prostaglandin-E2 on mucosal adaptation after massive distal small bowel resection in the rat. *Gut.* 1988;29(6):802–8.

39. Kollman-Bauerly KA, Thomas DL, Adrian TE, Lien EL, Vanderhoof JA. The role of eicosanoids in the process of adaptation following massive bowel resection in the rat. *J Parenter Enteral Nutr.* 2001;25(5):275–81.

40. Sukhotnik, I, Khateeb, K, Krausz, MM, et al. Sandostatin impairs postresection intestinal adaptation in a rat model of short bowel syndrome. *Dig Dis Sci.* 2002;47:2095.

41. Puolakkainen, PA, Ranchalis, JE, Gombotz, WR, et al. Novel delivery system for inducing quiescence in intestinal stem cells in rats by transforming growth factor beta 1. *Gastroenterology.* 1994;107:1319.
42. Krsek, M, Rosicka, M, Haluzik, M, et al. Plasma ghrelin levels in patients with short bowel syndrome. *Endocr Res.* 2002;28:27.
43. Feldman EJ, Dowling RH, McNaughton J, Peters TJ. Effects of oral versus intravenous nutrition on intestinal adaptation after small bowel resection in the dog. *Gastroenterology.* 1976;70(5 PT.1):712–9.
44. Weser E, Babbitt J, Hoban M, Vandeventer A. Intestinal adaptation. Different growth responses to disaccharides compared with monosaccharides in rat small bowel. *Gastroenterology.* 1986;91(6):1521–7.
45. Dworkin LD, Levine GM, Farber NJ, Spector MH. Small intestinal mass of the rat is partially determined by indirect effects of intraluminal nutrition. *Gastroenterology.* 1976;71(4): 626–30.
46. Weser E, Hernandez MH. Studies of small bowel adaptation after intestinal resection in the rat. *Gastroenterology.* 1971;60(1):69–75.
47. Wakabayashi, Y, Yamada, E, Yoshida, T, Takahashi, N. Effect of intestinal resection and arginine-free diet on rat physiology. *Am J Physiol.* 1995;269:G313.
48. Ding LA, Li JS. Effects of glutamine on intestinal permeability and bacterial translocation in TPN-rats with endotoxemia. *World J Gastroenterol.* 2003;9:1327–1332.
49. Tamada, H, Nezu, R, Matsuo, Y, et al. Alanyl glutamine-enriched total parenteral nutrition restores intestinal adaptation after either proximal or distal massive resection in rats. *JPEN J Parenter Enteral Nutr.* 1993;17:236.
50. Souba WW, Klimberg VS, Plumley DA, et al. The role of glutamine in maintaining a healthy gut and supporting the metabolic response to injury and infection. *J Surg Res.* 1990;48:383–391.
51. Alverdy JA, Aoys E, Weiss-Carrington P, Burke DA. The effect of glutamine-enriched TPN on gut immune cellularity. *J Surg Res.* 1992;52:34–38.
52. Michail, S, Mohammadpour, H, Park, JH, Vanderhoof, JA. Effect of glutamine-supplemented elemental diet on mucosal adaptation following bowel resection in rats. *J Pediatr Gastroenterol Nutr.* 1995;21:394.
53. Byrne TA, Morrissey TB, Nattakom TV, et al. Growth hormone, glutamine, and a modified diet enhance nutrient absorption in patients with severe short bowel syndrome. *J Parenter Enteral Nutr.* 1995;19:296.
54. Vanderhoof, JA, Park, JH, Herrington, MK, et al. Effects of dietary menhaden oil on mucosal adaptation after small bowel resection in rats. *Gastroenterology.* 1994;106:94.
55. Weizman Z, Schmueli A, Deckelbaum RJ. Continuous nasogastric drip elemental feeding: alternative for prolonged parenteral nutrition in severe prolonged diarrhea. *Am J Dis Child* 1983;137:253–255.
56. Ameen VZ, Powell GK, Jones LA. Qualitation of fecal carbohydrate excretion in patients with short bowel syndrome. *Gastroenterology.* 1987;92:493–500.
57. Hudson M, Pocknee R, Mowat NA. D-lactic acidosis in short bowel syndrome, an examination of possible mechanisms. *Q J Med.* 1990;74(274):157–63.
58. O'Keefe, SJ, Haymond, MW, Bennet, WM, et al. Long-acting somatostatin analog therapy and protein metabolism in patients with jejunostomies. *Gastroenterology.* 1994;107:379.
59. Hunt JB, Elliott EJ, Fairclough PD, et al. Water and solute absorption from hypotonic glucose-electrolyte solutions in human jejunum. *Gut.* 1992;33:479–483.
60. Shulman RJ. Zinc and copper balance studies in infants receiving total parenteral nutrition. *Am J Clin Nutr.* 1989;49(5):879–83.
61. Wessel JJ, Kocoshis SA. Nutritional management of infants with short bowel syndrome. *Semin Perinatol.* 2007;31(2):104–11.

62. Dudrick SJ, Wilmore DW, Vars HM, Rhoads JE. Long-term total parenteral nutrition with growth, development, and positive nitrogen balance. *Surgery* 1968;64:134–142.
63. Goulet O, Ruemmele F, Lacaille F, Colomb V. Irreversible intestinal failure. *J Pediatr Gastroenterol Nutri.* 2004;38:250–269.
64. Andorsky DJ, Lund DP, Lillehei CW, et al. Nutritional and other postoperative management of neonates with short bowel syndrome correlates with clinical outcomes. *J Pediatr.* 2001;139:27–33.
65. Watkins JB, Szczepanik P, Gould JB, Lester R. Bile salt metabolism in the human premature infant. *Gastroenterology.* 1975;69:706–713.
66. Beale EF, Nelson RM, Bucciarelli RL, Donnelly WH, Eitman DV. Intrahepatic cholestasis associated with parenteral nutrition in premature infants. *Pediatrics.* 1979;64: 342–7.
67. Watkins JB. Placental transport bile acid conjugation and sulphation in the fetus. *J Pediatr Gastroenterol Nutr.* 1983;2:365–373.
68. Palmer RH, Hruban Z. Production of bile duct hyperplasia and gallstones by lithocholic acid. *J Clin Invest.* 1964;45:1255–1267.
69. Beath SV, Davies P, Papadopolou P, Khan AR, Buick RG, Corkery JJ, Gornall P, Booth IW. Parenteral nutrition-related cholestasis in postsurgical neonates: multivariate analysis of risk factors. *J Pediatr Surg.* 1996;31:604–606.
70. Luman W, Shaffer JL. Prevalence, outcome and associated factors of deranged liver function tests in patients on home parenteral nutrition. *Clin Nutr.* 2002;21:337–343.
71. Cavicchi M, Beau P, Crenn P, Degott C, Messing B. Prevalence of liver disease and permanent intestinal failure. *Ann Intern Med.* 2000;132:525–532.
72. Colomb V, Goulet O, De Potter S, Ricour C. Liver disease associated with long-term parenteral nutrition in children. *Transplant Proc.* 1994;26:1467.
73. Clayton PT, Whitfield P, Iyer K. The role of phytosterols in the pathogenesis of liver complications of pediatric parenteral nutrition. *Nutrition.* 1998;14:158–164.
74. Meguid MM, Chen TY Yang ZJ, Campos ACL, Hich DC, Gleason JR. Effects of continuous graded total parenteral nutrition on feeding indexes and metabolic concomitants in rats. *Am J Physiol.* 1991;260:E126–E140.
75. Vromen A, Spira RM, Bercovier H, Berry E, Freund HR. Pentoxifyline and thalidomide fail to reduce hepatic steatosis during total parenteral nutrition and bowel rest in the rat *J Parenter Enteral Nutr.* 1997;21:233–234.
76. Sokol RJ, Taylor SF, Devereaux MW, et al. Hepatic oxidant injury and glutathione depletion during total parenteral nutrition in weanling rats. *Am J Physiol.* 1996;270:691–700.
77. Shronts EP. Essential nature of choline with implications for total parenteral nutrition. *J Am Diet Assoc.* 1997;6:639–646.
78. Silvers KM, Darlow BA, Winterbourn CC. Lipid peroxide and hydrogen peroxide formation in parenteral nutrition solutions containing multivitamins. *J Parenter Enteral Nutr.* 2001;25(1):14–7.
79. Tulikoura I, Huikuri K. Morphological fatty changes and function of the liver, serum free fatty acids and triglycerides during parenteral nutrition. *Scand J Gastroenterol.* 1982;17:177–185.
80. Greenberg G, Wolman S, Christofides N, Bloom SR, . JeeJeedhoy KN. Effect of total parenteral nutrition on gut hormone release in human. *Gastroenterology.* 1981;80:988–993.
81. Kaufman SS. Prevention of parenteral nutrition-associated liver disease in children. *Pediatr Transplant.* 2002;6:37–42.
82. Pierro A, van Saene HK, Jones MO, Brown D, Nunn AJ, Lloyd DA. Clinical impact of abnormal gut flora in infants receiving parenteral nutrition. *Am Surg.* 1998;227:547–552.

83. Heine RG, Bines JE. New approaches to parenteral nutrition in infants and children. *J Paediatr Child Health*. 2002;38:433–437.

84. Hodes JE, Grosseld JL, Webert R, Schreiner RO, Fitzgerald JF, Merkin DL. Hepatic failure in infants on total parenteral nutrition (TPN) clinical and histophathologic observations. *J Pediatr Surg*. 1982;17:463–468.

85. Roslyn JJ, Berquist WE, Pitt HA, et al. Increased risk of gall stones in children receiving total parenteral nutrition. *Pediatrics*. 1983;71:784–789.

86. Zlotkin SH, Anderton GH. The development of cystothianase activity during the first year of life. *Pediatr Res*. 1982;16:65–68.

87. Cooke RJ, Whitington PF, Kelts D. Effect of taurine supplementation on hepatic function during short-term parenteral nutrition in the premature infant. *J Pediatr Gastroenterol Nutr*. 1984;3:234–238.

88. Buchman AL, Ament ME, Sohel M, et al. Choline deficiency causes reversible hepatic abnormalities in patients receiving parenteral nutrition: proof of a human choline requirement: a placebo-controlled trial. *J Parenter Enteral Nutr*. 2001;25:260–268.

89. Moreno A, Guez C, Ballibriga A. Aluminium in the neonate related to parenteral nutrition. *Acta Pediatrica*. 1994;83:25–29.

90. Moukarzel AA, Song MK, Buchman A, et al. Excessive chromium intake in children receiving total parenteral nutrition. *Lancet*. 1992;15:385–389.

91. Fell JME, Reynolds AP, Meadows N, et al. Manganese toxicity in children receiving long-term parenteral nutrition, *Lancet*.1996;347(9010):1218–21.

92. Kafritsa Y, Fell J, Long S, Bynevelt S, Taylor W, Milla P. Long-term outcome of brain manganese deposition in patients on home parenteral nutrition. *Arch Dis Child*. 1998;79:263–265.

93. Toce SS, Keenan WJ. Lipid intolerance in newborns is associated with hepatic dysfunction but not infection. *Arch Pediatr Adolesc Med*. 1995;149:1249–1253.

94. Colomb V, Jobert-Giraud A, Lacaille F, Goulet O, Fournet JC, Ricour C. Role of lipid emulsions in cholestasis associated with long-term parenteral nutrition in children. *J Parenter Enteral Nutr*. 2000;24:345–350.

95. Doi F, Goya T, Torisu M. Potential role of hepatic macrophages in neutrophil-mediated liver injury in rats with sepsis. *Hepatology*. 1993;17:1086–1094.

96. Messing B, Bories C, Kunstlinger F, Bernier JJ. Does total parenteral nutrition induce gallbladder sludge formation and lithiasis? *Gastroenterology*, 1983;84:1012–1019.

97. Lucas A, Bloom SR, Ainsley-Green A. Metabolic and endocrine consequences of depriving preterm infants of enteral nutrition. *Acta Paediatr Scand*. 1983;72:245–249.

98. Nealon WH, Upp JR, Alexander RW, Gomez G, Townsend CR, Thompson JC. Intravenous amino acids stimulate human gallbladder emptying and hormone release. *Am J Physiol*. 1990;259:G173–G178.

99. Silberstein EE, Marcus CS. Unreported side effect of sincalide. *Radiology*. 1994;190: 902.

100. Beath SV, Booth IW, Murphy MS. Nutritional care in candidates for small bowel transplantation. *Arch Dis Child*. 1995;73:348–350.

101. Chan S, McCowen KC, Bistrian BR, et al., Incidence, prognosis and etiology of end-stage liver disease in patients receiving home total parenteral nutrition. *Surgery*. 1999;126:28–34.

102. Beath SV, Needham SJ, Kelly DA,et al. Clinical features and prognosis of children assessed for isolated small bowel (ISBTx) or combined small bowel and liver transplantation (CSBLTx). *J Pediatr Surg*. 1997;32:459–461.

103. Colomb BV, Goulet O, Rambau DC, et al. Long-term parenteral nutrition in children; liver and gall bladder disease. *Transplant Proc*. 1992;24:1054–1055.

104. Dahms BB, Halpin TC. Serial liver biopsies in parenteral nutrition associated cholestasis in early infancy. *Gastroenterology*. 1981;81:136–144.

105. Jawahweer G, Pierro A, Lloyd TA, Shaw NJ. Gall bladder contractility in neonates effect of parenteral and enteral feeding. *Arch Dis Child.* 1995;72: F200–F202.
106. Gura KM, Duggan CP, Collier SB, et al. Reversal of parenteral nutrition associated liver disease in two infants with short bowel syndrome using parenteral fish oil: implications for future management. *Pediatrics.* 2006;118:e197–e201.
107. Donnell SC, Taylor N, van Saene HK, Magnall VL, Pierro A, Lloyd DA. Infection rates in surgical neonates and infants receiving parenteral nutrition: a five-year prospective study. *J Hosp Infect.* 2002;52:273–280.
108. Spaeth G, Specian RD, Berg RD, Deitch EA. Bulk prevents bacterial translocation induced by the oral administration of total parenteral nutrition solution. *J Parenter Enteral Nutr.* 1990;14:442–447.
109. Markley MA, Pierro A, Eaton S. Hepatocyte mitochondrial metabolism is inhibited in neonatal rat endotoxaemia: effects of glutamine. *Clin Sci.* 2002;102:337–344.
110. Lacey JM, Crouch JB, Benfell K, et al.et al. The effects of glutamine supplemented parenteral nutrition in premature infants. *J Parenter Enteral Nutr.* 1996;20:74–80.
111. Neu J, Roig JC, Meetzer WH, et al. Enteral glutamine supplementation for very low birth weight infants decreases morbidity. *J Pediatr.* 1997;131:691–699.
112. Buts JP, Corthier G, Delmee M. Saccharomyces boulardii for clostridium difficile-associated enteropathies in infants. *J Parenter Enteral Nutr.* 1993;16:419–425.
113. Hwang TL, Lue MC, Chen LL. Early use of cyclic TPN prevents further deterioration of liver functions for the TPN patients with impaired liver function. *Hepatogastroenterology.* 2000;47:1347–1350.
114. Bianchi A. Intestinal loop lengthening: a technique for increasing small intestinal length. *J Pediatr Surg.* 1980;15:145–151.
115. Bianchi A. Longitudinal intestinal lengthening and tailoring: results in 20 children. *J R Soc Med.* 1997;90:429–432.
116. Kim HB, Fauza D, Garza J, et al. Serial transverse enteroplasty (STEP): a novel bowel lengthening procedure. *J Pediatr Surg.* 2003;38:425–429.
117. Modi BP, Javid PJ, Jaksic T, et al. First report of the international serial transverse enteroplasty data registry: indications, efficacy, and complications. *J Am Coll Surg.* 2007;204:365–371.
118. Horslen SP, Sudan DL, Iyer KR, et al. Isolated liver transplantation in infants with end-stage liver disease associated with short bowel syndrome. *Ann Surg.* 2002;235: 435–439.
119. Vianna R, Mangus RS, Tector AJ. Current status of small bowel and multivisceral transplantation. *Adv Surg.* 2008;42:129–150.
120. Fishbein TM. The current state of intestinal transplantation. *Transplantation.* 2004;78:175–178.
121. Levi DM, Tzakis AG, Kato T, et al. Transplantation of the abdominal wall. *Lancet.* 2003;361:2173–2176.
122. Starzl TE, Todo S, Tzakis A, et al. The many faces of multivisceral transplantation. *Surg Gynecol Obstet.* 1991;172:335–344.
123. Abu-Elmagd K, Todo S, Tazakis, et al. Three years clinical experience with intestinal transplantation. *J Am Coll Surg.* 1994;179:385–400.
124. Grant D, Wall W, Mimeault R, et al. Successful small bowel/liver transplantation. *Lancet.* 1990;335:181–184.
125. Fishbein T, Florman S, Gondolesi G, Decker R. Noncomposite simultaneous liver and intestinal transplantation. *Transplantation.* 2003;75:564–565.
126. Grant W, Langnas A. Pediatric small bowel transplantation: techniques and outcomes. *Curr Opin Organ Transplant.* 2002;7:202–207.
127. Tzakis A, Kato T, Levy D, et al. 100 multivisceral transplants at a single center. *Ann Surg.* 2005;242:480–490.

128. Carlsen B, Farmer D, Busuttil R, et al. Incidence and management of abdominal wall defects after intestinal and multivisceral transplantation. *Plast Reconstr Surg* 2007;119:1247–1255.

129. de Ville de Goyet J, Mitchell A, Mayer AD, et al. En block combined reduced-liver and small bowel transplants: from large donors to small children. *Transplantation.* 2000;69:555–559.

130. DiBenedetto F, Lauro A, Masetti M, et al. Use of prosthetic mesh in difficult abdominal wall closure after small bowel transplantation. *Transplant Proc.* 2005;37:2272–2274.

131. Asham E, Uknis ME, Rastellini C, et al. Acellular dermal matrix provides a good option for abdominal wall closure following small bowel transplantation: a case report. *Transplant Proc.* 2006;38:1770–1771.

132. Levi AG, Tzakis AG, Kato T, et al. Transplantation of the abdominal wall. *Lancet.* 2003;361:2173–2176.

133. Stepkowski S, Bitter-Suermann H, Duncan W. Evidence supporting an *in vivo* role of T suppressor cells in spleen allograft induced tolerance. *Transplant Proc.* 1986;18:207.

134. Kato T, Tzakis A, Selvaggi G, et al. Transplantation of the spleen. Effect of splenic allograft in human multivisceral transplantation. *Ann Surg.* 2007;246:436–446.

135. Gondolesi G, Fauda M. Technical refinements in small bowel transplantation. *Curr Opin Organ Transplant.* 2008;13(3):259–65.

136. Gruessner R, Sharp H. Living related intestinal transplantation: first report of a standardized surgical technique. *Transplantation.* 1997;11:271–274.

137. Testa G, Panaro F, Schena S, et al. Living related small bowel transplantation: donor surgical technique. *Ann Surg.* 2004;240:779–784.

138. Testa G, Holterman M, John E, et al. Combined living donor liver/small bowel transplantation. *Transplantation.* 2005;79:1401–1404.

139. Ruiz P, Kato T, Tzakis A. Current status of transplantation of the small intestine. *Transplantation.* 2007;83:1–6.

140. Grant D, Abu-Elmagd K, Reyes J, et al. On behalf of the Intestine Transplant Registry. 2003 report of the intestine transplant registry: a new era has dawned. *Ann Surg.* 2005;241:607.

141. Ruiz P, Soares MF, Garcia M, et al. Lymphoplasmacytic hyperplasia (possible pre-PTLD) has varied expression and appearance in intestinal transplant recipients receiving Campath immunosuppression. *Transplant Proc.* 2004;36:386.

142. Nishida S, Kato T, Burney T, et al. Rituximab treatment for posttransplantation lymphoproliferative disorder after small bowel transplantation. *Transplant Proc.* 2002;34:957.

143. Abu-Elmagd KM. Intestinal transplantation for short bowel syndrome and gastrointestinal failure: current consensus, rewarding outcomes, and practical guidelines. *Gastroenterology.* 2006;130(2 Suppl 1):S132–S137.

144. Matarese LE, Costa G, Bond G, et al. Therapeutic efficacy of intestinal and multivisceral transplantation: survival and nutrition outcome. *Nutr Clin Pract.* 2007;22:474–481.

145. Vianna RM, Mangus RS, Fridell JA, et al. Induction immunosuppression with thymoglobulin and rituximab in intestinal and multivisceral transplantation. *Transplantation.* 2008;85:1290–1293.

146. Fishbein TM, Florman S, Gondolesi G, et al. Intestinal transplantation before and after the introduction of sirolimus. *Transplantation.* 2002;73:1538–1542.

147. Garcia M, Delacruz V, Ortiz R, et al. Acute cellular rejection grading scheme for human gastric allografts. *Hum Pathol.* 2004;35:343.

148. Selvaggi G, Gaynor JJ, Moon J, et al. Analysis of acute cellular rejection episodes in recipients of primary intestinal transplantation: a single center, 11-year experience. *Am J Transplant.* 2007;7:1249.

149. Takahashi H, Kato T, Selvaggi G, et al. Subclinical rejection in the initial postoperative period in small intestinal transplantation: a negative influence on graft survival. *Transplantation*. 2007;84:689.

150. Ruiz P, Garcia M, Pappas P, et al. Mucosal vascular alterations in isolated small-bowel allografts: relationship to humoral sensitization. *Am J Transplant*. 2003;3:43.

151. Pascher A, Radke C, Dignass A, et al. Successful infliximab treatment of steroid and OKT3 refractory acute cellular rejection in two patients after intestinal transplantation. *Transplantation*. 2003;76: 615.

152. Tzakis AG, Kato T, Nishida S, et al. Alemtuzumab (Campath-1H) combined with tacrolimus in intestinal and multivisceral transplantation. *Transplantation*. 2003;75:1512.

153. Fishbein T, Novitskiy G, Mishra L, et al. NOD2-expressing bone marrow-derived cells appear to regulate epithelial innate immunity of the transplanted human small intestine. *Gut*. 2008;57(3):323–30. Epub 2007, Oct 26.

155. Testa, G, Simon, AJ, Benedetti, E. Intestinal transplantation: Cost analysis, pp. 718–720 in Gruessner RWG, Benedetti, E, Eds. Living donor organ transplantation. 2008. Columbus, OH: McGraw-Hill.

156. Sudan D. Cost and quality of life after intestinal transplantation. *Gastroenterology*. 2006; 130(2 Suppl. 1): S158.

16 Nutrition in Acute Pancreatitis

Rémy F. Meier and Robert Martindale

CONTENTS

16.1 INTRODUCTION

Acute pancreatitis can be a life-threatening inflammatory disease with an incidence of about 50 to 80 cases per 100,000 population per year.[1,2]

The clinical patterns of acute pancreatitis varies from mild disease to severe necrotizing pancreatitis with local and/or systemic complications. Classifying acute pancreatitis by the Atlanta criteria (definition of severity) of 1992, approximately 80% of patients will have a mild, self-limited disease with a mortality rate below 1%.[3,4] The morbidity and mortality increases up to 50% if the disease progresses to severe necrotizing pancreatitis and can further increase up to 80% if sepsis occurs.[5,6]

Severe acute pancreatitis is usually accompanied by systemic inflammatory response syndrome (SIRS), which results in hypermetabolism and significant protein catabolism. These patients often develop nutritional deficiencies during the prolonged and complicated course of the disease. This prolonged caloric and nutrient deficit can have fatal consequences especially in patients malnourished at the time of the initial episode of pancreatitis.[7]

Until recently, use of the gastrointestinal (GI) tract to deliver nutrients during an episode of pancreatitis has been relatively contraindicated as it was thought to further stimulate the exocrine pancreatic secretion and the exacerbation of autodigestive processes. These concerns were the basis of placing patients on bowel rest and using intravenous nutritional support to bypass the stimulatory effect of oral or enteral nutrition until the patients recovered.

There is still an ongoing debate on the optimal nutritional support in patients with acute pancreatitis, but today, nutritional support is guided by the nutritional status of the patients, the severity of the disease, and the tolerance to enteral nutrition.

16.2 OUTCOME PREDICTORS

There is evidence that not all patients need specific nutritional support.[8] In uncomplicated mild attacks, most patients recover rapidly and can start eating after a few days. Whether this is true for patients with preexisting malnutrition is not known.

Two main factors predict the outcome of acute pancreatitis: the nutritional status and the severity of the disease.

16.2.1 Nutritional Status

Malnutrition is a common problem in patients with acute pancreatitis. It has been estimated that 50 to 80% of chronic alcoholics are malnourished.[7] Protein calorie malnutrition can arise or worsen during the pancreatitis episode secondary to depletion of nutrients and the hypermetabolic state. In mild acute pancreatitis, the clinical course is usually uncomplicated. This form of acute pancreatitis has little impact on the nutritional status or on energy and substrate metabolism. Patients with severe acute necrotizing pancreatitis are hypermetabolic. Energy expenditure and protein catabolism is increased. Pain and inflammatory response modulated by numerous proinflammatory cytokines initiated by the autodigestive processes are involved. The inflammatory process results in a significant increased energy expenditure.[9] Patients with severe pancreatitis often have a nonsuppressible gluconeogenesis despite sufficient caloric intake, increased ureagenesis, and an accentuated net protein catabolism, which can be as high as 40 g nitrogen/day.[9,10] Exogenous glucose supply cannot completely inhibit intrinsic gluconeogenesis and the status of acute catabolism. Generally speaking, the increased metabolic demand increases linearly with the severity of pancreatitis. Despite this, resting energy expenditure in these patients can be 77 to 158% of what is predicted.[11] In severe acute pancreatitis, the Harris–Benedict equation is not sensitive enough to estimate caloric expenditure and indirect calorimetry is recommended to avoid over- or underfeeding. If energy expenditure is measured daily by indirect calorimetry, the values show a wide range according to the severity of acute pancreatitis.[11] If sepsis develops, 80% of patients have an elevation in protein catabolism with an increased nutrient requirement.[9,10] Protein catabolism and proteolysis of skeletal muscle increases by 80% (compared to healthy controls). The plasma levels of aromatic amino acids increase and the level of branched chain amino acids decrease. Negative nitrogen balance has an impact on the nutritional status and the clinical outcome. Sitzmann et al. reported a tenfold increased mortality rate when the nitrogen balance was negative compared to those patients with a positive balance.[12] It is not clear whether negative nitrogen balance is the principle factor that determines outcome. The relationship between nitrogen balance and the outcome may only reflect the association between nitrogen balance and the severity of the disease as none of the studies were stratified according to the disease severity.[13]

In clinical practice, therefore, it is crucial to assess the severity of the disease and to implement an optimal nutritional support in these patients to avoid severe nutritional depletion.

16.2.2 Assessment of the Severity of Acute Pancreatitis

Several scoring systems, clinical, laboratory, and radiological criteria are available to predict the course of this disease.[14–20]

The Atlanta classification for severity defines severe acute pancreatitis on the basis of standard clinical manifestation: a score of three or more Ranson criteria or a score of eight or more APACHE II criteria, and the evidence of organ failure and intrapancreatic pathological findings (necrosis or interstitial pancreatitis).[3]

The Balthazar score predicts severity based on computerized tomography (CT) appearance, including presence or absence of pancreatic necrosis. Failure of pancreatic parenchyma to enhance during the arterial phase of intravenous, contrast-enhanced CT indicates necrosis, which predicts the severity of the pancreatitis if more than 50% of the gland is involved.[17] Mortele and colleagues modified the CT severity index. Extrapancreatic complications, such as vascular or gastrointestinal tract involvement, were included in this modified score and the assessment of the extent of pancreatic necrosis was simplified.[21] It is generally recommended that a CT study should be performed with the aim of staging the severity of acute pancreatitis not earlier than 48 to 72 hours of the onset of symptoms. This time frame allows adequate time for the pancreatic necrosis to develop and increases the accuracy of prediction.

Other markers, such as concentration of serum C-reactive protein (CRP) or urinary trypsinogen activation peptide (TAP), are useful in clinical practice. CRP is the most widely used marker for inflammatory diseases. In acute pancreatitis, it reaches its peak serum concentration between 72 to 96 hours after symptom onset. There is general agreement that a cut-off level of 150 mg/l within the first 48 hours of onset of symptoms indicates acute necrotizing pancreatitis with a high specificity of >80% and an accuracy of 86%.[22–26] CRP is a useful marker to predict severity, but has limitations to detect infected necrosis. Procalcitonin seems to be a more suitable marker for detection of pancreatic infections.[27,28] The specificity is influenced by the fact that it also can be increased by other severe extrapancreatic infections. Urinary TAP, which is released during activation of trypsinogen to trypsin, has shown to accurately predict severity of acute pancreatitis 24 hours after onset. Urinary TAP is suggested to be used as a single marker for severity assessment, but it is still not used as a routine test today.[19] The sepsis-related organ failure assessment (SOFA) was also proposed to predict mortality. Mortality is higher if the SOFA score is >3.[20]

16.3 ARTIFICIAL NUTRITION IN ACUTE PANCREATITIS

Pancreatitis patients in the past were either fasted or the nutrients were given by the parenteral route supporting the concept of the day when it was felt the pancreas should be "rested" during inflammation. Oral or enteral nutrition was believed to have a negative impact on the progression of the disease due to stimulation of exocrine pancreatic secretion and the consequent worsening of the autodigestive processes. Oral feeding is also known to increase abdominal pain in patients with acute pancreatitis.

In the past 20 years, the opinion dramatically changed. Patients with mild to moderate acute pancreatitis can usually start with an oral diet within a few days of onset if their pain and the pancreatic enzymes return to normal. In this population of mild to moderate pancreatitis, there is no benefit from early enteral or total parenteral nutrition (TPN).[8] However, this is not the case in patients with severe acute pancreatitis, where adequate enteral or TPN has been shown to improve outcome.[8] The nutritional management has shifted from parenteral to enteral feeding. Enteral feeding can reduce catabolism and the loss of lean body mass. In addition, enteral feeding may modulate the acute phase response and preserve visceral protein metabolism with the potential to downregulate splanchnic cytokine response.[29]

16.3.1 SUBSTRATE METABOLISM DURING ACUTE PANCREATITIS

During acute pancreatitis, as in other patients with critical illness, the metabolism of the macronutrients can be altered.

16.3.1.1 Metabolism of Carbohydrates

Glucose metabolism in acute pancreatitis is determined by an increase in energy demand. Endogenous gluconeogenesis is increased as a consequence of the metabolic response to the severe inflammatory process. Glucose is an important source of energy and can only partially counteract the intrinsic gluconeogenesis from protein degradation. This can influence, to a certain degree, the deleterious and unwanted effect of protein catabolism.[30] During hypermetabolism, the maximum rate of glucose oxidation is approximately 4 mg/kg/min. The administration of glucose in excess can be harmful because of lipogenesis and glucose recycling. Furthermore, hyperglycemia and hyperkapnia can occur. Hyperglycemia is a major risk factor for infections and metabolic complications. Monitoring and blood glucose control, therefore, is essential.

16.3.1.2 Protein Metabolism

A negative nitrogen balance is often seen in severe acute pancreatitis. The protein losses and the muscle wasting should be minimized and the increased protein turnover must be compensated. Therefore, a protein supply of at least 1.2 to 1.5 g/kg/BW/d is highly recommended.

16.3.1.3 Lipid Metabolism

Hyperlipidemia is a common finding in acute pancreatitis. Increases in cholesterol and free fatty acid serum concentrations also have been reported. The mechanism associated with the changes in lipid metabolism is not entirely clear. Both altered lipid oxidation and lipid clearance may play a role. In the majority of cases developing hyperlipidemia following an acute episode of pancreatitis, serum lipid concentration returns to normal. It is also well reported that in some patients with severe hyperlipidemia acute pancreatitis can develop.[31] Several mechanisms have been described to explain the adverse influence of hyperlipidemia on the pancreas, but no single mechanism has been supported by significant scientific data.[32,33]

16.3.2 Exocrine Pancreatic Stimulation by Macronutrients

For nutritional intervention, the administration of glucose, protein, and fat are necessary; historically, enteral applications were considered to be harmful because of the potential stimulation of the exocrine pancreatic enzyme secretion.

Enteral glucose perfusion into the jejunum is a very weak stimulus for exocrine pancreatic secretory response. Jejunal perfusion of elemental diets containing defined amounts of protein or amino acids are well tolerated and do not stimulate exocrine pancreatic secretion.[34,35] Vu et al. studied the nutrient induced activation of pancreatic secretion in healthy volunteers.[36] They found no significant increase over basal duodenal outputs of pancreatic enzymes during the continuous administration of a mixed liquid meal when the tube was located 60 cm distal to the ligament of Treitz. These findings were confirmed by Kaushik et al. in a study of 36 healthy volunteers.[37] This group compared fasting, duodenal, jejunal, and intravenous nutrient delivery and reported that duodenal delivery stimulated trypsin secretion, whereas fasting, midjejunal, and intravenous feeding did not. These data are in contrast with another study by O'Keefe et al.[38] They studied the stimulatory effects of enteral or parenteral feeding on the synthesis and turnover of trypsin. Thirty healthy volunteers were studied during fasting, intravenous feeding, postpyloric enteral feeding into the duodenum (polymeric or elemental diet), and into the jejunum (elemental diet). Compared to fasting, enteral feeding increased the rate of appearance and secretion of newly labeled trypsin and expanded zymogen stores. These differences persisted whether the feedings were polymeric or elemental, duodenal, or jejunal. Only intravenous feeding had no effect on the trypsin synthesis and turnover. Whether these findings in healthy volunteers can be extrapolated to patients with severe acute pancreatitis is still not entirely clear. There is evidence that the secretion of pancreatic enzymes, especially trypsin and lipase, is decreased in patients with acute pancreatitis. This disease-induced alteration of pancreatic function would be another explanation for the observation that enteral feeding is well tolerated in patients with acute pancreatitis.

The stimulation of the exocrine pancreatic secretion by enteral administration of lipids depends on the anatomic side of administration. If the lipids are delivered into the distal jejunum, no stimulation of the exocrine pancreatic secretion occurs.[36] In addition, no negative side effects were reported in patients fed with lipid-containing diets by the jejunal route during a severe acute attack of pancreatitis.[8]

As discussed above in this section, intravenous administration of macronutrients (glucose, amino acids, and lipids) does not stimulate exocrine pancreatic function and appears safe in pancreatitis.[39,40] The main risk of intravenous glucose in acute pancreatitis is hyperglycemia. Hyperglycemia also can be aggravated by the insulin resistance, which is well described in critical ill patients.

All these findings have changed the nutritional concept in acute pancreatitis. In current critical care settings, enteral feeding in the jejunum is regarded to be safe and effective without major stimulation of autodigestive processes. Enteral nutritional support has now been shown to be important in maintaining the gut integrity by modulating the gastrointestinal tract systemic immunity.

16.3.3 TOTAL PARENTERAL NUTRITION OR ENTERAL NUTRITION?

Traditionally, TPN was used to avoid stimulation of the exocrine pancreatic secretion. In mild to moderate pancreatitis, two prospective studies comparing TPN with a naso-jejunal feeding regimen[41] or no nutritional support[42] showed no difference in outcome. However, TPN was more expensive[41] or was accompanied by an increase in catheter-related infections and longer hospital stay.[42] Furthermore, TPN was associated with more hyperglycemia and other metabolic disturbances. In the past 10 years, it has become clear that these complications were often the consequence of overfeeding and hyperglycemia.[43] In 2001, van den Berge et al. showed, irrespective of the route of nutritional support, that the control of hyperglycemia with insulin reduced mortality in critical ill patients.[44]

Several studies in patients with trauma, thermal injury, and major gastrointestinal surgery showed a reduction in septic complication with enteral feeding.[45,46] Enteral nutrition helps to maintain mucosal function and limits the absorption of endotoxin and cytokines from the gut.[47,48] In animals with experimentally induced pancreatitis, enteral nutrition prevents bacteria translocation.[49] Whether bacterial translocation is of clinical evidence in patients with acute pancreatitis is still unclear.[50] Following roughly 20 years in which TPN was considered the standard nutritional support in severe acute pancreatitis, enteral nutrition was introduced and is now the standard of care in the management of severe acute pancreatitis. Several prospective, randomized clinical trials have been performed comparing enteral with parenteral nutrition in patients with acute pancreatitis. In the first prospective study by McClave et al., patients with mild to moderate acute pancreatitis were randomized to either total parenteral nutrition or to total enteral nutrition via a naso-jejunal tube.[41] Both groups received an isocaloric, isonitrogenious enteral solution within 48 hours of admission to the hospital. The outcome in both groups revealed no statistical differences in infectious complications, length of intensive care unit stay, and length of hospital stay or days to oral food intake. In the TPN group, a significantly higher glucose concentration in the first five days was found. The caloric goal was reached in 82% of the patients with enteral feeding compared to 96% of patients with TPN.[41] A second prospective, randomized study compared either a naso-jejunal tube feeding with a semielemental diet or TPN within 48 hours of admissions in patients with severe necrotizing acute pancreatitis.[51] Enteral feeding was well tolerated without adverse effects on the course of the disease, but patients who received enteral feeding experienced fewer septic complications and fewer total complications compared to those receiving parenteral nutrition. Furthermore, the costs of nutritional support were three times higher in the patients receiving TPN. This study showed that, in severe acute pancreatitis, enteral nutrition support was beneficial compared to patients with mild or moderate pancreatitis.[41] These findings are supported by two other studies. Windsor et al.[52] compared parenteral nutrition with enteral nutrition in patients with acute pancreatitis with all levels of severity. This study demonstrated that enteral nutrition attenuates the acute phase response in pancreatitis, improves disease severity and clinical outcome, despite the fact that the pancreatic injuries were virtually unchanged on a CT scan. In the enteral feeding group, SIRS and sepsis were reduced, resulting in a beneficial clinical outcome (APACHE II-score and C-reactive protein). In this study, unfortunately, only a few patients had severe pancreatitis and the total amount of nutrient received revealed marked differences between the enteral and the parenteral group. Unfortunately, these positive results of the Windsor study could not be confirmed by Powell et al. on the inflammatory response in patients with prognostically severe acute pancreatitis.[53]

Abou-Assi et al. selected 156 patients with acute pancreatitis over a one-year period.[54] During the first 48 hours, all the patients were treated with intravenous (i.v.) fluid and analgesics. In this study, 87% of patients had mild, 10% moderate, and 3% severe disease. Those patients who improved during this first 48-hour period were fed orally. The nonresponders were randomized to receive nutrients either by a naso-jejunal tube or by TPN. Seventy-five percent of the initially enrolled patients improved with the oral regimen and were discharged within four days; 54% of the enteral group (n = 26) and 88% of the TPN group (n = 27) received inadequate energy intake. The patients in the enteral group were fed for a significantly shorter period (mean 6.7 days versus 10.8 days [TPN]), and had significantly fewer metabolic and septic complications. Hyperglycemia requiring insulin therapy was significantly higher in the parenteral fed patients. Despite fewer complications in the enteral group, the mortality was similar in the two groups. The authors concluded that hypocaloric enteral feeding is safer and less expensive than parenteral feeding and bowel rest in patients with acute pancreatitis.

Today, there is no doubt that enteral nutrition should be the first attempt to feed patients with severe acute pancreatitis. The first meta-analysis from McClave et al. showed that the use of enteral nutrition was associated with a significant reduction in infectious morbidity, a reduction of hospital length of stay, and a trend toward reduced organ failure when compared with the use of parenteral nutrition. There was no effect on mortality.[55] Compared to this meta-analysis, a new systemic review showed a reduction in mortality using enteral nutrition when only patients with severe acute pancreatitis were included.[56] This report emphasizes that the greater the severity of the disease, the greater is the benefit of the enteral nutrition.

16.3.4 ENERGY REQUIREMENTS

For enteral or parenteral nutrition, 25 to 35 kcal/kg/BW/d is recommended.[8] Overfeeding and hyperglycemia should be avoided. Blood glucose concentration should not exceed 10 mmol/l (180mg/dl). Insulin treatment is recommended, but the dose should not be higher than 4 to 6 units/h. The impaired glucose oxidation rate cannot be normalized by insulin administration. Normally, 3 to 6 g/kg/BW/d of carbohydrates can be recommended. The optimal goal of protein supply is between 1.2 to 1.5 g/kg/BW/d. Lower protein intake should only be given to patients with renal or severe hepatic failure. Fat can be given up to 2 g/kg/BW/d, but triglyceride levels must be carefully monitored. Triglycerides are tolerated up to 12 mmol/l (1068 mg/dl).[8]

In general, the nutrient recommendations are easier to reach with TPN than with enteral nutrition as intolerance is not an issue. Enteral solution contains fixed amounts of the macronutrients. The enteral intake of the different nutrients only can be regulated by changing the rate of delivery. Current recommendations support continuous jejunal feeding in severe acute pancreatitis.[8,57]

16.4 CLINICAL APPROACH FOR NUTRITIONAL SUPPORT IN ACUTE PANCREATITIS

If the patient meets criteria for supplemental enteral nutrition support, continuous jejunal feeding would be the first choice. Four prospective studies have shown that jejunal delivery is possible in most patients with acute pancreatitis.[41,58–60] Rarely, proximal migration of the feeding tube and the subsequent pancreatic stimulation has been reported to aggravate acute pancreatitis.[61] If the jejunal tube cannot be placed blindly at the bedside or with the aid of fluoroscopy, adequate endoscopic placement is usually feasible. A new approach was recently introduced by using a self-propelling naso-jejunal feeding tube. The tube was introduced into the stomach, and gastrointestinal motility was stimulated by metoclopramide. In 56 of 92 patients, the tube successfully migrated to the ligament of Treitz. Of the 36 patients with an initial failed placement, endoscopic placement of the tube was successful in 80%.[62]

Although tube feeding appears to be possible in most prospective trials, in more general studies, dealing with larger patient populations including all treated patients, this was not the case. Oleynikov et al. reported that tube feeding was not possible in most (25 out of 26) patients with severe acute pancreatitis (mean APACHE II-score 17.2 and mean Ranson score 4.3 on admission). This inability to successfully feed was thought to be secondary to severe retroperitoneal inflammatory changes.[63] On the other hand, tube feeding is possible in the presence of ascites and pancreatic fistulas.

Therefore, parenteral nutrition is indicated when side effects during tube feeding occur or the caloric goal cannot be reached. If parenteral nutrition is started, it also would be useful to combine it with small volumes of enteral feeds if tolerated. There is substantial evidence that enteral feeding in severe acute pancreatitis can downregulate the systemic inflammatory response and promote beneficial effects on gastrointestinal functions. The impaired gut motility may facilitate the colonization of the intestine with pathogenic bacteria and may contribute to bacterial translocation in the intestinal wall, with subsequent superinfection of the pancreatic necrosis. For this reason, if possible, a low volume of enteral feeding continuously perfused to the jejunum is recommended to supplement TPN when full enteral nutrition is not possible (e.g., prolonged paralytic ileus).[8]

16.4.1 NUTRITIONAL SUPPORT IN MILD TO MODERATE PANCREATITIS

There is no evidence that the nutritional support (enteral or parenteral) has a beneficial effect on outcome in patients with mild pancreatitis.[8] Enteral nutrition is unnecessary, if the patients can consume normal food within five to seven days of onset of the pancreatitis episode (ESPEN guidelines: grade B).[8] Enteral or parenteral nutrition within five to seven days has no positive effect on the course of the disease and, therefore, is not recommended (ESPEN guidelines: grade A).[8] Early enteral nutritional support can be of importance in patients with preexisting severe malnutrition or in patients when early refeeding in five to seven days is not possible. Figure 16.1 shows a frequently used approach for these patients.

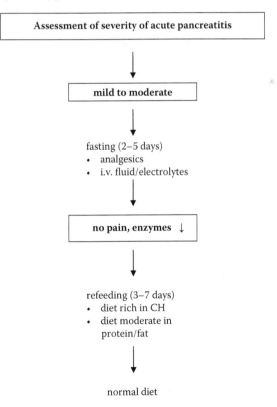

FIGURE 16.1 Management for mild to moderate acute pancreatitis.

16.4.2 Nutritional Support in Severe Acute Pancreatitis

In patients with severe pancreatitis, who have complications or need for surgery, early nutritional support is necessary to prevent the adverse effect of nutrient deprivation. In severe necrotizing pancreatitis, continuous early enteral nutrition over 24 hours is indicated as soon as possible (ESPEN Guidelines: Grade A).[8,57] Early enteral nutrition has been shown in many studies to be safe and well tolerated. In patients with severe necrotizing pancreatitis, intolerance to the enteral feeding commonly limits delivery of full nutrient requirements. If complete enteral nutrition is not possible, the enteral nutritional support should be supplemented with parenteral nutrition to meet caloric goals. Usually, the combined nutritional support allows that the patient reach the nutritional goals. The administration of lipids in parenteral nutrition can be regarded as safe, if hypertriglyceridemia (<12 mmol/l [1068 mg/dl]) is avoided.[8] A practical approach for nutrition in severe acute pancreatitis is outlined in Figure 16.2.

16.4.2.1 Route of Feeding

The route of nutrient delivery (parenteral/enteral) should be determined by patients' tolerance. Tube feeding is possible in the majority of patients, but some patients need a combination with parenteral nutrition (ESPEN Guideline: Grade A).[8] Placing

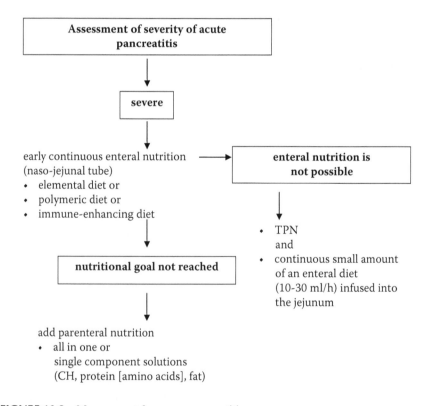

FIGURE 16.2 Management for severe pancreatitis.

a jejunal feeding tube distally to the ligament of Treitz can be performed safely and consistently. Several single or multilumen tubes are available. The tubes can be placed either with fluoroscopic help, using self-propelling tubes, or with the endoscope. Partial ileus is not a contraindication for enteral feeding because these patients frequently tolerate continuous low-volume jejunal nutrients. If surgery is required in pancreatitis, an intraoperative naso-jejunal tube can be directly placed into the jejunum by the surgeon by manipulating the tube passed into the stomach by the anesthesia provider, around the C-loop of the duodenum to the jejunum. A surgical jejunostomy for postoperative tube feeding is also feasible.[64]

Whether the jejunal feeding is absolutely necessary is not completely clear. Minimizing stimulation of the exocrine pancreatic secretion would support the jejunal feeding route. It is, however, controversial whether stimulation of pancreatic secretion is important for the outcome in this disease. Recently, two randomized studies comparing naso-gastric versus naso-jejunal feeding in severe acute pancreatitis were published.[65,66] In these studies, naso-gastric feeding was as safe as naso-jejunal feeding; little difference was documented between the two methods with respect to pain, analgesic requirements, serum CRP concentration, or clinical outcome. Also here, no clear recommendation can be given. If a multilumen tube is used for tube feeding, feeding through the gastric port can be initially attempted. If this is not possible, one can then switch to the jejunal port. More clinical trials using such concepts are warranted.

16.4.2.2 Choice of Optimal Formula

Most studies have been done using semielemental or peptide-based formulae. The use of peptide-based formulae showed beneficial effects (ESPEN Guidelines: Grade A).[8] Nowadays, in most institutions, polymeric formulae are used. A direct comparison of a peptide-based formula with the polymeric formula showed that there was no difference on outcome.[67] Today, it is common to start with a standard polymeric formula and, if this is not tolerated, a peptide-based formula is tried. Several published trials also used formulae containing immune-modulating substrates (glutamine, arginine, n-3 polyunsaturated fatty acids) or pre- and probiotics.[57] No specific formula can be recommended for pancreatitis as inadequate comparative studies have been done. The concept of using pre- and probiotics to prevent intestinal bacterial translocation is very attractive. Two studies by Oláh et al. examined the efficacy of enteral administration of probiotics in patients with severe acute pancreatitis.[68,69] In the first study, 22 patients received live lactobacillus plantarum and oat fiber, and 23 patients, the same formulation with heat-killed bacteria. In the group with live bacteria, they found fewer positive cultures (p = 0.23), reduced need for antibiotics, and a reduction in pancreatic infections requiring surgical intervention (p = 0.046). Furthermore, the length of hospital stay was shorter (13.7 days versus 21.4 days).[68] In the second study, 62 patients with acute pancreatitis who were fed with a naso-jejunal tube and randomized to receive enteral nutrition with fiber (29 patients) or enteral nutrition with fiber and a combination of four different lactobacilli (34 patients). The probiotic group again had significantly lower complication rates (p = 0.049) and the control group had higher rates of multiorgan failure, pancreatic septic complications, surgical intervention, and mortality.[69]

These observations were exciting until the large multicenter controlled trial by Besselink et al. was published.[70] They randomized 298 patients with severe acute pancreatitis with either a combination six probiotics (four strains lactobacilli and two strains bifidobacteria) or placebo. A multifiber enteral solution was given in both groups by a naso-jejunal tube. There were no differences in infectious complications between the probiotic and placebo group (30% versus 28%). Unfortunately, mortality was significantly higher in the probiotic group (16% versus 6%). Nine patients in the probiotic group developed bowel ischemia. At the moment, it is not clear if these complications are due to the combination of probiotics administered to the gut or if other underlying factors played a role and the two groups cannot be fully compared. Organ failure during admission was more common in the probiotic group than in the placebo group (27.0% versus 16.0%; p = 0.02). Intestinal ischemia also can be found more often during vasopressor treatment. In the probiotic group, more patients received vasopressor drugs than in the placebo group. This could be another explanation for the developing of bowel ischemia. In the Besselink study, no adverse events were shown in the group receiving only prebiotics. This is in line with a new study published by Karakan et al.[71] They found that naso-jejunal enteral nutrition with prebiotic fiber supplementation in patients with severe acute pancreatitis reduced hospital stay, duration of nutrition therapy, acute phase response, and overall complications compared to standard enteral nutrition. For the moment, probiotics in severe acute pancreatitis cannot be recommended until more trials have shown that pobiotics are effective and safe.

Several studies were done by supplementation of TPN with n-3 polyunsaturated fatty acids or glutamine. Wang et al. found that patients treated with n-3 polyunsaturated fatty acids had significantly higher eicosapentaenoic acid (EPA) plasma concentrations, lower CRP levels, and better oxygenation index after five days of TPN than the control group. In addition, the number of days of continuous renal replacement therapy was significantly decreased.[72] All of the glutamine studies demonstrated beneficial effects.[8,55] This was recently confirmed by the study from Fuentes-Orozco et al.[73] The group with glutamine supplementation had a significant increase in serum IL-10 levels, total lymphocyte and lymphocyte subpopulations counts, and albumin serum levels. Nitrogen balance improved to positive levels in the study group and remained negative in the control group. Infectious morbidity was more frequent in the control group. The duration of hospital stay and the mortality were similar between the two groups. It appears from this early work that in the future adding n-3 polyunsaturated fatty acids and/or glutamine to parenteral nutrition in patients with severe acute pancreatitis may prove beneficial.

16.4.2.3 Oral Refeeding

There are only few data available on oral refeeding. Oral feeding with normal food and/or oral supplements can be progressively attempted once gastric outlet obstruction has resolved, provided it does not result in pain, and if complications are under control. Tube feeding can be gradually withdrawn as intake improves. Currently, there are only two studies investigating oral refeeding.[74,75] In the study of Lévy et al., 21% of patients experienced a pain relapse on the first and second day of refeeding. Serum lipase concentration >3 times the upper limit of the normal range and higher Balthazar's CT-scores at the onset of refeeding were identified as risk factors for pain relapse.[74]

16.5 NUTRITIONAL SUPPORT IN PATIENTS WITH PANCREATIC SURGERY

After surgery, either a naso-jejunal tube or a needle catheter jejunostomy are used. Both types of feeding are safe, well tolerated and depend on the surgeon preference.

Postoperative feeding with a needle catheter jejunostomy was successful in several small studies.[59,64,76] Hernández-Aranda et al. found no difference between groups of patients who received postoperative parenteral nutrition or enteral nutrition via jejunostomy.[76] Furthermore, in patients undergoing surgery for severe acute pancreatitis, needle catheter jejunostomy for long-term enteral nutrition was safely applied with no nutritional risk.[64] In general, in these patients, nutritional support has to be planned before the operation according to the clinical situation and, the course, of the disease.

16.6 SUMMARY

Acute pancreatitis occurs in different clinical patterns ranging from a mild to severe necrotizing disease with local and systemic complications. The major pathological processes in acute pancreatitis are inflammation, edema, and necrosis of the pancreatic tissue as well as inflammation and injury of extrapancreatic organs; 75 to 80% have mild, edematous and about 20 to 25% experience severe necrotizing pancreatitis. The mortality rate for mild to moderate pancreatitis is less than 1%. The mortality rate for severe pancreatitis increases up to 30%, but can approach 50% if necrosis of the gland is greater than 50% and can further increase up to 80% if sepsis occurs.

For nutritional interventions, it is essential to assess the severity of the disease. Patients with severe acute pancreatitis are hypermetabolic. The more severe the acute pancreatitis is, the more excessive the hypermetabolism.

There is no evidence that a nutritional support (enteral or parenteral) has a beneficial effect on clinical outcome in patients with mild acute pancreatitis. Nutritional intervention is unnecessary if the patients can consume normal food within five to seven days of onset of disease. In patients with severe acute pancreatitis, who have complications or need surgery, early nutritional support is necessary to prevent the adverse effect of nutrient deprivation. Early continuous enteral nutrition by a naso-jejunal tube is recommended as the first line of support. If enteral nutrition is not possible, parenteral nutrition should be added. Peptide-based formula or polymeric formula can be used according to the tolerance of the patient. The use of enteral or parenteral formulae containing immune-modulating substrates (glutamine, arginine, n-3 polyunsaturated fatty acids) is promising, but more data are needed. Pre- and probiotics should not be used until new studies prove safety and efficacy.

REFERENCES

1. Clancy TE, Benoit EP, Ashley SW. Current management of acute pancreatitis. *J Gastrointest Surg* 2005;9:440–52.
2. Toouli J, Brooke-Smith M, Bassi C, et al. Guidelines for the management of acute pancreatitis. *J Gastroenterol Hepatol* 2002;17 Suppl:S15–39.
3. Bradley EL and Members of the Atlanta International Symposium. A clinically based classification system for acute pancreatitis: summary of the International Symposium on Acute Pancreatitis, Atlanta, Ga, September 11 through 13, 1992. *Arch of Surg* 193;128: 586–590.
4. Winslet MC, Hall C, London NJM, Neoptolemos JP. Relationship of diagnostic serum amylase to aetiology and prognosis in acute pancreatitis. *Gut* 1992;33:982–986.
5. Banks PA, Freeman ML, Practice Parameters Committee of the American College of Gastroenterology. Practice guidelines in acute pancreatitis. *Am J Gastroenterol* 2006;101:2379–400.
6. Whitcomb DC. Acute pancreatitis. *N Engl J Med* 2006;354:2142–50.
7. Robin AP, Campbell R, Palani CK, Liu K, Donahue PE, Nyhus LM. Total parenteral nutrition during acute pancreatitis: clinical experience with 156 patients. *World J Surg* 1990;14:572–9.
8. Meier R, Ockenga J, Pertkiewicz M, et al. ESPEN guidelines on enteral nutrition: pancreas. *Clin Nutr* 2006;25:275–84.
9. Shaw JH, Wolfe RR. Glucose, fatty acid, and urea kinetics in patients with severe pancreatitis: the response to substrate infusion and total parenteral nutrition. *Ann Surg* 1986;204:665–72.
10. Gupta R, Patel K, Calder PC, Yaqoob P, Primrose JN, Johnson CD. A randomised clinical trial to assess the effect of total enteral and total parenteral nutritional support on metabolic, inflammatory and oxidative markers in patients with predicted severe acute pancreatitis (APACHE II > or =6). *Pancreatology* 2003;3:406–13.
11. Dickerson RN, Vehe KL, Mullen JL, Feurer ID. Resting energy expenditure in patients with pancreatitis. *Crit Care Med* 1991;19:484–90.
12. Sitzmann JV, Steinborn PA, Zinner MJ, Cameron JL. Total parenteral nutrition and alternate energy substrates in treatment of severe acute pancreatitis. *Surg Gynecol Obstet* 1989;168:311–7.
13. Klein S, Kinney J, Jeejeebhoy K, et al. Nutrition support in clinical practice: review of published data and recommendations for future research directions. National Institutes of Health, American Society for Parenteral and Enteral Nutrition, and American Society for Clinical Nutrition. *JPEN J Parenter Enteral Nutr* 1997;21:133–56.
14. Blamey SL, Imrie CW, O'Neill J, Gilmour WH, Carter DC. Prognostic factors in acute pancreatitis. *Gut* 1984;25:1340–6.
15. Knaus WA, Draper EA, Wagner. D P, Zimmerman JE. APACHE II: a severity of disease classification system. *Crit Care Med* 1985;13:818–29.
16. Ranson JH, Rifkind KM, Roses DF, Fink SD, Eng K, Spencer FC. Prognostic signs and the role of operative management in acute pancreatitis. *Surg Gynecol Obstet* 1974;139:69–81.
17. Balthazar EJ, Robinson DL, Megibow AJ, Ranson JH. Acute pancreatitis: value of CT in establishing prognosis. *Radiology* 1990;174:331–6.
18. Wilson C, Heads A, Shenkin A, Imrie CW. C-reactive protein, antiproteases and complement factors as objective markers of severity in acute pancreatitis. *Br J Surg* 1989;76:177–81.
19. Neoptolemos JP, Kemppainen EA, Mayer JM, et al. Early prediction of severity in acute pancreatitis by urinary trypsinogen activation peptide: a multicentre study. *Lancet* 2000;355:1955–60.

20. De Campos T, Cerqueira C, Kuryura L, et al. Morbimortality indicators in severe acute pancreatitis. *JOP* 2008;9:690–7.
21. Mortele KJ, Wiesner W, Intriere L, et al. A modified CT severity index for evaluating acute pancreatitis: improved correlation with patient outcome. *AJR Am J Roentgenol* 2004;183:1261–5.
22. Uhl W, Büchler M, Malfertheiner P, Martini M, Beger HG. PMN-elastase in comparison with CRP, antiproteases, and LDH as indicators of necrosis in human acute pancreatitis. *Pancreas* 1991;6:253–9.
23. Mayer J, Rau B, Gansauge F, Beger HG. Inflammatory mediators in human acute pancreatitis: clinical and pathophysiological implications. *Gut* 2000;47:546–52.
24. Büchler M, Malfertheiner P, Schoetensack C, Uhl W, Beger HG. Sensitivity of antiproteases, complement factors and C-reactive protein in detecting pancreatic necrosis: results of a prospective clinical study. *Int J Pancreatol* 1986;1:227–35.
25. Rau B, Schilling MK, Beger HG. Laboratory markers of severe acute pancreatitis. *Dig Dis Sci* 2004;22:247–57.
26. Werner J, Hartwig W, Uhl W, Müller C, Büchler MW. Useful markers for predicting severity and monitoring progression of acute pancreatitis. *Pancreatology* 2003;3:115–27.
27. Purkayastha S, Chow A, Athanasiou T, et al. Does serum procalcitonin have a role in evaluating the severity of acute pancreatitis? A question revisited. *World J Surg* 2006;30:1713–21.
28. Rau BM, Kemppainen EA, Gumbs AA, et al. Early assessment of pancreatic infections and overall prognosis in severe acute pancreatitis by procalcitonin (PCT): a prospective international multicenter study. *Ann Surg* 2007;245:745–54.
29. Jabbar A, Chang WK, Dryden GW, McClave SA. Gut immunology and the differential response to feeding and starvation. *Nutr Clin Pract* 2003;18:461–82.
30. Alpers DH. Digestion and absorptoin of carbohydrats and protein. In: Jonson LR et al. (Eds.) *Physiology of the Gastrointestinal Tract* (2nd ed.) 1987; Raven Press, New York, 1469–87.
31. Greenberger NJ. Pancreatitis and hyperlipemia. *N Engl J Med* 1973;289:586–7.
32. Cameron JL, Capuzzi DM, Zuidema GD, Margolis S. Acute pancreatitis with hyperlipemia: evidence for a persistent defect in lipid metabolism. *Am J Med* 1974;56: 482–7.
33. Farmer RG, Winkelman EI, Brown HB, Lewis LA. Hyperlipoproteinemia and pancreatitis. *Am J Med* 1973;54:161–5.
34. McArdle AH, Echave W, Brown RA, Thompson AG. Effect of elemental diet on pancreatic secretion. *Am J Surg* 1974;128:690–2.
35. Grant JP, Davey-McCrae J, Snyder PJ. Effect of enteral nutrition on human pancreatic secretions. *JPEN J Parenter Enteral Nutr* 1987;11:302–4.
36. Vu MK, van der Veek PP, Frölich M, et al. Does jejunal feeding activate exocrine pancreatic secretion? *Eur J Clin Invest* 1999;29:1053–9.
37. Kaushik N, Pietraszewski M, Holst JJ, O'Keefe SJ. Enteral feeding without pancreatic stimulation. *Pancreas* 2005;31:353–9.
38. O'Keefe SJ, Lee RB, Anderson FP, et al. Physiological effects of enteral and parenteral feeding on pancreaticobiliary secretion in humans. *Am J Physiol Gastrointest Liver Physiol* 2003;284:G27–36.
39. Grant JP, Davey-McCrae J, Snyder PJ. Effect of enteral nutrition on human pancreatic secretions. *JPEN J Parenter Enteral Nutr* 1987;11:302–4.
40. Klein E, Shnebaum S, Ben-Ari G, Dreiling DA. Effects of total parenteral nutrition on exocrine pancreatic secretion. *Am J Gastroenterol* 1983;78:31–3.
41. McClave SA, Greene LM, Snider HL, et al. Comparison of the safety of early enteral vs parenteral nutrition in mild acute pancreatitis. *JPEN J Parenter Enteral Nutr* 1997;21:14–20.

42. Sax HC, Warner BW, Talamini MA, et al. Early total parenteral nutrition in acute pancreatitis: lack of beneficial effects. *Am J Surg* 1987;153:117–24.
43. Nordenström J, Thörne A. Benefits and complications of parenteral nutritional support. *Eur J Clin Nutr* 1994;48:531–7.
44. van den Berghe G, Wouters P, Weekers F, et al. Intensive insulin therapy in the critically ill patients. *N Engl J Med* 2001;345:1359–67.
45. Trice S, Melnik G, Page CP. Complications and costs of early postoperative parenteral versus enteral nutrition in trauma patients. *Nutr Clin Pract* 1997;12:114–9.
46. Heyland DK, Novak F, Drover JW, Jain M, Su X, Suchner U. Should immunonutrition become routine in critically ill patients? A systematic review of the evidence. *JAMA* 2001;286:944–53.
47. Buchman AL, Moukarzel AA, Bhuta S, et al. Parenteral nutrition is associated with intestinal morphologic and functional changes in humans. *JPEN J Parenter Enteral Nutr* 1995;19:453–60.
48. Lange JF, van Gool J, Tytgat GN. The protective effect of a reduction in intestinal flora on mortality of acute haemorrhagic pancreatitis in the rat. *Hepatogastroenterology* 1987;34:28–30.
49. Hallay J, Kovács G, Szatmári K, et al. Early jejunal nutrition and changes in the immunological parameters of patients with acute pancreatitis. *Hepatogastroenterology* 2001;48:1488–92.
50. Kotani J, Usami M, Nomura H, et al. Enteral nutrition prevents bacterial translocation but does not improve survival during acute pancreatitis. *Arch Surg* 1999;134:287–92.
51. Kalfarentzos F, Kehagias J, Mead N, Kokkinis K, Gogos CA. Enteral nutrition is superior to parenteral nutrition in severe acute pancreatitis: results of a randomized prospective trial. *Br J Surg* 1997;84:1665–9.
52. Windsor AC, Kanwar S, Li AG, et al. Compared with parenteral nutrition, enteral feeding attenuates the acute phase response and improves disease severity in acute pancreatitis. *Gut* 1998;42:431–5.
53. Powell JJ, Murchison JT, Fearon KC, Ross JA, Siriwardena AK. Randomized controlled trial of the effect of early enteral nutrition on markers of the inflammatory response in predicted severe acute pancreatitis. *Br J Surg* 2000;87:1375–81.
54. Abou-Assi S, Craig K, O'Keefe SJ. Hypocaloric jejunal feeding is better than total parenteral nutrition in acute pancreatitis: results of a randomized comparative study. *Am J Gastroenterol* 2002;97:2255–62.
55. McClave SA, Chang WK, Dhaliwal R, Heyland DK. Nutrition support in acute pancreatitis: a systematic review of the literature. *JPEN J Parenter Enteral Nutr* 2006;30:143–56.
56. Jafri NS, Mahid SS, Gopathi SK, et al. Enteral nutrition is superior to parenteral nutrition in severe acute pancreatitis: a systemic review and meta-analysis. *Gastroenterology* 2008;134:4:A141.
57. Meier R, Beglinger C, Layer P, et al. ESPEN guidelines on nutrition in acute pancreatitis. European Society of Parenteral and Enteral Nutrition. *Clin Nutr* 2002;21:173–83.
58. Cravo M, Camilo M, Marques A, Printo Correia J. Early tube feeding in acute pancreatitis: a prospective study. *Clin Nutr* 1989:A8–A14.
59. Kudsk KA, Campbell SM, O'Brien T, Fuller R. Postoperative jejunal feedings following complicated pancreatitis. *Nutr Clin Pract* 1990;5:14–7.
60. Nakad A, Piessevaux H, Marot JC, et al. Is early enteral nutrition in acute pancreatitis dangerous? About 20 patients fed by an endoscopically placed nasogastrojejunal tube. *Pancreas* 1998;17:187–93.
61. Scolapio JS, Malhi-Chowla N, Ukleja A. Nutrition supplementation in patients with acute and chronic pancreatitis. *Gastroenterol Clin North Am* 1999;28:695–707.

62. Joubert C, Tiengou LE, Hourmand-Ollivier I, Dao MT, Piquet MA. Feasibility of self-propelling nasojejunal feeding tube in patients with acute pancreatitis. *JPEN J Parenter Enteral Nutr* 2008;32:622–4. Epub 2008 Sept. 30.

63. Oleynikov D, Cook C, Sellers B, Mone MC, Barton R. Decreased mortality from necrotizing pancreatitis. *Am J Surg* 1998;176:648–53.

64. Weimann A, Braunert M, Müller T, Bley T, Wiedemann B. Feasibility and safety of needle catheter jejunostomy for enteral nutrition in surgically treated severe acute pancreatitis. *JPEN J Parenter Enteral Nutr* 2004;28:324–7.

65. Eatcock FC, Brombacher GD, Steven A, Imrie CW, McKay CJ, Carter R. Nasogastric feeding in severe acute pancreatitis may be practical and safe. *Int J Pancreatol* 2000;28:23–9.

66. Singh KA, Prakaeb S, et al. Early enteral nutrition in severe acute pancreatitis: a prospective randomized controlled trial comparing nasojejunal and nasogastric routes. *J Clin Gastroenterol* 2006;40:431–4.

67. Tiengou L, Gloro R, Pouzoulet J, et al. Semi-elemental formula or polymeric formula: is there a better choice for enteral nutrition in acute pancreatitis? Randomized comparative study. *JPEN J Parenter Enteral Nutr* 2006;30:1–5.

68. Oláh A, Belágyi T, Issekutz A, Gamal ME, Bengmark S. Randomized clinical trial of specific lactobacillus and fibre supplement to early enteral nutrition in patients with acute pancreatitis. *Br J Surg* 2002;89:1103–7.

69. Oláh A, Belágyi T, Pótó L, Romics LJ, Bengmark S. Synbiotic control of inflammation and infection in severe acute pancreatitis: a prospective, randomized, double blind study. *Hepatogastroenterology* 2007;54:590–4.

70. Besselink MG, van Santvoort HC, Buskens E, et al. Probiotic prophylaxis in predicted severe acute pancreatitis: a randomised, double-blind, placebo-controlled trial. *Lancet* 2008;371:651–9. ePub 2008 Feb. 14.

71. Karakan T, Ergun M, Dogan I, Cindoruk M, Unal S. Comparison of early enteral nutrition in severe acute pancreatitis with prebiotic fiber supplementation versus standard enteral solution: a prospective randomized double-blind study. *World J Gastroenterol* 2007;13:2733–7.

72. Wang X, Li W, Li N, Li J. Omega-3 fatty acids-supplemented parenteral nutrition decreases hyperinflammatory response and attenuates systemic disease sequelae in severe acute pancreatitis: a randomized and controlled study. *JPEN J Parenter Enteral Nutr* 2008;32:236–41.

73. Fuentes-Orozco C, Cervantes-Guevara G, Muciño-Hernández I, et al. L-alanyl-L-glutamine-supplemented parenteral nutrition decreases infectious morbidity rate in patients with severe acute pancreatitis. *JPEN J Parenter Enteral Nutr* 2008;32:403–11.

74. Lévy P, Heresbach D, Pariente EA, et al. Frequency and risk factors of recurrent pain during refeeding in patients with acute pancreatitis: a multivariate multicentre prospective study of 116 patients. *Gut* 1997;40:262–6.

75. Pandey SK, Ahuja V, Joshi YK, Sharma MP. A randomized trial of oral refeeding compared with jejunal tube refeeding in acute pancreatitis. *Indian J Gastroenterol* 2004;23:53–5.

76. Hernández-Aranda JC, Gallo-Chico B, Ramírez-Barba EJ. Nutritional support in severe acute pancreatitis. Controlled clinical trial [article in Spanish]. *Nutr Hosp* 1996;11:160–6.

17 Nutrition in Liver Disease

Mathias Plauth and Tatjana Schütz

CONTENTS

17.1 INTRODUCTION

Nutrition has long been recognized as a prognostic and therapeutic determinant in patients with chronic liver disease[1] and, therefore, has been included as one of the variables in the original prognostic score introduced by Child and Turcotte.[2] Yet, not all hepatologists consider nutrition issues in the management of their patients. In this chapter, the scientific and evidence base of nutrition management of patients with liver disease is reviewed to give recommendations for nutrition therapy.

17.2 NUTRITIONAL RISK IN LIVER DISEASE PATIENTS

Understanding adequate nutrition as a complex action that in healthy organisms is regulated in a condition-adapted way, the assessment of nutritional risk of patients must include variables indicative of the physiologic capabilities—the nutritional status—and the burden inflicted by the ongoing or impending disease and/or medical interventions. Thus, a meaningful assessment of nutritional status should encompass not only body weight and height, but information on energy and nutrient balance as well as body composition and tissue function reflecting the metabolic and physical fitness of the patient facing a vital contest. Furthermore, such information can best be interpreted only when available with a dynamic view (e.g., weight loss over time).

Numerous descriptive studies have shown higher rates of mortality and complications, such as refractory ascites, variceal bleeding, infection, and hepatic encephalopathy (HE) in cirrhotic patients with protein malnutrition as well as reduced survival when such patients undergo liver transplantation.[3–11] In malnourished cirrhosis patients, the risk of postoperative morbidity and mortality is increased after abdominal surgery.[12,13]

In cirrhosis or alcoholic steatohepatitis (ASH), poor oral food intake is a predictor of an increased mortality. In nutrition intervention trials, patients with the lowest spontaneous energy intake showed the highest mortality.[14–20] Dietary intake should be assessed by a skilled dietitian, and a three-day dietary recall can be used in outpatients. Appropriate tables for food composition should be used for the calculation of proportions of different nutrients. As a gold standard, food analysis by bomb calorimetry may be utilized.[18,21]

Simple bedside methods like the Subjective Global Assessment (SGA) or anthropometry have been shown to adequately identify malnutrition.[4,6,11] Composite scoring systems have been developed based on variables, such as actual/ideal weight, anthropometry, creatinine index, visceral proteins, absolute lymphocyte count, delayed type skin reaction, absolute CD8+ count, and handgrip strength.[14–16] Such systems, however, include unreliable variables, such as plasma concentrations of visceral proteins or 24-hour urine creatinine excretion and do not confer an advantage over SGA.

Accurate measurement of nutritional status is difficult in the presence of fluid overload or impaired hepatic protein synthesis (e.g., albumin) and necessitates sophisticated methods, such as total body potassium counting, dual energy x-ray absorptiometry (DEXA), *in vivo* neutron activation analysis (IVNAA)[22,23] and isotope dilution.[24] Among bedside methods, the measurement of phase angle alpha or determination of body cell mass (BCM) using bioimpedance analysis is considered superior to methods, such as anthropometry and 24-h creatinine excretion,[25–27] despite some limitations in patients with ascites.[28,29]

Muscle function is reduced in malnourished chronic liver disease patients[23,30,31] and, as monitored by handgrip strength, is an independent predictor of outcome.[16,32] Plasma levels of visceral proteins (albumin, prealbumin, retinol-binding protein) are highly influenced by liver synthesis, alcohol intake, or acute inflammatory conditions.[33,34] Immune status, which is often considered a functional test of malnutrition, may be affected by hypersplenism, abnormal immunologic reactivity, and alcohol abuse.[34]

17.3 EFFECT OF NUTRITIONAL STATE ON LIVER DISEASE

17.3.1 Undernutrition

Severe malnutrition in children can cause fatty liver,[35–37] which in general is fully reversible upon refeeding.[37] In children with kwashiorkor, there seems to be a maladaptation associated with less efficient breakdown of fat and oxidation of fatty acids[38,39] compared to children with marasmus. An impairment of fatty acid removal from the liver could not be observed.[40] Malnutrition impairs specific hepatic functions like phase-I xenobiotic metabolism,[41,42] galactose elimination capacity,[43] or plasma levels of c-reactive protein in infected children.[44,45] In nutritional intervention trials in cirrhotic patients, quantitative liver function tests improved more, or more rapidly in treatment groups. This included antipyrine,[19] aminopyrine,[46] and ICG clearance[47] as well as galactose elimination capacity.[48,49] It is unknown whether fatty liver of malnutrition can progress to chronic liver disease.

Quantitative liver function tests seem to be useful for monitoring the effects of nutritional intervention on liver function. They are not useful, however, for identification of patients who will benefit from nutritional intervention because none of the tests can distinguish between reduced liver function due to reduced hepatocellular mass versus reduced liver function due to lack of essential nutrients. A simple test is needed that can distinguish between these two alternatives, in analogy to the intravenous (i.v.) vitamin K test, in order to estimate the potential benefit of nutritional support in individual patients.

17.3.2 Overnutrition

In obese humans subjected to total starvation, or weight reducing diets or small-bowel bypass, the development of transient degenerative changes with focal necrosis has been described nearly four decades ago.[50] Nonalcoholic steatohepatitis (NASH) has initially been described in weight-losing individuals[51] and, to date, insulin resistance and obesity are the most common causes.[52] It is estimated that, in Europe, 20% of the population with moderate or no alcohol consumption have nonalcoholic fatty liver (NAFL) of whom 20% progress from NAFL to NASH.[53] Analyses of dietary habits in NASH patients do not show a uniform pattern. Increased consumption of fat and n-6 fatty acids[54,55] and increased consumption of carbohydrate and energy[56] have been observed. Body mass index and total body fat are predictors for the presence of NASH in the obese,[54,57] and, in patients undergoing bariatric surgery, the prevalence of NASH is 37% (24 to 98%).[58] Furthermore, the key role of obesity is illustrated by the observation that weight reduction, regardless of whether it is achieved by dietary counseling, bariatric surgery, or drug treatment, has the potential to ameliorate or even cure NASH.[59–63]

17.4   EFFECT OF LIVER DISEASE ON NUTRITIONAL STATE

17.4.1   ACUTE LIVER DISEASE

In general, acute liver disease induces the same metabolic effects as any disease associated with an acute phase response. The effect on nutritional status depends on the duration of the disease and on the presence of an underlying chronic liver disease, which may have already compromised the patients' nutritional status.

17.4.2   CIRRHOSIS

Mixed-type protein energy malnutrition with coexisting features of kwashiorkor-like malnutrition and marasmus is commonly observed in patients with cirrhosis.[64,65] Prevalence and severity of malnutrition are related to the clinical stage of chronic liver disease increasing from 20% of patients with well compensated disease up to more than 60% of patients with severe liver insufficiency.[66] Patients with cirrhosis frequently suffer from substantial protein depletion and the resulting sarcopenia is associated with impaired muscle function[23] and survival.[6] Recovery from this loss in BCM can be achieved by the control of complications, such as portal hypertension and adequate nutrition.[67,68] Etiology of liver disease, per se, does not seem to influence the prevalence and degree of malnutrition and protein depletion[23,65,66] and the higher prevalence and more profound degree of malnutrition in alcoholics obviously result from an unhealthy lifestyle and low socioeconomic conditions.

In hospitalized cirrhotics, fatigue, somnolence, or psychomotor dysfunction often lead to insufficient oral nutrition even in the absence of overt HE.[69,70]

17.4.3   SURGERY AND TRANSPLANTATION

A large number of patients, in whom normal liver function has been restored by liver transplantation show an enormous weight gain in the first year after surgery[71,72] and, unfortunately, a considerable number put their regained health in jeopardy by the development of full-blown metabolic syndrome.[73] In the first year after transplantation, patients expand their body fat mass while there is no gain in lean body mass[71,74] and there is persisting impairment of nonoxidative glucose disposal in skeletal muscle.[75,76] There is growing evidence that, in solid organ-transplanted patients, skeletal muscle deconditioning persists from the time of decreased physical performance prior to transplantation[31,77–79] that should be addressed by appropriate comprehensive rehabilitation programs including physiotherapy. Taken together, these observations indicate that upon restoration of hepatic function and cessation of portal hypertension full nutritional rehabilitation is possible.

17.5 PATHOPHYSIOLOGY AND NUTRIENT REQUIREMENT IN LIVER DISEASE

17.5.1 ENERGY

17.5.1.1 Acute Liver Failure (ALF)

In healthy individuals, hepatic energy expenditure contributes 25% to whole body energy expenditure[80] and, in ALF, one would expect a reduction in oxygen-consuming processes like hepatic ketone body production and lactate elimination[81,82] due to the loss of functional hepatocyte mass. Indirect calorimetry in patients with ALF, however, showed an increase in resting energy expenditure (REE) by 18 to 30% in comparison with healthy controls.[83] Most likely, the accompanying systemic inflammatory response syndrome has caused an increase in energy expenditure that more than outweighs the reduced oxygen consumption of hepatocytes. Thus, in terms of energy expenditure, patients with ALF are not different from critically ill patients with other etiologies.

17.5.1.2 Cirrhosis

On average, measured REE is of the same magnitude as energy expenditure predicted by use of formulae (Harris and Benedict).[84–87] Likewise, in ASH patients, one study showed the same relationship between measured REE and predicted REE as in healthy individuals.[88] Whenever available, indirect calorimetry should be used to measure REE because in the individual patient measured REE may differ considerably from estimated values.[89]

The question of hypermetabolism has been addressed in cirrhosis and ASH patients. ASH patients may be considered hypermetabolic when measured REE is related to their reduced muscle mass.[88] Measured REE is higher than predicted REE in up to 35% of cirrhotic patients (hypermetabolism) and below the predicted value in 18% of the patients.[85–87] In cirrhosis, hypermetabolism has been shown associated with reduced event-free survival and unfavorable outcome after transplantation[10,87] and seems to regress with improvement of body composition[68] and after liver transplantation.[90] For the diagnosis of hypermetabolism, however, indirect calorimetry is required so that in daily practice most clinicians cannot use this approach.

Measurements of total energy expenditure indicate that the 24-hour energy requirement of cirrhosis patients amounts to about 130% of the basal metabolic rate.[21,91] Diet-induced thermogenesis[92–94] and the energy cost of defined physical activity in stable cirrhosis patients[95–97] also show no deviation from values obtained in healthy patients. However, the spontaneous physical activity level is considerably lower in patients with cirrhosis. Obviously, the increased energy requirement in advanced illness is balanced by diminished physical activity reflecting the poor physical condition.[20,97]

In cirrhotics without ascites, the actual body weight should be used for the calculation of the basal metabolic rate using formulae, such as that proposed by Harris and Benedict.[84] In patients with ascites, the ideal weight according to body height should be used, despite the suggestion from a series of 10 patients with liver cirrhosis of whom only 4 were completely evaluated,[98] in which it was suggested that ascites mass should not be omitted when calculating energy expenditure by use of body weight.

17.5.1.3   Surgery and Transplantation

Liver transplant patients on average have the same energy requirements as the majority of patients undergoing major abdominal surgery. In general, nonprotein energy provision of $1.3 \times$ REE is sufficient.[99,100] In a longitudinal study, postoperative hypermetabolism peaked on day 10 after the transplantation at 124% of the predicted REE.[74] By 6 to 12 months posttransplant there was no longer a difference between the measured and predicted REE.[74,101]

17.5.2   Carbohydrate Metabolism

17.5.2.1   Acute Liver Failure

Hypoglycemia is a clinically relevant and common problem in ALF[102,103] resulting from a loss of hepatic gluconeogenetic capacity, lack of glycogen, and hyperinsulinism.[103] As a standard procedure, hypoglycemia is treated by infusing glucose at a rate of 1.5 to 2 g · kgBW^{-1} · d^{-1}.[104,105] Cerebral edema probably resulting from astrocyte swelling and infection are the two key factors in the prognosis of ALF. Therefore, the rigorous control of blood glucose and closer metabolic monitoring may prove beneficial in this condition where the central organ of metabolism is failing. Considering the facts: (1) glucose infusion is aimed to provide the critically ill with oxidative fuel essential for vital tissues, such as the central nervous system and erythrocytes; (2) exogenous insulin at rates above 4 IU/h cannot increase glucose oxidation;[106] and (3) in ALF there is insulin hypersecretion, hyperinsulinemia, and insulin resistance;[103] there seems to be little reason for insulin administration above 4 IU/h in order to control glycemia.

17.5.2.2   Cirrhosis

The utilization of oxidative fuels is characterized by an increased rate of lipid oxidation in the fasting state and the frequent occurrence of insulin resistance (even in Child–Pugh class A patients)[85,107–109] In the postabsorptive state, glucose oxidation rate is reduced and hepatic glucose production rate is low despite increased gluconeogenesis due to a depletion of hepatic glycogen.[110] Insulin resistance affects skeletal muscle metabolism: glucose uptake and nonoxidative glucose disposal, such as glycogen synthesis are reduced, while glucose oxidation and lactate production are normal after glucose provision.[75,93,110] It is not known to what extent glucose deposition as glycogen is impaired just in skeletal muscle or in both muscle and liver.[111,112] Some 15 to 37% of patients develop overt diabetes, indicating an unfavorable prognosis.[113,114]

17.5.2.3 Surgery and Transplantation

In the early postoperative phase, there is often a disturbance of glucose metabolism associated with insulin resistance. In this situation, hyperglycemia should be managed by reducing glucose intake because higher insulin doses are unable to increase glucose oxidation.[106]

17.5.3 FAT METABOLISM

17.5.3.1 Acute Liver Failure

The oxidation of fatty acids and ketogenesis are the main energy yielding processes for hepatocytes.[115] Thus, adequate provision of lipid would be a plausible therapeutic objective provided there is sufficient oxygen supply to the hepatic tissue. It must be kept in mind, however, that some cases of ALF, in particular those with microvesicular steatosis and mitochondrial dysfunction, are caused by an impairment of hepatic beta-oxidation. In such a case, exogenous lipid, even from administering propofol as a sedative, cannot be metabolized and may be harmful.[116,117] Unlike the situation in septic patients, the splanchnic organs of ALF patients do not take up, but rather release, free fatty acids.[81] This may result from either mobilization of mesenteric fat or, more likely, from the compromised hepatic utilization of fatty acids as a consequence of loss of parenchymal mass. Apart from these physiological data, there are no systematic studies available regarding the role of fat as a nutrient in ALF. Anecdotal data[118,119] and the European survey data[120] demonstrate that exogenous fat seems to be well tolerated by many patients. A word of caution, however, may be adequate regarding the use of fat in cases of ALF due to the group of microvesicular steatosis conditions, where mitochondrial dysfunction may be predominant. In the absence of data from systematic studies, it is recommended to use plasma triglyceride levels for monitoring fat utilization as the best variable currently available and to aim for levels no higher than 4 to 5 mmol/l.[120]

17.5.3.2 Cirrhosis

In the fasting state, the plasma levels of free fatty acids, glycerol, and ketone bodies are increased and free fatty acid and glycerol concentrations do not fully respond to low insulin infusion rates as in healthy subjects.[121] Lipids are oxidized as the preferential substrate and lipolysis is increased with active mobilization of lipid deposits.[107,109] There is insulin resistance with regard to the antilipolytic activity.

After a meal, the suppression of lipid oxidation is not uniformly impaired.[94,122] Plasma clearance and lipid oxidation rates are not reduced and, thus, the net capacity to utilize exogenous fat does not seem to be impaired.[123,124] Essential and polyunsaturated fatty acids are decreased in cirrhosis and this decrement correlates to nutritional status and severity of liver disease.[125,126]

17.5.3.3 Surgery and Transplantation

In hepatic transplant patients, improved functioning of the reticuloendothelial system was observed when using medium chain triglyceride/long chain triglyceride (MCT/LCT) emulsions with a lower content of n-6 unsaturated fatty acids compared to pure soy bean oil emulsions.[127]

17.5.4 Protein and Amino Acid Metabolism

17.5.4.1 Acute Liver Failure

The plasma levels of amino acids are raised three- to fourfold in ALF. The amino acid pattern is characterized by a decrease in branched chain amino acids (BCAAs) and an increase in tryptophan, aromatic and sulphur-containing amino acids.[128–130] More recent data show that in ALF the splanchnic organs do not take up amino acids in contrast to their net uptake in healthy humans and even in septic patients.[130] Ammonia released from the intestine can no more be extracted sufficiently by the failing liver, and, despite ammonia detoxification by skeletal muscle hyperammonemia ensues.[130–132] Since elevated arterial ammonia levels have been recognized as an independent predictor of poor outcome in ALF patients,[133–135] it seems prudent to adjust the provision of amino acids according to the ammonia levels (target: <100 μmol/l) monitored.[136]

17.5.4.2 Cirrhosis

Protein turnover in cirrhotic patients has been found to be normal or increased. Some authors mainly focused on the presence of increased protein breakdown, while others suggest that a reduced protein synthesis plays the main role.[137] Albumin, but not fibrinogen, synthesis rates correlate with quantitative liver function tests and clinical stages of cirrhosis.[138,139] Nevertheless, stable cirrhotics apparently are capable of efficient nitrogen retention and significant formation of lean body mass from increased protein intake during oral hyperalimentation.[21] Protein catabolism influences the amino acid imbalance of cirrhosis and indirectly causes nitrogen overload to the liver leading to hyperammonemia. In cirrhotics, after an overnight fast, glycogen stores are depleted and metabolic conditions are similar to prolonged starvation in healthy individuals. It has been shown that a late evening carbohydrate snack was associated with improved protein metabolism in cirrhotic patients.[140–142] Insulin resistance apparently is without effect on amino acid disposal.[143]

An explicit and systematic determination of the protein requirement of patients with liver cirrhosis has been carried out in only a few studies. Patients with stable cirrhosis were found to have an increased protein requirement leading to the recommendation of $1.2 \text{ g} \cdot \text{kgBW}^{-1} \cdot \text{d}^{-1}$ contrasting with the recommended minimal intake of $0.8 \text{ g} \cdot \text{kgBW}^{-1} \cdot \text{d}^{-1}$ in healthy humans.[20,21,43,144]

Similar to ALF, cirrhotic patients exhibit an altered pattern of plasma amino acids characterized by the elevation of aromatic (phenylalanine, tyrosine) and sulfur containing amino acids (methionine) and tryptophane on the one hand and the decrease in BCAA (leucine, isoleucine, valine) on the other hand.[129,145] Decreased metabolic clearance[146] by the failing liver of aromatic and sulfurous amino acids and increased breakdown in skeletal muscle of BCAA due to portal systemic shunting[147] and hyperammonemia[130,148–150] are discussed as causal.

Recently, it has been pointed out that, due to the absence of isoleucine from hemoglobin, blood is a protein source of low biologic value leading to BCAA antagonism after upper gastrointestinal hemorrhage.[151] This BCAA antagonism readily explains the long-known clinical observation that blood and vegetable protein represent the two extremes in the hierarchy of food proteins regarding their comagenic potential. Moreover, this antagonism leading to hyperammonemia could be overcome by the infusion of just isoleucine.[152]

17.5.4.3 Surgery and Transplantation

After transplantation there is a considerable nitrogen loss and patients remain in negative nitrogen balance for up to 28 days[74,99,153] necessitating an increase in the provision of protein or amino acids. Protein or amino acid intakes of 1.0 to 1.5 g · kgBW^{-1} · d^{-1} have been reported.[8,154] The determination of postoperative urea nitrogen excretion has proved helpful in the assessment of individual nitrogen requirements.

17.5.5 VITAMINS AND MINERALS

No recommendation on the requirement of micronutrients can be made on the basis of controlled studies. As in other diseases, the administration of micronutrients has no proven therapeutic effect apart from the prevention or correction of deficiency states.

Body composition of cirrhotics is altered profoundly and characterized by protein depletion and accumulation of total body water even in Child–Pugh class A patients.[22,23] This goes hand-in-hand with salt retention, which does not usually lead to hypernatremia. On the contrary, depletion of potassium, magnesium, phosphate, and other intracellular minerals frequently occurs. In an early study comparing parenteral nutrition versus oral diet in cirrhotic patients with ascites, the response to diuretics was poorer in those patients receiving parenteral nutrition.[155]

Zinc and selenium deficiencies have been observed in alcoholic and nonalcoholic liver disease.[156–159] An impressive association between HE and zinc deficiency has been described in case reports.[160,161] A deficiency in water soluble vitamins, mainly group B vitamins, is common in cirrhosis, especially that of alcoholic origin.[162,163] Deficiency in fat soluble vitamins has been observed in cholestasis-related steatorrhea, bile salt deficiency, and in alcoholics.[164,165]

Patients with hypophosphatemia after acetaminophen-induced liver damage have a better prognosis. Severe hypophosphatemia, however, results in respiratory insufficiency and dysfunction of the nervous system and erythrocytes[166] and, thus, serum phosphate levels should be monitored and corrected in order to support liver regeneration.

17.6   DISEASE-SPECIFIC NUTRITION THERAPY

17.6.1   ACUTE LIVER DISEASE

17.6.1.1   Acute Hepatitis

Acute viral hepatitis often is associated with a varying degree of anorexia and the sensation of abdominal fullness leading to reduced food intake and weight loss. Depending on the magnitude of cholestasis, there may be an impairment of fat malabsorption. Nutrition therapy is warranted in malnourished subjects and when inadequate food intake persists. Since no data from formal trials are available, nutritional management should adopt the strategies outlined for alcoholic steatohepatitis.

17.6.1.2   Acute Liver Failure

Without treatment, ALF results in death within days.[167] In the treatment of ALF, measures to stabilize the metabolism and vital functions and the treatment of brain edema are of utmost importance. Hypoglycemia is a clinically relevant and common problem in ALF[102] resulting from a loss of hepatic gluconeogenetic capacity, lack of glycogen, and hyperinsulinism.[103] As a standard procedure, hypoglycemia is treated by infusing glucose at a rate of 1.5 to 2 g · kgBW^{-1} · d^{-1}.[104,105] In ALF, nutritional therapy has two objectives:

1. Ensuring the adequate provision of energy, especially assuring euglycemia by giving glucose, lipid, vitamins, and trace elements.
2. Ensuring optimal rates of protein synthesis by providing an adequate intake of protein or amino acids, respectively.

In the absence of data from clinical trials, it is difficult to give recommendations. In recognition of this deficit, a survey was carried out in European hepatology centers on issues of parenteral nutrition in patients with ALF.[120] One important result was that centers with a high caseload favor nasoduodenal tube feeding, which could be carried out successfully in the majority of cases. Therefore, it is recommended that patients with ALF should receive enteral nutrition via nasoduodenal tube. No recommendations concerning a disease-specific composition of enteral formulae can currently be given. The recommended amount of enteral formula is based on the dosage in critical illness.

Also, when using parenteral nutrition, sufficient glucose provision (2 to 3 g · kg BW^{-1} · d^{-1}) is mandatory for the prophylaxis and treatment of hypoglycemia. Xylitol or sorbitol in exchange for glucose are of no proven benefit in acute ALF; moreover, both have to be metabolized by the liver before they can be utilized. Ensuring euglycemia has been shown to confer a survival and morbidity benefit to critically ill patients regardless of etiology.[168,169] Great care, however, must be taken to avoid hypoglycemia.[170]

There are no systematic data on the role of lipid as a nutrient in this context. Exogenously applied, lipid seems to be well tolerated by most patients.[118,119] According to the European survey, two-thirds of participating hepatology centers give parenteral lipid to patients with acute liver failure, the majority opting for an LCT/MCT emulsion.[120] In clinical practice, glucose and lipid (0.8 to 1.2 g · kgBW^{-1} · d^{-1}) can be given simultaneously; the use of lipid may be especially advantageous in the presence of insulin resistance.

Amino acid administration is not mandatory in hyperacute liver failure. In acute or subacute liver failure, however, amino acids (0.8 to 1.2 g · kgBW^{-1} · d^{-1} in parenteral nutrition) or protein (0.8 to 1.2 g · kgBW^{-1} · d^{-1} in enteral nutrition) should be used in order to support protein synthesis. The use of amino acid infusions has often been omitted for fear of aggravating existing hyperammonemia and hyperaminoacidemia and causing cerebral edema and HE. In the survey, however, the majority reported giving i.v. amino acids.[120] Some clinicians reported use of standard amino acid solutions while the majority prescribed BCAA-enriched solutions aiming for a correction of the deranged plasma amino acid pattern.[171–173] Because elevated arterial ammonia levels have been recognized as an independent predictor of poor outcome in ALF patients,[133–135] it seems prudent to adjust the provision of amino acids according to the ammonia levels monitored. While pathophysiological considerations provide a rationale for the use of liver-adapted solutions rich in BCAA, no clinical trial in acute ALF has shown an outcome benefit in comparison to standard solutions. Adequate metabolic monitoring is necessary in order to adapt nutrient provision to substrate utilization in order to prevent substrate overload due to inadequate intake. Strict control of the plasma levels of glucose (target: 5 to 8 mmol/l), lactate (target: <5.0 mmol/l), triglycerides (target: <3.0 mmol/l), and ammonia (target: <100 μmol/l) is necessary for this purpose.[120,136]

17.6.2 Chronic Liver Disease

17.6.2.1 Alcoholic Steatohepatitis (ASH)

Supplementary enteral nutrition is indicated when ASH patients cannot meet their caloric requirements through normal food and when there are no contraindications like ileus. Clinical trials[14–17,174,175] in ASH patients show that supplementary enteral nutrition either by oral nutritional supplement or by tube feeding ensures adequate energy and protein intake without the risk of complications, such as HE. Enteral nutrition appears preferable to parenteral nutrition, but there has been no large randomized trial comparing the feeding regimens in ASH patients.

Enteral nutrition was as effective as steroids in patients with severe alcoholic hepatitis. Survivors of the 28-day treatment period who had been treated with enteral nutrition showed a lower mortality rate in the following year.[175] Severely malnourished ASH patients who achieve an adequate intake of oral nutrition supplements have an improved survival rate, regardless of whether or not additional anabolic steroids are used.[15] Malnourished ASH patients are at great risk of developing refeeding syndrome and additional phosphate, potassium, and magnesium will be required, together with water soluble vitamins.

In general, oral nutrition supplements are recommended, but if patients are not able to maintain adequate oral intake, tube feeding should be used. There is no evidence that the use of fine bore nasogastric tubes poses an undue risk in patients with esophageal varices.[18,19,176] Placement of a percutaneous endoscopic gastrostomy

(PEG) is associated with a higher risk of complications (due to ascites or varices) and is not recommended.[177]

As a standard approach, standard whole protein formulae should be used aiming for an energy intake of 35 kcal · kgBW^{-1} · d^{-1} and a protein intake of 1.2 to 1.5 g · kg BW^{-1} · d^{-1}.[14–17,175] Formulae with high energy density (1.5 to 2.4 kcal · ml^{-1}) are preferable in patients with ascites to avoid positive fluid balance. When patients develop HE during enteral nutrition, BCAA-enriched formulae should be used.[177] A direct comparison between standard formula and BCAA-enriched formula has not yet been made in ASH patients. It should be kept in mind that in ASH patients as in cirrhotics, a low protein intake can worsen HE.[19,178]

Parenteral nutrition should be commenced immediately in ASH patients with moderate or severe malnutrition who cannot be fed sufficiently either orally or enterally. Parenteral nutrition supplemental to oral nutrition *ad libitum* did not improve survival, but did not negatively affect the mental state.[47–49,174,179–182] It has been shown that a late evening carbohydrate snack is associated with improved protein metabolism in cirrhotic patients.[140–142] Therefore, it is recommended that patients with ASH and/or cirrhosis who need to be managed nil by mouth (nothing through the mouth) for more than 12 hours (including nocturnal fasting) should be given i.v. glucose at 2 to 3 g · kgBW^{-1} · d^{-1}. When this fasting period lasts longer than 72 hours, total parenteral nutrition should be implemented.

Parenteral nutrition should be formulated and administered as in liver cirrhosis patients (176.2.3). All water soluble vitamins, in particular thiamine (vitamin B$_1$), pyridoxine (vitamin B$_6$), nicotinamide (vitamin PP), and folic acid, and fat soluble vitamins should be administered daily in a standard total parenteral nutrition (TPN) dosage. Due to the high risk of Wernicke's encephalopathy, vitamin B$_1$ must be administered prior to starting i.v. glucose in alcoholic patients. Recently, high doses for both prophylaxis (250 mg i.m. daily for three to five days) and treatment (500 mg i.v. t.i.d. for two to three days) of Wernicke's encephalopathy have been advocated.[183] In jaundiced patients, vitamin K deficiency due to cholestasis-induced fat malabsorption may require i.v. vitamin K for correction.

17.6.2.2 Nonalcoholic Steatohepatitis (NASH)

In overweight individuals with NASH, weight reduction is the key to the successful treatment of this condition. The histopathologic changes of NASH can be ameliorated or even fully regress by weight reduction regardless of whether it is achieved by dietary counseling,[59] bariatric surgery,[60–62] or inhibition of intestinal fat absorption by orlistat.[63] Likewise, insulin resistance[59,63] and lipid metabolism[59,62] can be improved.

Targeting insulin resistance by use of insulin-sensitizing drugs like pioglitazone or rosiglitazone, the beneficial effects on liver histology[184,185] seem to be offset by a considerable gain in body weight and body fat mass.[184,186]

Taken together, overweight NASH patients benefit from effective long-term weight reduction regardless of the therapeutic strategy implemented.

17.6.2.3 Liver Cirrhosis

In patients with cirrhosis, the primary goal is to ensure a quantitatively adequate nutrient intake.[16–19,187–189] Increasing protein intake by nutrition therapy can decrease mortality,[20] and adequate nutrition after successful treatment of portal hypertension by transjugular intrahepatic portosystemic stent-shunt (TIPS) has the potential to improve body composition.[67,68]

Regarding the method of nutritional intervention, nutritional counseling alone[187] or in combination with oral nutrition supplements[16,17,189] will often prove successful. Supplemental enteral nutrition should be given when patients with liver cirrhosis cannot meet their nutritional requirements from normal food despite adequate individualized nutritional counseling. Very often, the spontaneous food intake of these patients is overestimated and the therapeutic gain[18,19,69,70] by timely use of tube feeding is missed. Due to somnolence and psychomotor dysfunction, oral nutrition is often insufficient even in mild HE (I°-II°).[69,70] Therefore, tube feeding may be required to ensure adequate nutrient provision. The risk of aspiration in uncooperative patients and those with advanced HE should be considered when deciding on whether to feed by the enteral or the parenteral route. As already discussed for ASH patients, tube feeding is not contraindicated in the presence of esophageal varices, but the use of PEGs in cirrhotics is discouraged. Ascites, impairment of the coagulation system, and portosystemic collateral circulation due to portal hypertension have been reported as contraindications to PEG placement.[190]

Cirrhotic patients should achieve an energy intake of 35 kcal $\cdot$ kgBW^{-1} $\cdot$ d^{-1} and a protein intake of 1.2 to 1.5 g $\cdot$ kgBW^{-1} $\cdot$ d^{-1} [24] using a standard whole protein formula. The appropriateness of this recommendations has been tested recently. Diets containing 1.2 g $\cdot$ kgBW^{-1} $\cdot$ d^{-1} protein could safely be administered to patients with cirrhosis suffering from episodic HE. Even transient protein restriction did not confer any benefit to patients during an episode of encephalopathy.[191] In stable cirrhotics, formulae enriched in BCAA are not necessary. Such formulae are helpful in the very select subgroup of protein intolerant patients with HE.[192] In stable patients with cirrhosis, long-term (12 and 24 months) nutritional supplementation with oral BCAA granulate as oral nutrition supplement has the potential to slow the progression of hepatic failure and prolong event-free survival,[193–195] but this treatment is not reimbursed in many countries. When patients develop HE during enteral nutrition, BCAA-enriched formulae should be used.[177]

Regarding trace elements and vitamins, in a pragmatic approach, liberal supplementation is recommended in the first two weeks of nutritional support because the laboratory diagnosis of a specific deficiency may be more costly and would delay provision. Oral zinc supplementation as a treatment of HE has been disappointing in controlled trials,[196–208] despite encouraging case reports.[160,161] Urea production capacity increased after oral zinc application when previously subnormal plasma levels were normalized.[199] Supplementing zinc and vitamin A may indirectly improve food intake and nutritional state by improving dysgeusia.[200,201] Supplementation with calcium and vitamin D is recommended for patients with osteopenia, although this did not result in any improvement in bone density in patients with primary biliary cirrhosis; estrogen substitution proved to be much more effective in female patients.[164,165,202] Vitamin B$_1$ must be provided to all patients with alcoholic liver disease before providing glucose as outlined in Section 17.6.2.1.

Parenteral nutrition is a valuable second line option and must be implemented immediately when moderately or severely malnourished cirrhotics cannot be nourished sufficiently by either the oral or enteral route. Parenteral nutrition should be considered in patients with unprotected airways and advanced HE when swallow and cough reflexes are compromised.

Patients with liver cirrhosis suffer from a depletion of hepatic glycogen stores and thus are less prepared to adequately master periods of even short-term food deprivation. A late evening carbohydrate snack can improve protein metabolism in cirrhotics[140–142] and, thus, every patient with cirrhosis who needs to be managed nil by mouth for more than 12 hours (including nocturnal fasting) should be given i.v. glucose at 2 to 3 g · kgBW^{-1} · d^{-1} as the minimum metabolic intervention. When this fasting period lasts longer than 72 hours, TPN should be implemented and, as an intermediary measure, hypocaloric peripheral parenteral nutrition may be used when fasting periods are expected to last for less than 72 hours.

If parenteral nutrition is used as the exclusive form of nutrition, then the i.v. provision of all macro- and micronutrients must be ensured from the beginning of TPN. Carbohydrates should be given as glucose to cover 50 to 60% of nonprotein energy requirements. Ensuring euglycemia has been shown to confer a survival and morbidity benefit to critically ill patients regardless of etiology.[168,169] Great care, however, must be taken to avoid hypoglycemia.[170] In case of hyperglycemia, glucose infusion should be reduced to 2 to 3 g · kgBW^{-1} · d^{-1} and i.v. insulin infusion should be used.

The simultaneous infusion of lipid and glucose provides a better metabolic profile than glucose alone.[203] Plasma clearance and oxidation of infused lipids are normal in cirrhosis patients.[123,124] Regarding the optimal composition of i.v. oxidative fuels fat and carbohydrate, only limited information is available.[204,205] European guidelines recommend fat provision to cover 40 to 50% of nonprotein energy requirements using emulsions with a content of n-6 unsaturated fatty acids lower than in traditional pure soy bean oil emulsions.[177] Compared to the traditional soy bean-based long-chain triglycerides (LCT) emulsions (n-6:n-3 = 8:1), new fat emulsions have a lower content of n-6 unsaturated fatty acids due to the admixture of medium-chain triglycerides (MCT) and/or olive oil and/or fish oil rendering them less suppressive to leukocyte and immune function and less stimulant of proinflammatory modulators.[206–210]

The infusion of amino acids should provide an amount of 1.2 g · kgBW^{-1} · d^{-1} in compensated cirrhosis without malnutrition and 1.5 g · kgBW^{-1} · d^{-1} in decompensated cirrhosis with severe malnutrition. In clinical trials, studying patients with liver cirrhosis and severe HE, the provision of protein or amino acids ranged from 0.6 to 1.2 g · kgBW^{-1} · d^{-1}.[211] In patients with alcoholic hepatitis or alcoholic cirrhosis with or without low-grade HE, the provision ranged from 0.5 to 1.6 g · kgBW^{-1} · d^{-1}.[17–19,48,49,179–182,212] For parenteral nutrition in compensated cirrhosis amino acid solutions with a special "hepatic formula," composition are not required.

For parenteral nutrition of cirrhotics with overt HE amino acid solutions with a special "hepatic formula" high in BCAA (35% to 45%) but low in tryptophan, aromatic and sulfur-containing amino acids were developed.[171,213,214] Such solutions help to correct the amino acid imbalance in liver cirrhosis. The efficacy of BCAAs in the treatment of hepatic encephalopathy has been studied[215–219] and a meta-analysis showed an improvement in mental state by the BCAA-enriched solutions, but no definite benefit in survival.[211] Hepatic encephalopathy of cirrhotic patients, however, is precipitated by serious and life-threatening complications, such as infection or hemorrhage, which are more potent determinants of survival than HE. Therefore, it is not surprising that BCAA-based parenteral nutrition failed to improve short-term survival. Likewise, in a Cochrane analysis of seven randomized controlled trials studying 397 patients with acute HE, the parenteral BCAA administration had a significant, positive effect on the course of HE, but not on survival.[220] A liver-adapted complete amino acid solution should be given in more severe HE (III°–IV°). Blood from gastrointestinal hemorrhage is a protein source of low biologic value leading to BCAA antagonism.[151] This antagonism leads to hyperammonemia, but HE could be overcome by the infusion of just isoleucine.[152] Isoleucine solutions for i.v. infusions, however, are not commercially available. Special hepatic formula amino acid solutions (c.f. above) contain high amounts of isoleucine and of the other BCAAs, leucine, and valine.

For parenteral nutrition, water, electrolytes, water- and fat-soluble vitamins, and trace elements should be given daily in order to cover daily requirements. Trace elements should be administered daily in a standard TPN dose. In a pragmatic approach, routine administration of twice the normal daily requirement of zinc (= 2×5 mg · d^{-1}) is recommended. Malnourished cirrhotic patients are in danger of developing refeeding syndrome and additional phosphate, potassium, and magnesium may be required.[136]

17.7 PERIOPERATIVE NUTRITION

Nutrition therapy prior to elective surgery should be managed according to the recommendations given for the underlying disease, which most likely is liver cirrhosis in the majority of cases. Cirrhotic patients have a reduced rate of complications and an improved nitrogen economy after abdominal surgery if they receive nutritional support instead of just fluid and electrolytes.[221–223] It may safely be assumed that enteral nutrition in the early postoperative period yields even better results; however, no studies have compared the two regimens in liver cirrhosis. A beneficial effect on gut permeability of sequential parenteral/enteral nutrition (via jejunostomy) as compared to parenteral nutrition alone and no postoperative nutrition has been reported.[223]

Cirrhotic patients should receive early postoperative (additional) parenteral nutrition after surgery if they cannot be nourished sufficiently by the oral/enteral route. In cirrhotic patients undergoing liver resection, esophageal transection and splenectomy or splenorenal shunt, the rate of HE was not increased when a conventional rather than a BCAA-enriched amino acid solution was used.[222]

17.8 LIVER TRANSPLANTATION

Although the prognostic relevance of undernutrition in transplant candidates is well recognized, it has not yet been shown that preoperative nutritional intervention improves clinically relevant outcomes. However, nutritional therapy in undernourished cirrhotic patients is clearly indicated as outlined above. In the only randomized trial addressing this question, there was no advantage of oral nutrition supplements over nutritional counseling and normal food in adults.[187] Since normal food and nutritional counseling lead to the same adequate intake as when oral nutrition supplements are added, both regimens are considered similarly effective. Pediatric transplant patients with predominantly cholestatic liver disease show a better increase in body cell mass if they receive BCAA-enriched formula.[224]

After liver transplantation, normal food and/or enteral nutrition should be initiated within 12 to 24 hours postoperatively in order to achieve lower rates of morbidity and complications and cost than during parenteral nutrition.[154,225] Whole protein formulae with[226] or without pre- and probiotics[225,227] or peptide-based formulae via catheter jejunostomy[228,229] have been used for early enteral nutrition of adult liver transplant recipients. Nasogastric or nasoduodenal tubes after endoscopic placement[227] or via catheter jejunostomy[223,228,229] placed during laparotomy are used.

In hepatic transplant patients, the principles of parenteral nutrition are no different from those in abdominal surgery. In the early postoperative phase, hyperglycemia (due to disturbed glucose metabolism and insulin resistance) should be managed by reducing glucose intake because higher insulin doses are unable to increase glucose oxidation.[106] The diabetogenic potential of the immunosuppressant tacrolimus can be lowered by reducing its dose, aiming for trough levels of 3 to 8 ng · ml^{-1} without undue risk of rejection.[230] Regarding lipid emulsions, an improved functioning of the reticuloendothelial system was observed when using MCT/LCT emulsions with a lower content of n-6 unsaturated fatty acids compared to pure soy bean oil emulsions.[127]

After transplantation, there is a considerable nitrogen loss and patients remain in negative nitrogen balance for up to 28 days[74,99,153] necessitating an increase in the provision of protein or amino acids. Protein or amino acid intakes of 1.0 to 1.5 g · kg BW^{-1} · d^{-1} have been reported.[8,154] There is no need to use a BCAA-enriched amino acid solution after liver transplantation.[154]

In transplanted patients, the often preexisting chronic dilutional hyponatremia should be corrected carefully in order to avoid pontine myelinolysis.[231] Magnesium levels need to be monitored in order to detect and treat ciclosporin- or tacrolimus-induced hypomagnesemia.[232] Postoperative hypophosphatemia and its possible relation to parenteral nutrition following right hemihepatectomy in living donors has been reported by some, but not all study groups.[233–235]

At present, no specific recommendations can be made with regard to optimal organ donor conditioning. Fatty liver is known to be a risk factor for primary graft malfunction. No data are available addressing the role of nutritional management of the organ donor. Animal data indicate that the balanced nutrition of a brain dead liver donor, using moderate amounts of carbohydrate, lipid (long-chain fatty acids and possibly fish oil), and amino acids, is associated with improved function of the transplanted organ.[236] The value of donor or organ conditioning, which aims to reduce ischemia/reperfusion damage in man by provision of high doses of arginine or glutamine, is unclear.

REFERENCES

1. Patek AJ Jr, Post J. Treatment of cirrhosis of the liver by a nutritious diet and supplements rich in vitamin B complex. *J Clin Invest* 1941, 20: 481–505.

2. Child CG, Turcotte JG. Surgery and portal hypertension. In: Child CG, Ed. *The Liver and Portal Hypertension*. Philadelphia: Saunders, 1964: 50–51.

3. Alberino F, Gatta A, Amodio P et al. Nutrition and survival in patients with liver cirrhosis. *Nutrition* 2001, 17: 445–450.

4. Caregaro L, Alberino F, Amodio P et al. Malnutrition in alcoholic and virus-related cirrhosis. *Am J Clin Nutr* 1996, 63: 602–609.

5. Harrison J, McKiernan J, Neuberger JM. A prospective study on the effect of recipient nutritional status on outcome in liver transplantation. *Transpl Int* 1997, 10: 369–374.

6. Merli M, Riggio O, Dally L, and PINC. What is the impact of malnutrition on survival in liver cirrhosis: Does malnutrition affect survival in cirrhosis?. *Hepatology* 1996, 23: 1041–1046.

7. Moukarzel AA, Najm I, Vargas J, McDiarmid SV, Busuttil RW, Ament ME. Effect of nutritional status on outcome of orthotopic liver transplantation in pediatric patients. *Transplant Proc* 1990, 22: 1560–1563.

8. Pikul J, Sharpe MD, Lowndes R, Ghent CN. Degree of preoperative malnutrition is predictive of postoperative morbidity and mortality in liver transplant recipients. *Transplantation* 1994, 57: 469–472.

9. Selberg O, Böttcher J, Pirlich M, Henkel E, Manns M, Müller M. Clinical significance and correlates of whole body potassium status in patients with liver cirrhosis. *Hepatology* 2006, 16: 36–48.

10. Selberg O, Böttcher J, Tusch G, Pichlmayr R, Henkel E, Müller MJ. Identification of high- and low-risk patients before liver transplantation: a prospective cohort study of nutritional and metabolic parameters in 150 patients. *Hepatology* 1997, 25: 652–657.

11. Gunsar F, Raimondo ML, Jones S, Terreni N, Wong C, Patch D, Sabin C, Burroughs AK. Nutritional status and prognosis in cirrhotic patients. *Aliment Pharmacol Ther* 2006, 24: 563–72.

12. Garrison RN, Cryer HM, Howard DA, Polk HC, Jr. Clarification of risk factors for abdominal operations in patients with hepatic cirrhosis. *Ann Surg* 1984, 199: 648–655.

13. Merli M, Nicolini G, Angeloni S, Riggio O. Malnutrition is a risk factor in cirrhotic patients undergoing surgery. *Nutrition* 2002, 18: 978–86.

14. Mendenhall CL, Tosch T, Weesner RE et al. VA cooperative study on alcoholic hepatitis. II: Prognostic significance of protein-calorie malnutrition. *Am J Clin Nutr* 1986, 43: 213–218.

15. Mendenhall CL, Moritz TE, Roselle GA et al. A study of oral nutritional support with oxandrolone in malnourished patients with alcoholic hepatitis: results of a Department of Veterans Affairs cooperative study. *Hepatology* 1993, 17: 564–576.

16. Mendenhall CL, Moritz TE, Roselle GA et al. Protein energy malnutrition in severe alcoholic hepatitis: diagnosis and response to treatment. The VA Cooperative Study Group #275. *J Parenter Enteral Nutr* 1995, 19: 258–265.

17. Bunout D, Aicardi V, Hirsch S et al. Nutritional support in hospitalized patients with alcoholic liver disease. *Eur J Clin Nutr* 1989, 43: 615–621.

18. Cabré E, González-Huix F, Abad A et al. Effect of total enteral nutrition on the short-term outcome of severely malnourished cirrhotics: a randomized controlled trial. *Gastroenterology* 1990, 98: 715–720.

19. Kearns PJ, Young H, Garcia G et al. Accelerated improvement of alcoholic liver disease with enteral nutrition. *Gastroenterology* 1992, 102: 200–205.

20. Kondrup J, Müller MJ. Energy and protein requirements of patients with chronic liver disease. *J Hepatol* 1997, 27: 239–247.

21. Nielsen K, Kondrup J, Martinsen L, et al. Long-term oral refeeding of patients with cirrhosis of the liver. *Br J Nutr* 1995, 74: 557–567.

22. Prijatmoko D, Strauss BJ, Lambert JR et al. Early detection of protein depletion in alcoholic cirrhosis: role of body composition analysis. *Gastroenterology* 1993, 105: 1839–45.

23. Peng S, Plank LD, McCall JL, Gillanders LK, McIlroy K, Gane EJ. Body composition, muscle function, and energy expenditure in patients with liver cirrhosis: a comprehensive study. *Am J Clin Nutr* 2007, 85: 1257–66.

24. Plauth M, Merli M, Kondrup J, Ferenci P, Weimann A, Muller MJ. ESPEN guidelines for nutrition in liver disease and transplantation. *Clin Nutr* 1997, 16: 43–55.

25. Pirlich M, Selberg O, Böker K, Schwarze M, Muller MJ. The creatinine approach to estimate skeletal muscle mass in patients with cirrhosis. *Hepatology* 1996, 24: 1422–7.

26. Pirlich M, Schütz T, Spachos T et al. Bioelectrical impedance analysis is a useful bedside technique to assess malnutrition in cirrhotic patients with and without ascites. *Hepatology* 2000, 32: 1208–15.

27. Selberg O, Selberg D. Norms and correlates of bioimpedance phase angle in healthy human subjects, hospitalized patients, and patients with liver cirrhosis. *Eur J Appl Physiol* 2002, 86: 509–16.

28. Guglielmi FW, Contento F, Laddaga L, Panella C, Francavilla A. Bioelectric impedance analysis: experience with male patients with cirrhosis. *Hepatology* 1991 13: 892–895.

29. Panella C, Guglielmi FW, Mastronuzzi T, Francavilla A. Whole-body and segmental bioelectrical parameters in chronic liver disease: effect of gender and disease stages. *Hepatology* 1995, 21: 352–358.

30. Andersen H, Borre M, Jakobsen J, Andersen PH, Vilstrup H. Decreased muscle strength in patients with alcoholic liver cirrhosis in relation to nutritional status, alcohol abstinence, liver function, and neuropathy. *Hepatology* 1998, 27: 1200–6.

31. Beyer N, Aadahl M, Strange B, Kirkegaard P, Hansen BA, Mohr T, Kjaer M. Improved physical performance after orthotopic liver transplantation. *Liver Transplant Surg* 1999, 5: 301–309.

32. Alvares-da-Silva MR, Reverbel da Silveira T. Comparison between handgrip strength, subjective global assessment, and prognostic nutritional index in assessing malnutrition and predicting clinical outcome in cirrhotic outpatients. *Nutrition* 2005, 21: 113–7.

33. Merli M, Romiti A, Riggio O, Capocaccia L. Optimal nutritional indexes in chronic liver disease *J Parenter Enteral Nutr* 1987, 11: 130S–134S.

34. Crawford DHG, Cuneo RC, Shepherd RW. Pathogenesis and assessment of malnutrition in liver disease. *J Gastroenterol Hepatol* 1993, 8: 89–94.

35. McLean AE. Hepatic failure in malnutrition. *Lancet* 1962, II: 1292–4.

36. Webber BL, Freiman I. The liver in kwashiorkor: a clinical and electron microscopical study. *Arch Pathol* 1974, 98: 400–8.

37. Waterlow JC. Amount and rate of disappearance of liver fat in malnourished infants in Jamaica. *Am J Clin Nutr* 1975, 28: 1330–6.

38. Manary MJ, Broadhead RL, Yarasheski KE. Whole-body protein kinetics in marasmus and kwashiorkor during acute infection. *Am J Clin Nutr* 1998, 67: 1205–9.

39. Badaloo AV, Forrester T, Reid M, Jahoor F. Lipid kinetic differences between children with kwashiorkor and those with marasmus. *Am J Clin Nutr* 2006, 83: 1283–8.

40. Badaloo A, Reid M, Soares D, Forrester T, Jahoor F. Relation between liver fat content and the rate of VLDL apolipoprotein B-100 synthesis in children with protein-energy malnutrition. *Am J Clin Nutr* 2005, 81: 1126–32.

41. Pantuck EJ, Pantuck CB, Weissman C, Gil KM, Askanazi J. Stimulation of oxidative drug metabolism by parenteral refeeding of nutritionally depleted patients. *Gastroenterology*1985, 89: 241–5.

42. Tranvouez JL, Lerebours E, Chretien P, Fouin-Fortunet H, Colin R. Hepatic antipyrine metabolism in malnourished patients: influence of the type of malnutrition and course after nutritional rehabilitation. *Am J Clin Nutr* 1985, 41: 1257–64.

43. Nielsen K, Kondrup J, Martinsen L, Stilling B, Vikman B Nutritional assessment and adequacy of dietary intake in hospitalized patients with alcoholic liver cirrhosis. *Br J Nutr* 1993, 69: 665–679.
44. Reid M, Badaloo A, Forrester T, Morlese JF, Heird WC, Jahoor F. The acute-phase protein response to infection in edematous and nonedematous protein-energy malnutrition. *Am J Clin Nutr* 2002, 76: 1409–15.
45. Manary MJ, Yarasheski KE, Berger R, Abrams ET, Hart CA, Broadhead RL. Whole-body leucine kinetics and the acute phase response during acute infection in marasmic Malawian children. *Pediatr Res* 2004, 55: 940–6.
46. O'Keefe SJ, El-Zayadi AR, Carraher TE, Davis M, Williams R. Malnutrition and immunoincompetence in patients with liver disease. *Lancet* 1980 ii: 615–617.
47. Mezey E, Caballería J, Mitchell MC, Parés A, Herlong HF, Rodés J. Effect of parenteral amino acid supplementation on short-term and long-term outcomes in severe alcoholic hepatitis: a randomized controlled trial. *Hepatology* 1991, 14: 1090–1096.
48. Achord JL. A prospective randomized clinical trial of peripheral amino acid-glucose supplementation in acute alcoholic hepatitis. *Am J Gastroenterol* 1987, 82: 871–875.
49. Bonkovsky HL, Fiellin DA, Smith GS, Slaker DP, Simon D, Galambos JT. A randomized controlled trial of treatment of alcoholic hepatitis with parenteral nutrition and oxandrolone.I. Short-term effects on liver function. *Am J Gastroenterol* 1991, 86: 1200–1208.
50. Drenick EJ, Simmons F, Murphy JF. Effect on hepatic morphology of treatment of obesity by fasting, reducing diets and small-bowel bypass. *N Eng J Med* 1970, 282: 829–834.
51. Ludwig J, Viggiano TR, McGill DB, Oh BJ. Nonalcoholic steatohepatitis: Mayo Clinic experiences with a hitherto unnamed disease. *Mayo Clin Proc* 1980, 55: 434–438.
52. Sanyal AJ. AGA technical review on nonalcoholic fatty liver disease. *Gastroenterology* 2002, 123: 1705–1725.
53. Bellentani S, Saccoccio G, Masutti F, Crocé RS, Brandi G, Sasso F, Cristianini G, Tiribelli C. Prevalence of and risk factors for hepatic steatosis in Northern Italy. *Ann Intern Med* 2000, 132: 112–117.
54. Vilar L, Oliveira CP, Faintuch J, Mello ES, Nogueira MA, Santos TE, Alves VA, Carrilho FJ. High-fat diet: a trigger of non-alcoholic steatohepatitis? Preliminary findings in obese subjects. *Nutrition* 2008, 24: 1097–102.
55. Cortes-Pinto ClinNutr 2006 Cortez-Pinto H, Jesus L, Barros H, Lopes C, Moura MC, Camilo ME. How different is the dietary pattern in non-alcoholic steatohepatitis patients? *Clin Nutr* 2006, 25: 816–23.
56. Toshimitsu K, Matsuura B, Ohkubo I, Niiya T, Furukawa S, Hiasa Y, Kawamura M, Ebihara K, Onji M. Dietary habits and nutrient intake in non-alcoholic steatohepatitis. *Nutrition* 2007, 23: 46–52.
57. Harnois F, Msika S, Sabaté JM, Mechler C, Jouet P, Barge J, Coffin B. Prevalence and predictive factors of non-alcoholic steatohepatitis (NASH) in morbidly obese patients undergoing bariatric surgery. *Obes Surg* 2006, 16: 183–8.
58. Machado M, Marques-Vidal P, Cortez-Pinto H. Hepatic histology in obese patients undergoing bariatric surgery. *J Hepatol* 2006, 45: 600–6.
59. Huang MA, Greenson JK, Chao C, Anderson L, Peterman D, Jacobson J, Emick D, Lok AS, Conjeevaram HS. One-year intense nutritional counseling results in histological improvement in patients with non-alcoholic steatohepatitis: a pilot study. *Am J Gastroenterol* 2005, 100: 1072–81.
60. Stratopoulos C, Papakonstantinou A, Terzis I, Spiliadi C, Dimitriades G, Komesidou V, Kitsanta P, Argyrakos T, Hadjiyannakis E. Changes in liver histology accompanying massive weight loss after gastroplasty for morbid obesity. *Obes Surg* 2005, 15: 1154–60.

61. Dixon JB, Bhathal PS, O'Brien PE. Weight loss and non-alcoholic fatty liver disease: falls in gamma-glutamyl transferase concentrations are associated with histologic improvement. *Obes Surg* 2006, 16: 1278–86.

62. Barker KB, Palekar NA, Bowers SP, Goldberg JE, Pulcini JP, Harrison SA. Non-alcoholic steatohepatitis: effect of Roux-en-Y gastric bypass surgery. *Am J Gastroenterol* 2006, 101: 368–73.

63. Harrison SA, Fecht W, Brunt EM, Neuschwander-Tetri BA. Orlistat for overweight subjects with nonalcoholic steatohepatitis: a randomized, prospective trial. *Hepatology* 2009, 49: 80–6.

64. Mendenhall CL, Anderson S, Weesner RE, Goldberg SJ, Crolic KA. Protein calorie malnutrition associated with alcoholic hepatitis. *Am J Med* 1984, 76: 211–221.

65. Lautz HU, Selberg O, Körber J, Bürger M, Müller MJ. Protein calorie malnutrition in liver cirrhosis. *Clin Investig* 1992, 70: 478–486.

66. Italian Multicentre Cooperative Project on nutrition in liver cirrhosis. Nutritional status in cirrhosis. *J Hepatol* 1994, 21: 317–325.

67. Allard JP, Chau J, Sandokji K, Blendis LM, Wong F. Effects of ascites resolution after successful TIPS on nutrition in cirrhotic patients with refractory ascites. *Am J Gastroenterol* 2001, 96: 2442–7.

68. Plauth M, Schütz T, Buckendahl DP et al. Weight gain after transjugular intrahepatic portosystemic shunt is associated with improvement in body composition in malnourished patients with cirrhosis and hypermetabolism. *J Hepatol* 2004, 40: 228–233.

69. Keohane PP, Attrill H, Grimble G, Spiller R, Frost P, Silk DB. Enteral nutrition in malnourished patients with hepatic cirrhosis and acute encephalopathy. *J Parenter Enteral Nutr* 1983, 7: 346–350.

70. Davidson HI, Richardson R, Sutherland D, Garden OJ. Macronutrient preference, dietary intake, and substrate oxidation among stable cirrhotic patients. *Hepatology* 1999, 29: 1380–6.

71. Hussaini SH, Oldroyd B, Stewart SP, Soo S, Roman F, Smith MA, Pollard S, Lodge P, O'Grady JG, Losowsky MS. Effects of orthotopic liver transplantation on body composition. *Liver* 1998, 18: 173–9.

72. Richards J, Gunson B, Johnson J, Neuberger J. Weight gain and obesity after liver transplantation. *Transpl Int* 2005, 18: 461–6.

73. Laryea M, Watt KD, Molinari M, Walsh MJ, McAlister VC, Marotta PJ, Nashan B, Peltekian KM. Metabolic syndrome in liver transplant recipients: prevalence and association with major vascular events. *Liver Transpl* 2007, 13: 1109–14.

74. Plank LD, Metzger DJ, McCall JL, Barclay KL, Gane EJ, Streat SJ, Munn SR, Hill GL. Sequential changes in the metabolic response to orthotopic liver transplantation during the first year after surgery. *Ann Surg* 2001, 234: 245–55.

75. Selberg O, Burchert W, van den Hoff J et al. Insulin resistance in liver cirrhosis. Positron-emission tomography scan analysis of skeletal muscle glucose metabolism. *J Clin Invest* 1993, 91: 1897–1902.

76. Tietge UJF, Selberg O, Kreter A, Bahr M, Pirlich M, Burchert W, Müller MJ, Manns MP, Böker KWW. Alterations in glucose metabolism associated ith liver cirrhosis persist in the clinically stable long-term course after liver transplantation. *Liver Transpl* 2004, 10: 1030–1040.

77. Walldorf K, Ewert R, Witt C, Böhm M, Rogalla P, Reibis R, Lochs H, Plauth M. Impaired lung function after liver transplantation: Role of the membrane factor and reduced function of respiratory muscles. *J Hepatol* 2000, 32(Suppl 2): 58.

78. van den Ham EC, Kooman JP, Christiaans MH, van Hooff JP. Relation between steroid dose, body composition and physical activity in renal transplant patients. *Transplantation* 2000, 69: 1591–8.

79. Ewert R, Wensel R, Bruch L, Mutze S, Bauer U, Plauth M, Kleber F-X. Relationship between impaired pulmonary diffusion and cardiopulmonary exercise capacity after heart transplantation. *Chest* 2000, 117: 968–975.

80. Ganong W F. *Review of Medical Physiology.* East Norwalk: Appleton & Lange, 1991, 563.

81. Clemmesen JO, Hoy C-E, Kondrup J, Ott P. Splanchnic metabolism of fuel substrates in acute liver failure. *J Hepatol* 2000, 33: 941–948.

82. Murphy ND, Kodakat SK, Wendon JA, Jooste CA, Muiesan P, Rela M, Heaton ND. Liver failure and intestinal lactate metabolism in patients with acute hepatic failure undergoing liver transplantation. *Crit Care Med* 2001, 29: 2111–2118.

83. Schneeweiss B, Pammer J, Ratheiser K et al. Energy metabolism in acute hepatic failure. *Gastroenterology* 1993, 105: 1515–1521.

84. Harris JA, Benedict FG. A biometric study of basal metabolism in man. 270. Washington, DC: Carnegie Institute. 1919.

85. Müller MJ, Lautz HU, Plogmann B, Burger M, Korber J, Schmidt FW. Energy expenditure and substrate oxidation in patients with cirrhosis: the impact of cause, clinical staging and nutritional state. *Hepatology* 1992, 15: 782–794.

86. Müller MJ, Böttcher J, Selberg O et al. Hypermetabolism in clinically stable patients with liver cirrhosis. *Am J Clin Nutr* 1999, 69: 1194–1201.

87. Mathur S, Peng S, Gane EJ, McCall JL, Plank LD. Hypermetabolism predicts reduced transplant-free survival independent of MELD and Child-Pugh scores in liver cirrhosis. *Nutrition* 2007, 23: 398–403.

88. John WJ, Phillips R, Ott L, Adams LJ, McClain CJ. Resting energy expenditure in patients with alcoholic hepatitis. *J Parenter Enteral Nutr* 1989, 13: 124–127.

89. Madden AM, Morgan MY. Resting energy expenditure should be measured in patients with cirrhosis, not predicted. *Hepatology* 1999, 30: 655–64.

90. Richardson RA, Garden OJ, Davidson HI. Reduction in energy expenditure after liver transplantation. *Nutrition* 2001, 17: 585–589.

91. Nielsen K, Martinsen L, Dossing H, Stilling B, Kondrup J. Energy expenditure measured by the doubly labeled water method during hyperalimentation of patients with liver cirrhosis. *J Hepatol* 1991, 13: S151.

92. Campillo B, Bories PN, Devanlay M, Sommer F, Wirquin E, Fouet P. The thermogenic and metabolic effects of food in liver cirrhosis: consequences on the storage of nutrients and the hormonal counterregulatory response. *Metabolism* 1992, 41: 476–482.

93. Müller MJ, Willmann O, Rieger A et al. Mechanism of insulin resistance associated with liver cirrhosis. *Gastroenterology* 1992, 102: 2033–2041.

94. Riggio O, Merli M, Romiti A et al. Early postprandial energy expenditure and macronutrient use after a mixed meal in cirrhotic patients. *J Parenter Enteral Nutr* 1992, 16: 445–450.

95. Campillo B, Fouet P, Bonnet JC, Atlan G. Submaximal oxygen consumption in liver cirrhosis: evidence of severe functional aerobic impairment. *J Hepatol* 1990, 10: 163–167.

96. De Lissio M, Goodyear LJ, Fuller S, Krawitt EL, Devlin JT. Effects of treadmill exercise on fuel metabolism in hepatic cirrhosis. *J Appl Physiol* 1991, 70: 210–215.

97. Müller MJ, Dettmer A, Tettenborn M et al. Metabolic, endocrine, haemodynamic and pulmonary responses to different types of exercise in individuals with normal or reduced liver function. *Eur J Appl Physiol Occup Physiol* 1996, 74: 246–257.

98. Dolz C, Raurich JM, Ibanez J, Obrador A, Marse P, Gaya J. Ascites increases the resting energy expenditure in liver cirrhosis. *Gastroenterology* 1991, 100: 738–744.

99. Plevak DJ, DiCecco SR, Wiesner RH et al. Nutritional support for liver transplantation: identifying caloric and protein requirements. *Mayo Clin Proc* 1994, 69: 225–230.

100. Weimann A, Kuse ER, Bechstein WO, Neuberger JM, Plauth M, Pichlmayr R. Perioperative parenteral and enteral nutrition for patients undergoing orthotopic liver transplantation: results of a questionnaire from 16 European transplant units. *Transpl Int* 1998, 11 Suppl 1: S289–S291.

101. Perseghin G, Mazzaferro V, Benedini S et al. Resting energy expenditure in diabetic and nondiabetic patients with liver cirrhosis: relation with insulin sensitivity and effect of liver transplantation and immunosuppressive therapy. *Am J Clin Nutr* 2002, 76: 541–548.

102. Samson R L, Trey C, Timme AH, Saunders SJ. Fulminating hepatitis with recurrent hypoglycemia and hemorrhage. *Gastroenterology* 1967, 53: 291–300.

103. Vilstrup H, Iversen J, Tygstrup N. Glucoregulation in acute liver failure. *Eur J Clin Invest* 1986, 16: 193–197.

104. Bernuau J, Rueff B, Benhamou JP. Fulminant and subfulminant liver failure: definitions and causes. *Semin Liver Dis* 1986, 6: 97–106.

105. O'Grady JG, Portmann B, Williams R. Fulminant hepatic failure. In: Schiff L, Schiff ER (Eds.). *Diseases of the Liver*. Philadelphia: Lippincott, 1993: 1077–1090.

106. Wolfe RR, Allsop JR, Burke JF. Glucose metabolism in man: responses to intravenous glucose infusion. *Metabolism* 1979, 28: 210–220.

107. Merli M, Erikson S, Hagenfeldt H, Wahren J. Splanchnic and peripheral exchange of FFA in patients with liver cirrhosis. *Hepatology* 1986, 3: 348–355.

108. Merli M, Riggio O, Romiti A et al. Basal energy production rate and substrate use in stable cirrhotic patients. *Hepatology* 1990, 12: 106–112.

109. Owen OE, Trapp VE, Reichard GA, Jr. et al. Nature and quantity of fuels consumed in patients with alcoholic cirrhosis. *J Clin Invest* 1983, 72: 1821–1832.

110. Petrides AS, De Fronzo RA. Glucose and insulin metabolism in cirrhosis. *J Hepatol* 1989, 8: 107–114.

111. Kruszynska Y, Williams N, Perry M, Home P. The relationship between insulin sensitivity and skeletal muscle enzyme activity in hepatic cirrhosis. *Hepatology* 1988, 8: 1615–1619.

112. Selberg O, Radoch E, Walter GF, Müller MJ. Skeletal muscle glycogen content in patients with cirrhosis. *Hepatology* 1994, 20: 135–141.

113. Bianchi G, Marchesini G, Zoli M, Bugianesi E, Fabbri A, Pisi E. Prognostic significance of diabetes in patients with cirrhosis. *Hepatology* 1994, 20: 119–125.

114. Müller MJ, Pirlich M, Balks HJ, Selberg O. Glucose intolerance in liver cirrhosis: role of hepatic and non-hepatic influences. *Eur J Clin Chem Clin Biochem* 1994, 32: 749–758.

115. Ohyanagi H, Nomura H, Nishimatsu S, Usami M, Kasahara H. The liver and nutrient metabolism. In: Payne-James J, Grimble G, Silk D (Hrsg.). *Artificial Nutrition and Support in Clinical Practice*. London: Edward Arnold, 1995: 59–71.

116. Mahler H, Pasi A, Kramer JM et al. Fulminant liver failure in association with the emetic toxin of *Bacillus cereus*. *N Engl J Med* 1997, 336: 1142–1148.

117. Schafer DF, Sorrell MF. Power failure, liver failure. *N Engl J Med* 1997, 336: 1173–1174.

118. Kleinberger G. Parenterale ernährung bei leberinsuffizienz. *Schweiz Med WSchr* 1986, 116: 545–549.

119. Forbes A, Wicks C, Marshall W, Johnson P, Forsey P, Williams R. Nutritional support in fulminant hepatic failure: the safety of lipid solutions. *Gut* 1987, 28: 1347–1349.

120. Schütz T, Bechstein WO, Neuhaus P, Lochs H, Plauth M. Clinical practice of nutrition in acute liver failure—a European survey. *Clin Nutr* 2004, 23: 975–982.

121. Petrides SA, Groop LC, Riely CA, De Fronzo RA. Effect of physiologic hyperinsulinemia on glucose and lipid metabolism in cirrhosis. *J Clin Invest* 1991, 88: 561–570.

122. Müller MJ, Fenk A, Lautz HU, et al. Energy expenditure and substrate metabolism in ethanol-induced liver cirrhosis. *Am J Physiol* 1991, 260: E338–E344.
123. Müller M, Rieger A, Willmann O, Lautz HU, Balks H, von zur Mühlen A. Metabolic responses to lipid infusions in patients with liver cirrhosis. *Clin Nutr* 1992, 11: 193–206.
124. Druml W, Fischer M, Pidlich J, Lenz K. Fat elimination in chronic hepatic failure: long-chain vs medium-chain triglycerides. *Am J Clin Nutr* 1995, 61: 812–817.
125. Cabré E, Nunez MC, Gonzalez-Huix F, et al. Clinical and nutritional factors predictive of plasma lipid unsaturation deficiency in advanced liver cirrhosis: a logistic regression analysis. *Am J Gastroenterol* 1993, 88: 1738–1743.
126. Cabré E, Abad-Lacruz A, Nunez MC, et al. The relationship of plasma polyunsaturated fatty acid deficiency with survival in advanced liver cirrhosis: Multivariate analysis. *Am J Gastroenterol* 1993, 88: 718–722.
127. Kuse ER, Kotzerke J, Müller S, Nashan B, Lück R, Jaeger K. Hepatic reticuloendothelial function during parenteral nutrition including an MCT/LCT or LCT emulsion after liver transplantation— a double-blind study. *Transpl Int* 2002, 15: 272–7.
128. Record CO, Buxton B, Chase RA, Curzon G, Murray-Lyon IM, Williams R. Plasma and brain amino acids in fulminant hepatic failure and their relationship to hepatic encephalopathy. *Eur J Clin Invest* 1976, 6: 387–394.
129. Rosen HM, Yoshimura N, Hodgman JM, Fischer JE. Plasma amino acid patterns in hepatic encephalopathy of differing etiology. *Gastroenterology* 1977, 72: 483–487.
130. Clemmesen JO, Kondrup J, Ott P. Splanchnic and leg exchange of amino acids and ammonia in acute liver failure. *Gastroenterology* 2000, 118: 1131–1139.
131. Plauth M, Roske A-E, Romaniuk P, Roth E, Ziebig R, Lochs H. Post-feeding hyperammonemia in patients with transjugular intrahepatic portosystemic shunt and liver cirrhosis: role of small intestinal ammonia release and route of nutrient administration. *Gut* 2000, 46: 849–855.
132. Olde Damink SWM, Jalan R, Redhead D, Hayes PC, Deutz NEP, Soeters PB. Interorgan ammonia and amino acid metabolism in metabolically stable patients with liver cirrhosis and a TIPSS. *Hepatology* 2002, 36: 1163–1171.
133. Clemmesen JO, Larsen FS, Kondrup J, Hansen BA, Ott P. Cerebral herniation in patients with acute liver failure is correlated with arterial ammonia concentration. *Hepatology* 1999, 29: 648–53.
134. Bhatia V, Singh R, Acharya SK. Predictive value of arterial ammonia for complications and outcome in acute liver failure. *Gut* 2006, 55: 98–104.
135. Bernal W, Hall C, Karvellas CJ, Auzinger G, Sizer E, Wendon J. Arterial ammonia and clinical risk factors for encephalopathy and intracranial hypertension in acute liver failure. *Hepatology* 2007, 46: 1844–52.
136. Plauth M, Cabré E, Campillo B, Kondrup J, Marchesini G, Schütz T, Shenkin A, Wendon J. ESPEN guidelines parenteral nutrition. liver disease. *Clin Nutr* 2009, 28: 436–444.
137. McCullough AJ, Tavill AS. Disordered Energy and protein metabolism in liver disease. *Semin Liver Dis* 1991, 11: 265–273.
138. Ballmer PE, Walshe D, McNurlan MA, Watson H, Brunt PW, Garlick PJ. Albumin synthesis rates in cirrhosis: correlation with Child-Turcotte classification. *Hepatology* 1993, 18: 292–297.
139. Ballmer PE, Reichen J, McNurlan MA, Sterchi A-B, Anderson SE, Garlick PJ. Albumin but not fibrinogen synthesis correlates with galactose elimination capacity in patients with liver cirrhosis. *Hepatology* 1996, 24: 53–59.
140. Swart GR, Zillikens MC, van Vuure JK, van den Berg JW. Effect of a late evening meal on nitrogen balance in patients with cirrhosis of the liver. *Br Med J* 1989, 299: 1202–1203.

141. Verboeket-van de Venne WP, Westerterp KR, van Hoek B, Swart GR. Energy expenditure and substrate metabolism in patients with cirrhosis of the liver: effects of the pattern of food intake. *Gut* 1995, 36: 110–116.

142. Zillikens MC, van den Berg JW, Wattimena JL, Rietveld T, Swart GR. Nocturnal oral glucose supplementation. The effects on protein metabolism in cirrhotic patients and in healthy controls. *J Hepatol* 1993, 17: 377–383.

143. Petrides AS, Luzi L, Reuben A, Riely C, DeFronzo RA. Effect of insulin and plasma amino acid concentration on leucine metabolism in cirrhosis. *Hepatology* 1991, 14: 432–441.

144. Swart GR, van den Berg JW, van Vuure JK, Tietveld T, Wattimena D, Frenkel M. Minimum protein requirements in liver cirrhosis determined by nitrogen balance measurements at three levels of protein intake. *Clin Nutr* 1989, 8: 329–336.

145. Iob V, Coon WW, Sloan M. Free amino caids in liver, plasma, and muscle of patients with cirrhosis of the liver. *J Surg Res* 1967, 7: 41–43.

146. O'Keefe SJD Abraham R, El-Zayadi A, Marshall W, Davis M, Williams R. Increased plasma tyrosine concentrations in patients with cirrhosis and fulminant hepatic failure associated with increased plasma tyrosine flux and reduced hepatic oxidation capacity. *Gastroenterology* 1981, 81: 1017–1024.

147. Iwasaki Y, Sato H, Ohkubo A, Sanjo T, Futagawa S, Sugiura M, Tsuji S. Effect of spontaneous portal-systemic shunting on plasma insulin and amino acid concentrations. *Gastroenterology* 1980, 78: 677–683.

148. Ganda OP, Ruderman NB. Muscle nitrogen metabolism in chronic hepatic insufficiency. *Metabolism* 1976, 25: 427–435.

149. Hayashi M, Ohnishi H, Kawade Y et al. Augmented utilisation of branched-chain amino acids by skeletal muscle in decompensated cirrhosis in special relation to ammonia detoxification. *Gastroenterol Japon* 1981, 16: 64–70.

150. Leweling H, Breitkreutz R, Behne F, Staedt U, Striebel JP, Holm E. Hyperammonemia-induced depletion of glutamate and branched-chain amino acids in muscle and plasma. *J Hepatol* 1996, 25: 756–62.

151. Olde Damink SW, Dejong CH, Deutz NE, van Berlo CL, Soeters PB. Upper gastrointestinal bleeding: an ammoniagenic and catabolic event due to the total absence of isoleucine in the haemoglobin molecule. *Med Hypotheses* 1999, 52: 515–9.

152. Olde Damink SWM, Jalan R, Deutz NEP, de Jong CHC, Redhead DN, Hynd P, Hayes PC, Soeters PB. Isoleucine infusion during "simulated" upper gastrointestinal bleeding improves liver and muscle protein synthesis in cirrhotic patients. *Hepatology* 2007, 45: 560-568.

153. Plank LD, McCall JL, Gane EJ et al. Pre- and postoperative immunonutrition in patients undergoing liver transplantation: a pilot study of safety and efficacy. *Clin Nutr* 2005, 24: 288–296.

154. Reilly J, Mehta R, Teperman L et al. Nutritional support after liver transplantation: a randomized prospective study. *J Parenter Enteral Nutr* 1990, 14: 386–391.

155. Naveau S, Pelletier G, Poynard T et al. A randomized clinical trial of supplementary parenteral nutrition in jaundiced alcoholic cirrhotic patients. *Hepatology* 1986, 6: 270–274.

156. Aggett P. Severe Zinc defiency. In: Mills C (Ed.). Zinc in Human Biology. Berlin: Springer, 1989: 259–274.

157. Barry M, Keeling PW, Feely J. Tissue zinc status and drug elimination in patients with chronic liver disease. *Clin Sci* 1990, 78: 547–549.

158. Halsted JA, Hackley B, Rudzki C, Smith JC, Jr. Plasma zinc concentration in liver diseases. Comparison with normal controls and certain other chronic diseases. *Gastroenterology* 1968, 54: 1098–1105.

159. Thuluvath PJ, Triger DR. Selenium in chronic liver disease. *J Hepatol* 1992, 14: 176–182.
160. Grüngreiff K, Abicht K, Kluge M et al. Clinical studies on zinc in chronic liver diseases. *Z Gastroenterol* 1988, 26: 409–415.
161. van der Rijt CC, Schalm SW, Schat H, Foeken K, De Jong G. Overt hepatic encephalopathy precipitated by zinc deficiency. *Gastroenterology* 1991, 100: 1114–1118.
162. Mills PR, Shenkin A, Anthony RS et al. Assessment of nutritional status and *in vivo* immune responses in alcoholic liver disease. *Am J Clin Nutr* 1983, 38: 849–859.
163. Shenker S, Halff G. Nutritional therapy in alcoholic liver disease. *Sem Liver Dis* 1993, 13: 196–209.
164. Lieber CS. Alcohol, liver, and nutrition. *J Am Coll Nutr* 1991, 10: 602–632.
165. Lindor KD. Management of osteopenia of liver disease with special emphasis on primary biliary cirrhosis. *Semin Liver Dis* 1993, 13: 367–373.
166. Schmidt LE, Dalhoff K. Serum phosphate is an early predictor of outcome in severe acetaminophen-induced hepatotoxicity. *Hepatology* 2002, 36: 659–665.
167. O'Grady JG, Schalm SW, Williams R. Acute liver failure: redefining the syndromes. *Lancet* 1993, 342: 273–275.
168. van den Berghe G, Wouters P, Weekers F et al. Intensive insulin therapy in the critically ill patients. *N Engl J Med* 2001, 345: 1359–1367.
169. van den Berghe G, Wilmer A, Hermans G, Meersseman W, Wouters P, Milants I, van Wijngaerden E, Bobbaers H, Bouillon R. Intensive insulin therapy in the medical ICU. *N Engl J Med* 2006, 354: 449–61.
170. Brunkhorst FM, Engel C, Bloos F et al. Intensive insulin therapy and pentastarch in severe sepsis. *N Engl J Med* 2008, 358: 125–139.
171. Fischer JE, Rosen HM, Ebeid AM, James JH, Keane JM, Soeters PB. The effect of normalization of plasma amino acids on hepatic encephalopathy in man. *Surgery* 1976, 80: 77–91.
172. Fryden A, Weiland O, Martensson J. Successful treatment of hepatic coma probably caused by acute infectious hepatitis with balanced solution of amino acids. *Scand J Infect Dis* 1982, 14: 177–180.
173. Hensle T, Blackburn GL, O'Donnell T, McDermott WV, Jr. Intravenous feeding in hepatic failure. *Surg Forum* 1973, 24: 388–391.
174. Calvey H, Davis M, Williams R. Controlled trial of nutritional supplementation, with and without branched chain amino acid enrichment, in treatment of acute alcoholic hepatitis. *J Hepatol* 1985, 1: 141–51.
175. Cabré E., Rodriguez-Iglesias, Caballeria J. et al. Short- and long-term outcome of severe alcohol-induced hepatitis treated with steroids or enteral nutrition: a multicenter randomized trial. *Hepatology* 2000, 32: 36–42.
176. De Ledinghen V, Beau P, Mannant PR et al. Early feeding or enteral nutrition in patients with cirrhosis after bleeding from esophageal varices? A randomized controlled study. *Dig Dis Sci* 1997, 42: 536–41.
177. Plauth M, Cabré E, Riggio O et al. ESPEN guidelines on enteral nutrition: liver disease. *Clin Nutr* 2006, 25: 285–294.
178. Morgan TR, Moritz TE, Mendenhall CL, Haas R. Protein consumption and hepatic encephalopathy in alcoholic hepatitis. VA Cooperative Study Group #275. *J Am Coll Nutr* 1995, 14: 152–8.
179. Bonkovsky HL, Singh RH, Jafri IH et al. A randomized, controlled trial of treatment of alcoholic hepatitis with parenteral nutrition and oxandrolone. II. Short-term effects on nitrogen metabolism, metabolic balance, and nutrition. *Am J Gastroenterol* 1991, 86: 1209–1218.
180. Diehl AM, Boitnott JK, Herlong HF et al. Effect of parenteral amino acid supplementation in alcoholic hepatitis. *Hepatology* 1985, 5: 57–63.

181. Nasrallah SM, Galambos JT. Aminoacid therapy of alcoholic hepatitis. *Lancet* 1980, 2: 1276–1277.
182. Simon D, Galambos JT. A randomized controlled study of peripheral parenteral nutrition in moderate and severe alcoholic hepatitis. *J Hepatol* 1988, 7: 200–207.
183. Sechi G, Serra A. Wernicke's encephalopathy: new clinical settings and recent advances in diagnosis and management. *Lancet Neurol* 2007, 6: 442–455.
184. Neuschwander-Tetri BA, Brunt EM, Wehmeier KR, Sponseller CA, Hampton K, Bacon BR. Interim results of a pilot study demonstrating the early effects of the PPAR-gamma ligand rosiglitazone on insulin sensitivity, aminotransferases, hepatic steatosis and body weight in patients with non-alcoholic steatohepatitis. *J Hepatol* 2003, 38: 434–40.
185. Idilman R, Mizrak D, Corapcioglu D, Bektas M, Doganay B, Sayki M, Coban S, Erden E, Soykan I, Emral R, Uysal AR, Ozden A. Clinical trial: insulin-sensitizing agents may reduce consequences of insulin resistance in individuals with non-alcoholic steatohepatitis. *Aliment Pharmacol Ther* 2008, 28: 200–8.
186. Balas B, Belfort R, Harrison SA, Darland C, Finch J, Schenker S, Gastaldelli A, Cusi K. Pioglitazone treatment increases whole body fat but not total body water in patients with non-alcoholic steatohepatitis. *J Hepatol* 2007, 47: 565–70.
187. Le Cornu KA, McKiernan FJ, Kapadia SA, Neuberger JM. A prospective randomized study of preoperative nutritional supplementation in patients awaiting elective orthotopic liver transplantation. *Transplantation* 2000, 69: 1364–9.
188. Smith J, Horowitz J, Henderson JM, Heymsfield S. Enteral hyperalimentation in undernourished patients with cirrhosis and ascites. *Am J Clin Nutr* 1982, 35: 56–72.
189. Hirsch S, Bunout D, de la MP et al. Controlled trial on nutrition supplementation in outpatients with symptomatic alcoholic cirrhosis. *J Parenter Enteral Nutr* 1993, 17: 119–24.
190. Löser C, Folsch UR. Guidelines for treatment with percutaneous endoscopic gastrostomy. German Society of Digestive and Metabolic Diseases. *Z Gastroenterol* 1996, 34: 404–8.
191. Córdoba J, López-Hellín J, Planas M, Sabín P, Sanpedro F, Castro F, Esteban R, Guardia J. Normal protein for episodic hepatic encephalopathy: results of a randomized trial. *J Hepatol* 2004, 41: 38–43.
192. Horst D, Grace ND, Conn HO et al. Comparison of dietary protein with an oral, branched chain-enriched amino acid supplement in chronic portal-systemic encephalopathy: a randomized controlled trial. *Hepatology* 1984, 4: 279–87.
193. Yoshida T, Muto Y, Moriwaki H, Yamato M. Effect of long-term oral supplementation with branched-chain amino acid granules on the prognosis of liver cirrhosis. *Gastroenterol Japon* 1989, 24: 692–698.
194. Marchesini G, Bianchi G, Merli M, Amodio P, Panella C, Loguercio C, Rossi Fanelli F, Abbiati R and the Italian BCAA Study Group. Nutritional supplementation with branched-chain amino acids in advanced cirrhosis: a double-blind, randomized trial. *Gastroenterology* 2003, 124: 1792–1801.
195. Muto Y, Sato S, Watanabe A, Moriwaki H, Suzuki K, Kato A, Kato M, Nakamura T, Higuchi K, Nishiguchi S, Kumada H, for the LOTUS group. Effects of oral branched chain amino acid granules on event-free survival in patients with liver cirrhosis. *Clin Gastroenterol Hepatol* 2005, 3: 705–713.
196. Bresci G, Parisi G, Banti S. Management of hepatic encephalopathy with oral zinc supplementation: a long-term treatment. *Eur J Med* 1993, 2: 414–416.
197. Reding P, Duchateau J, Bataille C. Oral zinc supplementation improves hepatic encephalopathy: results of a randomised controlled trial. *Lancet* 1984, 2: 493–495.
198. Riggio O, Ariosto F, Merli M et al. Short-term oral zinc supplementation does not improve chronic hepatic encephalopathy. Results of a double-blind crossover trial. *Dig Dis Sci* 1991, 36: 1204–1208.

199. Marchesini G, Fabbri A, Bianchi G, Brizi M, Zoli M. Zinc supplementation and amino acid-nitrogen metabolism in patients with advanced cirrhosis. *Hepatology* 1996, 23: 1084–1092.

200. Garrett-Laster M, Russell RM, Jacques PF. Impairment of taste and olfaction in patients with cirrhosis: the role of vitamin A. *Hum Nutr Clin Nutr* 1984, 38: 203–214.

201. Weismann K, Christensen E, Dreyer V. Zinc supplementation in alcoholic cirrhosis: a double-blind clinical trial. *Acta Med Scand* 1979, 205: 361–366.

202. Crippin JS, Jorgensen RA, Dickson ER, Lindor KD. Hepatic osteodystrophy in primary biliary cirrhosis: effects of medical treatment. *Am J Gastroenterol* 1994, 89: 47–50.

203. Holm E, Leweling H, Saeger H, Arnold V, Gladisch R. Exogenous lipids as a caloric support in hepatic failure. In: Francavilla A, Panella C, Di Leo A, van Thiel D (Hrsg.). *Liver and Hormones.* New York: Raven Press, 1987: 125–144.

204. Michel H, Bories P, Aubin JP, Pomier-Layrargues G, Bauret P, Bellet-Herman H. Treatment of acute hepatic encephalopathy in cirrhotics with a branched-chain amino acids enriched versus a conventional amino acids mixture: a controlled study of 70 patients. *Liver* 1985, 5: 282–289.

205. Wahren J, Denis J, Desurmont P et al. Is intravenous administration of branched chain amino acids effective in the treatment of hepatic encephalopathy? A multicenter study. *Hepatology* 1983, 3: 475–480.

206. Battistella FD, Widergren JT, Anderson JT, Siepler JK, Weber JC, MacColl K. A prospective, randomized trial of intravenous fat emulsion administration in trauma victims requiring total parenteral nutrition. *J Trauma* 1997, 43: 52–58.

207. Granato D, Blum S, Rossle C, Boucher J Le, Malnoe A, Dutot G. Effects of parenteral lipid emulsions with different fatty acid composition on immune cell functions in vitro. *J Parenter Enteral Nutr* 2000, 24: 113–118.

208. Mayer K, Meyer S, Reinholz–Muhly M et al. Short-time infusion of fish oil-based lipid emulsions, approved for parenteral nutrition, reduces monocyte proinflammatory cytokine generation and adhesive interaction with endothelium in humans. *J Immunol* 2003, 171: 4837–4843.

209. Mayer K, Gokorsch S, Fegbeutel C, Hattar K, Rosseau S, Walmrath D, Seeger W, Grimminger F. Parenteral nutrition with fish oil modulates cytokine response in patients with sepsis. *Am J Respir Crit Care Med* 2003, 167: 1321–8.

210. Mayer K, Seeger W. Fish oil in critical illness. *Curr Opin Clin Nutr Metab Care* 2008, 11: 121–7.

211. Naylor CD, O'Rourke K, Detsky AS, Baker JP. Parenteral nutrition with branched-chain amino acids in hepatic encephalopathy: a meta-analysis. *Gastroenterology* 1989, 97: 1033–1042.

212. Mendenhall C, Bongiovanni G, Goldberg S et al. VA Cooperative Study on Alcoholic Hepatitis. III: Changes in protein-calorie malnutrition associated with 30 days of hospitalization with and without enteral nutritional therapy. *J Parenter Enteral Nutr* 1985, 9: 590–596.

213. Freund H, Dienstag J, Lehrich J et al. Infusion of branched-chain enriched amino acid solution in patients with hepatic encephalopathy. *Ann Surg* 1982, 196: 209–220.

214. Holm E, Striebel K, Meisinger E, Haux P, Langhans W, Becker H. [Amino-acid mixtures for parenteral feeding in liver insufficiency.] Article in German. *Infusionsther Klin Ernähr* 1978, 5: 274–292.

215. Cerra FB, Cheung NK, Fischer JE et al. Disease-specific amino acid infusion (F080) in hepatic encephalopathy: a prospective, randomized, double-blind, controlled trial. *J Parenter Enteral Nutr* 1985, 9: 288–295.

216. Fiaccadori F, Ginelli F, Pedretti G, Pelosi G, Sacchini D, Zeneroli M. Branched-chain enriched amino acid solutions in the treatment of hepatic encephalopathy: a controlled trial. *Ital J Gastroenterol* 1985, 17: 5–10.

217. Rossi-Fanelli F, Riggio O, Cangiano C et al. Branched-chain amino acids vs lactulose in the treatment of hepatic coma: a controlled study. *Dig Dis Sci* 1982, 27: 929–935.

218. Strauss E, Dos Santos W, Da Silva E. Treatment of hepatic encephalopathy: a randomized clinical trial comparing a branched chain enriched amino acid solution to oral neomycin. *Nutr Supp Services* 1986, 6: 18–21.

219. Vilstrup H, Gluud C, Hardt F et al. Branched chain enriched amino acid versus glucose treatment of hepatic encephalopathy: a double-blind study of 65 patients with cirrhosis. *J Hepatol* 1990, 10: 291–296.

220. Als-Nielsen B, Koretz RL, Kjaergard LL, Gluud C. Branched-chain amino acids for hepatic encephalopathy. *Cochrane Database Syst Rev* 2003; CD001939.

221. Fan ST, Lo CM, Lai EC, Chu KM, Liu CL, Wong J. Perioperative nutritional support in patients undergoing hepatectomy for hepatocellular carcinoma. *N Engl J Med* 1994, 331: 1547–52.

222. Kanematsu T, Koyanagi N, Matsumata T, Kitano S, Takenaka K, Sugimachi K. Lack of preventive effect of branched-chain amino acid solution on postoperative hepatic encephalopathy in patients with cirrhosis: a randomized, prospective trial. *Surgery* 1988, 104: 482–8.

223. Hu Q-G, Zheng G-C. The influence of enteral nutrition in postoperative patients with poor liver function. *World J Gastroenterol* 2003, 9: 843–846.

224. Chin SE, Shepherd RW, Thomas BJ et al. Nutritional support in children with end-stage liver disease: a randomized crossover trial of a branched-chain amino acid supplement. *Am J Clin Nutr* 1992, 56: 158–63.

225. Hasse JM, Blue LS, Liepa GU et al. Early enteral nutrition support in patients undergoing liver transplantation. *J Parenter Enteral Nutr* 1995, 19: 437–43.

226. Rayes N, Seehofer D, Hansen S et al. Early enteral supply of lactobacillus and fiber versus selective bowel decontamination: a controlled trial in liver transplant recipients. *Transplantation* 2002, 74: 123–7.

227. Wicks C, Somasundaram S, Bjarnason I et al. Comparison of enteral feeding and total parenteral nutrition after liver transplantation. *Lancet* 1994, 344: 837–40.

228. Pescovitz MD, Mehta PL, Leapman SB, Milgrom ML, Jindal RM, Filo RS. Tube jejunostomy in liver transplant recipients. *Surgery* 1995, 117: 642–7.

229. Mehta PL, Alaka KJ, Filo RS, Leapman SB, Milgrom ML, Pescovitz MD. Nutrition support following liver transplantation: comparison of jejunal versus parenteral routes. *Clin Transplant* 1995, 9: 364–9.

230. Golling M, Lehmann T, Senninger N, Herfarth C, Otto G. Tacrolimus reduction improves glucose metabolism and insulin secretion after liver transplantation. *Transplant Proc* 1996, 28: 3180–3182.

231. Lundbom N, Laurila O, Laurila S. Central pontine myelinolysis after correction of chronic hyponatraemia. *Lancet* 1993, 342: 247–248.

232. McDiarmid SV, Colonna JO, Shaked A, Ament ME, Busuttil RW. A comparison of renal function in cyclosporine- and FK-506-treated patients after primary orthotopic liver transplantation. *Transplantation* 1993, 56: 847–853.

233. Pomposelli JJ, Pomfret EA, Burns DL et al. Life-threatening hypophosphatemia after right hepatic lobectomy for live donor adult liver transplantation. *Liver Transpl* 2001, 7: 637–642.

234. Smyrniotis V, Kostopanagiotou G, Katsarelias D, Theodoraki K, Hondros K, Kouskouni E. Changes of serum phosphorus levels in hepatic resections and implications on patients' outcomes. *Int Surg* 2003, 88: 100–104.

235. Tan HP, Madeb R, Kovach SJ et al. Hypophosphatemia after 95 right-lobe living-donor hepatectomies for liver transplantation is not a significant source of morbidity. *Transplantation* 2003, 76: 1085–1088.
236. Singer P, Cohen J, Cynober L. Effect of nutritional state of brain-dead organ donor on transplantation. *Nutrition* 2001, 17: 948–952.

18 Nonalcoholic Fatty Liver Disease

Kevin M. Korenblat

CONTENTS

18.1 INTRODUCTION

The modern history of nonalcoholic fatty liver disease (NAFLD) as a distinct clinical entity has its origins with three independent publications 30 years ago describing liver disease with histologic features similar to those seen with alcohol-related injury, but in patients reliably lacking excessive alcohol consumption.[1–3] Many of these patients were obese, glucose intolerant, or had hypertriglyceridemia. In the years that followed, NAFLD has emerged as a substantial cause of liver disease and progress made into understanding the natural history, mechanisms, and treatments of this condition.

Hepatic steatosis with varying degrees of inflammation is a recognized histologic pattern in liver diseases that include Wilson's Disease, kwashiorkor, and some medication-related liver injuries.[4,5] These unrelated diseases are often referred to

301

as secondary causes of NAFLD and distinguished from the bulk of patients with primary NAFLD:

Wilson's disease
Abetalipoproteinemia
Total parenteral nutrition (TPN)
Kwashiorkor
Celiac disease
Jejunal-ileal bypass
Medications
    Tamoxifen
    Antiretroviral protease inhibitors
    Amiodarone
    Methotrexate

Precise data on the prevalence of NAFLD remains elusive. There are currently over 50 population-based studies of the prevalence of NAFLD from 15 countries.[6] In these studies, the rates of NAFLD in the general population vary from 2.8 to 46%. Among high-risk populations, those with diabetes or obesity, the prevalence is 7 to 99%. These ranges illustrate the difficulties of studying a process that reflects a spectrum of disease and lacks a dispositive screening test applicable at the population level.

Despite these limitations, common themes have emerged. In the third U.S. National Health and Nutritional Examination Survey (1988–1994) (NHANES III), 7.9% of the study population had aminotransferase elevations.[7] The percentage narrows to 5.5% if individuals with daily alcohol consumption or serologic evidence of hepatitis B, hepatitis C, and iron overload are excluded. In this subset of both men and women, abnormal aminotransferases were strongly associated with markers of the metabolic syndrome.

The reliance on aminotransferase elevations as a metric for NAFLD is problematic because the prevalence rates will be dependent on the threshold used to define the reference range and current reference ranges may fail to capture all patients with NAFLD.[8,9]

An alternate approach utilizes hepatic imaging and many population-based studies have used ultrasonographic imaging of the liver to gauge steatosis. In the largest population-based application of ultrasound performed in Japan, the prevalence of hepatic steatosis was estimated at 14%.[10] As a screening tool, however, ultrasound has limitations. Ultrasound is unable to discern features of necroinflammation or fibrosis and a threshold of steatosis—estimated as >30%—is cited for the detection of steatosis.[11]

A promising noninvasive imaging technique is magnetic resonance spectroscopy (MRS) to quantify intrahepatic fat content. In a large, ethically diverse group of subjects from Dallas County (Texas), MRS was applied in 2,287 participants of the Dallas Heart Study. The range of intrahepatic triglyceride (IHTG) content went from 0 to 47.5% and followed a nonnormalized distribution. The median IHTG was 4.69% in the entire cohort. Within a subset of lean, nondiabetics with low levels of alcohol consumption and normal aminotransferases, the median IHTG was 1.9% and 5.6%

defined the 95th percentile. When this upper limit of normal is applied to the entire cohort, 30.7% had hepatic steatosis.[12]

The population-based estimates have been further refined in groups at high-risk for NAFLD. Among subjects eligible for bariatric surgery, approximate rates of steatosis are 76% of which 5.8% have cirrhosis. NAFLD is also overrepresented in type 2 diabetics with rates of NAFLD estimated between 40 to 70%.[13]

18.2 CLINICAL MANIFESTATIONS

NAFLD is most commonly described as a spectrum of disease ranging from hepatic steatosis alone to steatohepatitis.[14] The latter is also known as nonalcoholic steatohepatitis (NASH) and is the form of NAFLD that is associated with progressive liver disease and risk of cirrhosis. The major component of intrahepatic fat is triglyceride, which can exist within the hepatocyte cytoplasm as macrovascular droplets that enlarge displacing the nucleus to the cell membrane or microvesicular fat, numerous small droplets of fat that separate the cytoplasm from the nucleus. The former is more typical of NAFLD, while the latter is seen in metabolic disorders that affect mitochondrial oxidative phosphorylation (e.g., Reye's syndrome).

Patients with steatosis are frequently identified only by abdominal imaging undertaken for reasons other than a directed study of the liver. In individuals with NASH, abnormal aminotransferases uncovered as part of a yearly medical evaluation or a preinsurance evaluation may be the first clue of disease. NAFLD can present in all ages and can be found in all ethnic groups; however, NAFLD tends to be less frequent in African Americans despite similar or greater levels of obesity than in Hispanic and non-Hispanic Caucasians. In a study of patients enrolled in a large health maintenance organization in Alameda County in California, African Americans comprised 9% of HMO enrollees though only 3% met a case definition for probable NAFLD with an average body mass index (BMI) of 36.6 kg/m². Hispanics, in comparison, comprised 10% of enrollees, but 28% of those who met the case definition of NAFLD and the BMI of suspected cases was 34 kg/m².[15]

As in the original description of the disease, individuals with NAFLD tend to be centrally obese though excessive body weight is not a requirement.[16] Most patients will present without symptoms of liver disease unless more advanced fibrosis sufficient to result in either hepatic dysfunction or portal hypertension is present. Constitutional symptoms, such as fatigue or a vague right upper quadrant discomfort, may be elicited though it may not be obvious that these symptoms are from liver disease. Elevated aminotransferases are the most common clinical finding in NAFLD. Alanine aminotransferase (ALT) elevations are typically less than 5 times the upper limits of the reference range and typically greater in magnitude than elevations in aspartate aminotransferase (AST) unless cirrhosis is present, in which case the ratio of AST to ALT may be greater than 1. Isolated alkaline phosphatase elevations may be present in 10% of subjects with NAFLD.[17]

The strictly biochemical approach to NAFLD has its limitations. Aminotransferases elevations may be intermittent and there are ample reports of NAFLD occurring despite normal aminotransferases. In a group of 80 patients with the metabolic syndrome but normal aminotransferases referred for abdominal surgery, 58 had nonalcoholic steatohepatitis and 8 had cirrhosis.[9] The recognized limitations in aminotransferase elevations have given voice to those who have encouraged lowering of the reference range for the aminotransferases.

Auto-antibodies, particularly antinuclear antibodies and antismooth muscle actin antibodies, may be present in one-third of subjects with NAFLD and serum ferritin elevations are common. Elevated serum ferritin, however, does not necessarily imply parenchymal iron overload and there is no clear association between disease causing alleles in the HFE gene responsible for hemochromatosis with either hepatic fibrosis or hyperferritinemia.[18]

18.3 PATHOLOGY

Liver biopsy remains an essential diagnostic tool in the evaluation of NAFLD. Liver biopsy permits exclusion of other pathologic conditions and can assess the severity of steatosis, necroinflammation, and fibrosis. The degree of steatosis is variable and may be discordant with the inflammatory changes. Typical inflammatory features of NAFLD include a mixed lobular infiltrate with polymorphonuclear leukocytes, acidophil bodies, and hepatocyte ballooning.[19] Acidophil bodies are hepatocytes that have either undergone or are in the process of undergoing apoptotic cell death. Hepatocyte ballooning describes swollen-appearing hepatocytes from microtubular disruption. Neither ballooning nor acidophil bodies are unique to NAFLD; however, the presence of ballooning in the appropriate context is sufficient for the diagnosis of steatohepatitis.[20]

The histologic features of steatosis, lobular inflammation and hepatocyte ballooning, comprise the essential feature that determine the NAFLD activity score (NAS), a validated histology scoring system for NAFLD that is used to distinguish steatosis from steatohepatitis.[21] Fibrosis in NAFLD, as in other forms of liver disease, reflects collagen deposition by activated hepatic stellate cells within the space of Disse. Early fibrosis in NAFLD is frequently perisinusoidal within acinar zone 3. This is often described as a "chicken wire" fibrosis for its delicate lace-like pattern. Progression of disease gives way to periportal fibrosis that can eventually bridge and cirrhosis is established. Though biopsy is a critical component to the evaluation of NAFLD, a shortcoming that requires acknowledgment is sampling variability that may influence the precision of grading and staging hepatic histology.[22]

18.4 NATURAL HISTORY

Emerging data from a combination of longitudinal and cross-sectional studies have helped to delineate the natural history of NAFLD. The longest longitudinal study to date is of 129 Swedish subjects followed for 13 years.[23] Individuals with steatosis alone progressed at a variable rate to NASH though symptomatic liver disease was rare. However, among patients with NASH at baseline, 41% developed progressive fibrosis.

In both the Swedish and a cross-sectional study from Olmstead County, Minnesota, mortality rates within the NAFLD cohort were higher than in reference populations. Death from cardiovascular disease in the NAFLD cohort ranged from 5 to 25% and occurred at a higher rate than liver disease-associated mortality

(2 to 13%) with NAFLD groups when compared to their respective reference populations.[24]

Symptomatic liver disease developed in 5% of patient in the Swedish study, though this may underestimate the true risk of progressive liver disease. Cryptogenic cirrhosis is the fourth most common indication for liver transplantation and studies in subgroup have identified features of obesity and diabetes in 73% leading to speculation that a sizeable number of subjects with cryptogenic cirrhosis may reflect progression of liver disease resulting from NAFLD.[25,26]

18.5 MECHANISMS OF DISEASE DEVELOPMENT

The cause of NAFLD is the subject of intensive investigation at many levels. Two early paradigm were first to emerge. The first was a separation of the steatosis formation from necroinflammation leading to the "two-hit" hypothesis.[27] This theory posits accumulation of hepatic fat as an initial inciting step. The second step is the injury elicited by the fat, also known as lipotoxicity from a combination of cytokine induced injury, lipid peroxidation, and reactive oxygen species.

The second organizing principle is that of NAFLD as the hepatic manifestation of the metabolic syndrome.[28,29] The metabolic syndrome is a disorder characterized by decreased insulin sensitivity and often coexisting with proinflammatory states. Accepted criteria used in its diagnosis involve the finding of three or more of the following: central obesity, hypertriglyceridemia, low HDL cholesterol, hypertension, and increased fasting plasma glucose.[30] The full metabolic syndrome can be identified in as many as 88% of those with biopsy-proven NAFLD and this observation led to many studies of the organ-level metabolic changes associated with NAFLD.

18.5.1 ORGAN-LEVEL METABOLIC CHANGES

Euglycemic-hyperinsulinemic glucose clamps are the gold standard for assessment of insulin sensitivity. Application of this technique in clinical studies has established insulin resistance in obese nondiabetics with NASH and steatosis, nonobese nondiabetics with steatosis, and nonobese diabetics with steatosis.[31–34] Insulin signaling is impaired in the muscle, adipose tissue, and liver, and the degree of impairment increases in a monotonic fashion with the degree of hepatic steatosis.[35] Though both intrahepatic triglyceride content and visceral adipose tissue volume correlated with each other and tissue insulin sensitivity, in multivariate analysis, intrahepatic triglyceride content is a superior predictor of insulin resistance than visceral adipose tissue volume. Whether hepatic fat is the cause or result of insulin resistance is not known. Hepatic steatosis is common in type 2 diabetes, but not universal. Thus, hepatic steatosis is not universal in all cases where insulin resistance is dominant.

One of insulin's actions in adipose tissue is the suppression of release of free fatty acids that are eventually taken up by the liver and reesterified to triglycerides and increased free fatty acid delivery to the liver could account for one mechanism to promote an increase in hepatic steatosis. Hepatic triglycerides not consumed in the process of mitochondrial, peroxisomal, or microsomal fatty acid oxidation are secreted as apoB-100 containing very low density lipoproteins (VLDL). An imbalance between the intrahepatic accumulation of triglycerides and its removal would provide another potential mechanism for hepatic steatosis. ApoB-100 production is the rate-limiting step in VLDL synthesis and decreased apolipoprotein synthesis in subjects with NASH compared to lean and body mass index matched controls with NASH has been reported.[36]

A more comprehensive study of obese subjects found similar rates of VLDL-apoB-100 secretion rates, but increased VLDL-triglyceride secretion rates linearly related to increases IHTG content. Nonsystemic fatty acids, presumably derived from intraabdominal fat, intrahepatic fat, and *de novo* hepatic lipogenesis were the principle source for the increase in VLDL-triglyceride secretion that plateaus at hepatic triglyceride contents above >10%. These findings provide experimental support to the hypothesis of an imbalance in free fatty acid delivery relative to its hepatic secretion as a mechanism for hepatic triglyceride accumulation.[37]

18.6   MOLECULAR MECHANISMS IN THE DEVELOPMENT OF NAFLD

Hepatic lipid uptake, metabolism, and its *de novo* synthesis are regulated by a myriad molecules of which transcription factors, cytokines, and adipokines appear most relevant to NAFLD.

18.6.1   TRANSCRIPTION FACTORS

The mammalian sterol response, element-binding proteins 1c (SREBP-1c) is one of three isoforms of a class of transcription factors that upon its nuclear translocation activates hepatic lipogenesis. Overexpression of SREBP-1c in mouse models leads to the development of hepatic steatosis.[38] Conversely, ob/ob mice that harbor mutations in the leptin receptor and are both obese and insulin-resistance experience a 50% reduction in hepatic triglyceride when SREBP-1c is inactivate.[39] SREBP-1c is able to achieve this effect by activation of genes involve in lipogenesis, such as fatty acid synthase, and acyl-coA carboylase 1.[40] Whether upregulation of lipogenesis through SREBP-1c is a mechanism in human cases of NAFLD is unclear, though there is preliminary data that supports the relevance of this pathway.[41]

SREBP-1c can also transcriptionally activate the perioxisome proliferator-activated receptor gamma (PPAR γ). PPAR γ consists of three isoforms (γ1, γ2, and γ3) created by alternate splicing. Activation of this transcription factor expressed largely, but not exclusively, in adipose tissue, increases the expression of genes associated with fatty acid uptake and the storage of triglycerides. PPAR γ2 is exclusively expressed in adipocytes, exhibits a correlation with body mass index[42] and rare heterozygous mutations of PPAR γ result in a syndrome of severe insulin resistance and hepatic steatosis.[43,44] Perhaps the strongest evidence for a role for PPAR γ in NAFLD comes from emerging data on treatment of NAFLD with thiazolidinediones, agonists of the PPARs.

18.6.2 Cytokines and Adipokines

Adipose tissue was historically considered to be site of fat deposition only; however, it is now accepted that it is a metabolically active tissue that can influence insulin sensitivity and lipid metabolism in adipose and other tissues. Two adipokines that have been well studied in NAFLD are TNF-alpha and adiponectin. TNF-alpha is secreted by both adipocytes and hepatocytes and promotes insulin resistance though there was no difference in circulating levels of TNF-alpha in subjects with NASH relative to weight matched controls.[45] Adiponectin, by comparison, promotes insulin sensitivity.[46] In the same study that evaluated TNF-alpha, the expression of adiponectin was dramatically higher in controls than NASH subjects and the low serum adiponectin levels correlated with the severity of hepatic histology in NASH. In response to an oral fat load, adiponectin increased in control subjects, but showed a slight decrease in NASH subjects.[45]

18.6.3 Lipotoxicity

Necroinflammation resulting from hepatic steatosis comprises the second of the "two hits" resulting in liver damage from NAFLD. How precisely steatosis contributes to cellular damage is unknown. The generation of reactive oxygen species in response to the oxidation of free fatty acids (FFAs) is one hypothesized mechanism. FFAs undergo oxidation in mitochondria, peroxisomes, and microsomes. Cytochrome P4502E1 is a member of the P450 mixed function oxidase system and is involved in the metabolism of xenobiotics. The activity of CYP2E1 is greater in patients with NASH and has been associated with disordered insulin signaling and hepatic lipid peroxidation.[47]

An additional source of inflammation and injury is suggested to occur with macrophage infiltration of white adipose tissue. Central adiposity, of which omental fat is a major contributor, exhibits a strong correlation with hepatic fat content. In obese humans, omental fat becomes infiltrated with CD68-positive macrophages to a much greater extent than subcutaneous adipose tissue and the degree of infiltration correlates with scores of necroinflammation. The presence of these macrophages is postulated to contribute to the necroinflammatory injury, possibly through the elaboration of soluble factors that gain access to the liver by direct secretion into the portal circulation.[48,49]

18.7 TREATMENT

To date, all treatment strategies proffered for NAFLD appear to address either the issue of insulin resistance or oxidative stress. Therapies that have been tried include lifestyle modification, bariatric surgery, antioxidant therapy, insulin sensitizing agents, and lipid-lowering medications. Therapies used in clinical trials include:

Diet
Exercise
Weight loss medications
    Orlistat
    Sibutramine
    Endocannabinoid antagonists

Bariatric Surgery
Antioxidants
   Vitamin E
   N-acetylcysteine
Cytoprotective agents
   Ursodeoxycholic acid
Anticytokine agents
   Pentoxifylline
Insulin sensitizing agents
   Metformin
   Thiazolidinediones
Lipid lowering medications
   Atorvastatin
   Fenofibrate

Despite the increasing volume of literature in this area, no single therapy has yet to emerge that would satisfy the requirement of rigorous evidence-based processes. The reasons for this are many and include small study populations and the use of endpoints, such as aminotransferases, that are unreliable predictors of hepatic histology. Though some studies have used pre- and postintervention liver biopsy to address this latter concern, even histologic changes are at best surrogates for what ultimately are the most informative of endpoints of liver disease-related morbidity, need for liver transplantation, and mortality. To date, the most promising therapies focus on weight loss or improvements in insulin sensitivity.

18.7.1 LIFESTYLE MODIFICATION/WEIGHT REDUCTION

Nutritional assessment of subjects with NAFLD reveal greater than average consumption of meat (both lean and nonlean meats), increased carbohydrate consumption from sweetened liquids, and low-nutrient and high sodium foodstuffs.[50,51] Weight reduction by a combination of increased energy expenditure (exercise) and decreased caloric intake makes intuitive sense for a disease so closely linked to insulin resistance. Support for this approach can be drawn from the Diabetes Prevention Program in which over 3,000 prediabetics were randomized to receive either metformin with written recommendations for healthier diets and exercise or an intensive lifestyle modification program that included 150 minutes of moderate activity weekly and a goal to lose 7% of body weight. Intensive lifestyle modification proved to be far more effective in reducing the incidence of diabetes than metformin-treated subjects.[52] The outcome of the study is even more sobering in light of the fact that an arm of the study that used troglitazone as a treatment was discontinued after some study subjects developed life-threatening medication-induced liver injury.

This success notwithstanding, most weight loss studies through lifestyle modifications in NAFLD have substantial methodologic issues. Intensive nutritional counseling has been shown to decrease steatosis and inflammation in one small study and a widely accepted recommendation is for those with obesity and NAFLD to target a 10% reduction in body weight.[53]

18.7.2 BARIATRIC SURGERY

Bariatric surgery is indicated in the treatment of obesity when the body mass index is at least 40 kg/m^2 or in those at least 35 kg/m^2 and coexisting weight-related morbidities (e.g., type 2 diabetes, arterial hypertension, and obstructive sleep apnea). Contemporary surgical procedures include the Roux-en-Y gastric bypass, biliopancreatic diversion with and without duodenal switch, laparoscopic adjustable gastric banding, and vertically banded gastroplasty. These surgical procedures are very effective at achieving and maintaining weight loss. On average, a 61.2% reduction in weight can be achieved with bariatric surgery with concomitant improvements of associated weight-related comorbidities.[54]

The efficacy of weight loss surgery with respect to NAFLD has been evaluated in retrospective and prospective observational studies. The majority of studies that have included pre- and postoperative liver biopsies have demonstrated improvements in steatosis and inflammation and either no significant change or an improvement in fibrosis over a period of follow up ranging from 1 to 3.5 years.[55]

These promising data notwithstanding, concern persists about the potential risks of bariatric surgery. Historically, these concerns were engendered from experience with jejunal–ileal bypass, which resulted in the development of cirrhosis in 5 to 40% of patients[56] and acute liver failure. In comparison, neither Roux-en-Y gastric bypass nor laparoscopic adjustable gastric banding have been reported to cause either acute or chronic liver disease. Transient elevations in aminotransferases and portal vein thrombosis have been observed with these surgeries, though are believed to arise from complications of the operative procedure.[57–60] Transient elevations in aminotransferases with and without hyperbilirubinemia have been observed following biliopancreatic diversion and, in rare cases, death from liver failure has been reported.[61]

18.7.3 INSULIN SENSITIZING AGENTS

18.7.3.1 Metformin

Metformin is a commonly prescribed oral antidiabetic medication of the biguanide class. Its mechanism of action involves the activation of the kinase LKB1 to phosphorylate adenosine monophosphate activated protein kinase (AMPK), which is a key regulator of glucose and fatty acid metabolism.[62] Treatment of NAFLD with metformin has been evaluated in at least seven clinical trials of which only four report follow-up histology.[63–69] In a pilot study of 26 patients who completed 48 weeks of treatment, 30% showed improvement in liver histology and ALT levels. All of the histologic responders also were those who lost more than 5 kg of body weight during the trial.[65]

18.7.3.2 Thiazolidinediones

The thiazolidinediones (TZDs) are agonist of the peroxisome proliferator-activated receptor gamma and result in improved insulin sensitivity in adipose tissue, skeletal muscle, and liver. Troglitazone was the first TZD approved for the treatment of diabetes; however, this medication was withdrawn after numerous reports surfaced of severe drug-induced liver injury. Clinical trials of TZDs in NAFLD have used rosiglitazone and pioglitazone, two other agent in the class for which medication-induced liver injury is rare. All of the six clinical trials with these agents have documented improvements in aminotransferases, hepatic fat content, and necroin-flammatory activity.[70–75] In a placebo-controlled trial of pioglitazone in subjects with NASH, six months of treatment resulted in a 54% reduction of hepatic fat content with concomitant improvements in hepatocyte ballooning and inflammation, but not fibrosis.[74] These successes notwithstanding, these agents have important side effects that include weight gain and risk of increased mortality from cardiovascular disease.[76] TZDs are also contraindicated in patients with heart failure. Most importantly, response to TZDs is incomplete and, in a one-year trial with rosiglitazone, only 47% had an improvement in steatosis.[75] These issues notwithstanding, TZDs are emerging as the leading agent in the treatment of NAFLD. Though not currently a standard of care in the management of NAFLD, compelling arguments could be made for their use in type 2 diabetics with concomitant NAFLD.

18.8   PEDIATRIC NAFLD

Though historically considered a disease of adults, there is a growing awareness and concern for the NAFLD in pediatric populations reflecting the epidemic of child-hood obesity. A study from Japan using ultrasound imaging reported an incidence of fatty liver in 2.6% of school age children.[77] The more recent Study of Child and Adolescent Epidemiology (SCALE) reported a prevalence of 9.6% in San Diego, California, based on autopsy performed on children from age 2 to 19 years over a 10-year period.[78] Fatty liver is present in 38% of obese children and shows a striking heritability. Parents and siblings of children with NAFLD have greater rates of excessive intrahepatic triglyceride content than overweight children without NAFLD.[79] And similar to findings regarding race and ethnicity in adults, Hispanic children have been observed to have five times the odds of having fatty liver than African American children after controlling for the severity of obesity.

Akin to adult NAFLD, the disease is strongly associated with insulin resistance.[80] Where a difference with the adults disease does exist is in the association with hypo-thalamic or pituitary disease[81] and histologic findings. Children with NAFLD have two distinct histologic patterns. The adult pattern (steatosis, hepatocyte ballooning, and perisinusoidal fibrosis) is present, but a minority of the time. More commonly, liver biopsies in children have steatosis with a prominence of portal inflammation and varying degrees of fibrosis.[82] The mechanisms that determine which pattern will occur are not known nor are the clinical import of having one or the other of the pattern.

18.9   CONCLUSION

Over the past three decades, NAFLD has emerged as a substantial cause of liver disease-related morbidity and mortality in both children and adults. A growing body of literature suggests that the disease should be considered as the hepatic manifestation of insulin resistance and the metabolic syndrome. No definitive treatment for

NAFLD has been established; yet, strategies that improve obesity (lifestyle modification, bariatric surgery) or improve insulin resistance appear to hold the most promise for effective treatment of this disorder.

REFERENCES

1. Adler, M. and F. Schaffner, *Fatty liver hepatitis and cirrhosis in obese patients.* Am J Med, 1979. **67**(5): 811–6.
2. Miller, D., H. Ishimaru, and G. Klatskin, *Non-alcoholic liver disease mimicking alcoholic hepatitis and cirrhosis.* Gastroenterology, 1979. **77**: A27.
3. Ludwig, J., et al., *Nonalcoholic steatohepatitis: Mayo Clinic experiences with a hitherto unnamed disease.* Mayo Clin Proc, 1980. **55**(7): 434–8.
4. Chanda, N.K., *Pathological study of the liver in kwashiorkor.* Br Med J, 1958. **1**(5082): 1263–6.
5. Roberts, E.A. and M.L. Schilsky, *A practice guideline on Wilson disease.* Hepatology, 2003. **37**(6): 1475–92.
6. Lazo, M. and J.M. Clark, *The epidemiology of nonalcoholic fatty liver disease: a global perspective.* Semin Liver Dis, 2008. **28**(4): 339–50.
7. Clark, J.M., F.L. Brancati, and A.M. Diehl, *The prevalence and etiology of elevated aminotransferase levels in the United States.* Am J Gastroenterol, 2003. **98**(5): 960–7.
8. Chang, Y., et al., *Higher concentrations of alanine aminotransferase within the reference interval predict nonalcoholic fatty liver disease.* Clin Chem, 2007. **53**(4): 686–92.
9. Sorrentino, P., et al., *Silent non-alcoholic fatty liver disease-a clinical-histological study.* J Hepatol, 2004. **41**(5): 751–7.
10. Nomura, H., et al., *Prevalence of fatty liver in a general population of Okinawa, Japan.* Jpn J Med, 1988. **27**(2): 142–9.
11. Saadeh, S., et al., *The utility of radiological imaging in nonalcoholic fatty liver disease.* Gastroenterology, 2002. **123**(3): 745–50.
12. Szczepaniak, L.S., et al., *Magnetic resonance spectroscopy to measure hepatic triglyceride content: prevalence of hepatic steatosis in the general population.* Am J Physiol Endocrinol Metab, 2005. **288**(2): E462–8.
13. Targher, G., et al., *Prevalence of nonalcoholic fatty liver disease and its association with cardiovascular disease among type 2 diabetic patients.* Diabetes Care, 2007. **30**(5): 1212–8.
14. Matteoni, C.A., et al., *Nonalcoholic fatty liver disease: a spectrum of clinical and pathological severity.* Gastroenterology, 1999. **116**(6): 1413–9.
15. Weston, S.R., et al., *Racial and ethnic distribution of nonalcoholic fatty liver in persons with newly diagnosed chronic liver disease.* Hepatology, 2005. **41**(2): 372–9.
16. Bacon, B.R., et al., *Nonalcoholic steatohepatitis: an expanded clinical entity.* Gastroenterology, 1994. **107**(4): 1103–9.
17. Pantsari, M.W. and S.A. Harrison, *Nonalcoholic fatty liver disease presenting with an isolated elevated alkaline phosphatase.* J Clin Gastroenterol, 2006. **40**(7): 633–5.
18. Younossi, Z.M., et al., *Hepatic iron and nonalcoholic fatty liver disease.* Hepatology, 1999. **30**(4): 847–50.
19. Brunt, E.M., *Nonalcoholic steatohepatitis.* Semin Liver Dis, 2004. **24**(1): 3–20.
20. Brunt, E.M., *Pathology of nonalcoholic steatohepatitis.* Hepatol Res, 2005. **33**(2): 68–71.
21. Kleiner, D.E., et al., *Design and validation of a histological scoring system for nonalcoholic fatty liver disease.* Hepatology, 2005. **41**(6): 1313–21.
22. Ratziu, V., et al., *Sampling variability of liver biopsy in nonalcoholic fatty liver disease.* Gastroenterology, 2005. **128**(7): 1898–906.

23. Ekstedt, M., et al., *Long-term follow-up of patients with NAFLD and elevated liver enzymes.* Hepatology, 2006. **44**(4): 865–73.

24. Adams, L.A., et al., *The natural history of nonalcoholic fatty liver disease: a population-based cohort study.* Gastroenterology, 2005. **129**(1): 113–21.

25. Caldwell, S.H., et al., *Cryptogenic cirrhosis: clinical characterization and risk factors for underlying disease.* Hepatology, 1999. **29**(3): 664–9.

26. Maheshwari, A. and P.J. Thuluvath, *Cryptogenic cirrhosis and NAFLD: are they related?* Am J Gastroenterol, 2006. **101**(3): 664–8.

27. James, O. and C. Day, *Non-alcoholic steatohepatitis: another disease of affluence.* Lancet, 1999. **353**(9165): 1634–6.

28. Marchesini, G., et al., *Nonalcoholic fatty liver, steatohepatitis, and the metabolic syndrome.* Hepatology, 2003. **37**(4): 917–23.

29. Pagano, G., et al., *Nonalcoholic steatohepatitis, insulin resistance, and metabolic syndrome: further evidence for an etiologic association.* Hepatology, 2002. **35**(2): 367–72.

30. Eckel, R.H., S.M. Grundy, and P.Z. Zimmet, *The metabolic syndrome.* Lancet, 2005. **365**(9468): 1415–28.

31. Bugianesi, E., et al., *Insulin resistance in non-diabetic patients with non-alcoholic fatty liver disease: sites and mechanisms.* Diabetologia, 2005. **48**(4): 634–42.

32. Gastaldelli, A., et al., *Relationship between hepatic/visceral fat and hepatic insulin resistance in nondiabetic and type 2 diabetic subjects.* Gastroenterology, 2007. **133**(2): 496–506.

33. Kelley, D.E., et al., *Fatty liver in type 2 diabetes mellitus: relation to regional adiposity, fatty acids, and insulin resistance.* Am J Physiol Endocrinol Metab, 2003. **285**(4): E906–E916.

34. Seppala-Lindroos, A., et al., *Fat accumulation in the liver is associated with defects in insulin suppression of glucose production and serum free fatty acids independent of obesity in normal men.* J Clin Endocrinol Metab, 2002. **87**(7): 3023–8.

35. Korenblat, K.M., et al., *Liver, muscle, and adipose tissue insulin action is directly related to intrahepatic triglyceride content in obese subjects.* Gastroenterology, 2008. **134**(5): 1369–75.

36. Charlton, M., et al., *Apolipoprotein synthesis in nonalcoholic steatohepatitis.* Hepatology, 2002. **35**(4): 898–904.

37. Fabbrini, E., et al., *Alterations in adipose tissue and hepatic lipid kinetics in obese men and women with nonalcoholic fatty liver disease.* Gastroenterology, 2008. **134**(2): 424–31.

38. Shimano, H., et al., *Isoform 1c of sterol regulatory element binding protein is less active than isoform 1a in livers of transgenic mice and in cultured cells.* J Clin Invest, 1997. **99**(5): 846–54.

39. Yahagi, N., et al., *Absence of sterol regulatory element-binding protein-1 (SREBP-1) ameliorates fatty livers but not obesity or insulin resistance in Lep(ob)/Lep(ob) mice.* J Biol Chem, 2002. **277**(22): 19353–7.

40. Browning, J.D. and J.D. Horton, *Molecular mediators of hepatic steatosis and liver injury.* J Clin Invest, 2004. **114**(2): 147–52.

41. Higuchi, N., et al., *Liver X receptor in cooperation with SREBP-1c is a major lipid synthesis regulator in nonalcoholic fatty liver disease.* Hepatol Res, 2008. **38**(11): 1122–9.

42. Vidal-Puig, A.J., et al., *Peroxisome proliferator-activated receptor gene expression in human tissues: effects of obesity, weight loss, and regulation by insulin and glucocorticoids.* J Clin Invest, 1997. **99**(10): 2416–22.

43. Barroso, I., et al., *Dominant negative mutations in human PPARgamma associated with severe insulin resistance, diabetes mellitus and hypertension.* Nature, 1999. **402**(6764): 880–3.

44. Savage, D.B., et al., *Human metabolic syndrome resulting from dominant-negative mutations in the nuclear receptor peroxisome proliferator-activated receptor-gamma.* Diabetes, 2003. **52**(4): 910–7.

45. Musso, G., et al., *Adipokines in NASH: postprandial lipid metabolism as a link between adiponectin and liver disease.* Hepatology, 2005. **42**(5): 1175–83.

46. Yamauchi, T., et al., *The mechanisms by which both heterozygous peroxisome proliferator-activated receptor gamma (PPARgamma) deficiency and PPARgamma agonist improve insulin resistance.* J Biol Chem, 2001. **276**(44): 41245–54.

47. Schattenberg, J.M., et al., *Hepatocyte CYP2E1 overexpression and steatohepatitis lead to impaired hepatic insulin signaling.* J Biol Chem, 2005. **280**(11): 9887–94.

48. Cancello, R. and K. Clement, *Is obesity an inflammatory illness? Role of low-grade inflammation and macrophage infiltration in human white adipose tissue.* BJOG, 2006. **113**(10): 1141–7.

49. Cancello, R., et al., *Increased infiltration of macrophages in omental adipose tissue is associated with marked hepatic lesions in morbid human obesity.* Diabetes, 2006. **55**(6): 1554–61.

50. Kim, C.H., et al., *Nutritional assessments of patients with non-alcoholic fatty liver disease.* Obes Surg, 2010. **20**(2): 154–160.

51. Zelber-Sagi, S., et al., *Long term nutritional intake and the risk for non-alcoholic fatty liver disease (NAFLD): a population based study.* J Hepatol, 2007. **47**(5): 711–7.

52. Knowler, W.C., et al., *Reduction in the incidence of type 2 diabetes with lifestyle intervention or metformin.* N Engl J Med, 2002. **346**(6): 393–403.

53. Thomas, E.L., et al., *Effect of nutritional counselling on hepatic, muscle and adipose tissue fat content and distribution in non-alcoholic fatty liver disease.* World J Gastroenterol, 2006. **12**(36): 5813–9.

54. Buchwald, H., et al., *Bariatric surgery: a systematic review and meta-analysis.* JAMA, 2004. **292**(14): 1724–37.

55. de Freitas, A.C., A.C. Campos, and J.C. Coelho, *The impact of bariatric surgery on non-alcoholic fatty liver disease.* Curr Opin Clin Nutr Metab Care, 2008. **11**(3): 267–74.

56. Hocking, M.P., et al., *Long-term consequences after jejunoileal bypass for morbid obesity.* Dig Dis Sci, 1998. **43**(11): 2493–9.

57. De Roover, A., et al., *Pylephlebitis of the portal vein complicating intragastric migration of an adjustable gastric band.* Obes Surg, 2006. **16**(3): 369–71.

58. Denne, J.L. and C. Kowalski, *Portal vein thrombosis after laparoscopic gastric bypass.* Obes Surg, 2005. **15**(6): 886–9.

59. Lohlun, J.C., A. Guirguis, and L. Wise, *Elevated liver enzymes following open Roux-en-Y gastric bypass for morbid obesity—does timing of liver retraction affect the rise in the levels of transaminases?* Obes Surg, 2004. **14**(4): 505–8.

60. Pigeyre, M., et al., *Laparoscopic gastric bypass complicated by portal venous thrombosis and severe neurological complications.* Obes Surg, 2008. **18**(9): 1203–7.

61. Baltasar, A., et al., *Clinical hepatic impairment after the duodenal switch.* Obes Surg, 2004. **14**(1): 77–83.

62. Shaw, R.J., et al., *The kinase LKB1 mediates glucose homeostasis in liver and therapeutic effects of metformin.* Science, 2005. **310**(5754): 1642–6.

63. Bugianesi, E., et al., *A randomized controlled trial of metformin versus vitamin E or prescriptive diet in nonalcoholic fatty liver disease.* Am J Gastroenterol, 2005. **100**(5): 1082–90.

64. Duseja, A., et al., *Metformin is effective in achieving biochemical response in patients with nonalcoholic fatty liver disease (NAFLD) not responding to lifestyle interventions.* Ann Hepatol, 2007. **6**(4): 222–6.

65. Loomba, R., et al., *Clinical trial: Pilot study of metformin for the treatment of nonalcoholic steatohepatitis.* Aliment Pharmacol Ther, 2008. **29**: 172–82

66. Marchesini, G., et al., *Metformin in non-alcoholic steatohepatitis.* Lancet, 2001. **358**(9285): 893–4.
67. Nair, S., et al., *Metformin in the treatment of non-alcoholic steatohepatitis: a pilot open label trial.* Aliment Pharmacol Ther, 2004. **20**(1): 23–8.
68. Schwimmer, J.B., et al., *A phase 2 clinical trial of metformin as a treatment for non-diabetic paediatric non-alcoholic steatohepatitis.* Aliment Pharmacol Ther, 2005. **21**(7): 871–9.
69. Uygun, A., et al., *Metformin in the treatment of patients with non-alcoholic steatohepatitis.* Aliment Pharmacol Ther, 2004. **19**(5): 537–44.
70. Neuschwander-Tetri, B.A., et al., *Improved nonalcoholic steatohepatitis after 48 weeks of treatment with the PPAR-gamma ligand rosiglitazone.* Hepatology, 2003. **38**(4): 1008–17.
71. Promrat, K., et al., *A pilot study of pioglitazone treatment for nonalcoholic steatohepatitis.* Hepatology, 2004. **39**(1): 188–96.
72. Sanyal, A.J., et al., *A pilot study of vitamin E versus vitamin E and pioglitazone for the treatment of nonalcoholic steatohepatitis.* Clin Gastroenterol Hepatol, 2004. **2**(12): 1107–15.
73. Tiikkainen, M., et al., *Effects of rosiglitazone and metformin on liver fat content, hepatic insulin resistance, insulin clearance, and gene expression in adipose tissue in patients with type 2 diabetes.* Diabetes, 2004. **53**(8): 2169–76.
74. Belfort, R., et al., *A placebo-controlled trial of pioglitazone in subjects with nonalcoholic steatohepatitis.* N Engl J Med, 2006. **355**(22): 2297–307.
75. Ratziu, V., et al., *Rosiglitazone for nonalcoholic steatohepatitis: one-year results of the randomized placebo-controlled Fatty Liver Improvement with Rosiglitazone Therapy (FLIRT) trial.* Gastroenterology, 2008. **135**(1): 100–10.
76. Nissen, S.E. and K. Wolski, *Effect of rosiglitazone on the risk of myocardial infarction and death from cardiovascular causes.* N Engl J Med, 2007. **356**(24): 2457–71.
77. Tominaga, K., et al., *Prevalence of fatty liver in Japanese children and relationship to obesity: an epidemiological ultrasonographic survey.* Dig Dis Sci, 1995. **40**(9): 2002–9.
78. Schwimmer, J.B., et al., *Prevalence of fatty liver in children and adolescents.* Pediatrics, 2006. **118**(4): 1388–93.
79. Schwimmer, J.B., et al., *Heritability of nonalcoholic fatty liver disease.* Gastroenterology, 2009. **136**(5): 1585–92.
80. Deivanayagam, S., et al., *Nonalcoholic fatty liver disease is associated with hepatic and skeletal muscle insulin resistance in overweight adolescents.* Am J Clin Nutr, 2008. **88**(2): 257–62.
81. Nakajima, K., et al., *Pediatric nonalcoholic steatohepatitis associated with hypopituitarism.* J Gastroenterol, 2005. **40**(3): 312–5.
82. Schwimmer, J.B., et al., *Histopathology of pediatric nonalcoholic fatty liver disease.* Hepatology, 2005. **42**(3): 641–9.

19 Weight Management Strategies

Shelby Sullivan

CONTENTS

19.1 INTRODUCTION

We are currently experiencing an epidemic of overweight and obesity both in the United States and abroad. The most current National Health and Nutrition Examination Survey (NHANES) data as of the writing of this chapter was from 2005–2006, which showed that more than one third of U.S. adults (33.3% of men and 35.3% of women) were obese as defined by a body mass index (BMI) of >30 kg/m²[1]. Obesity is associated with increased risks for diabetes, hypertension, cardiovascular disease, and certain cancers as well as an increase in relative risk of mortality. A study of over one million healthy, nonsmoking U.S. adults found that obese white men and white women had a 2.58 and 2.00 relative risk of death, respectively, compared to lean men and women.[2]

The health risks of obesity and the need for weight loss are well known and even small reductions in weight are associated with significant health benefits.[3] However, successful weight loss continues to be a challenge for patients and clinicians. This chapter will review the fundamentals of energy balance and detail weight management strategies.

19.2   ASSESSING BODY MASS

The body is divided into lean body mass and fat mass. Lean body mass includes bone, muscle, and organs. Lean body mass can be further divided into intracellular and extracellular mass; however, for the purposes of this section we are focusing on the differentiation between lean mass (or fat free mass) and fat mass. Body composition can be measured using densitometry, bioelectrical impedance, underwater weighing, and with total body water techniques using deuterium oxide (heavy water). While these measures are commonly used in research, they are not practical in the hospital setting.

We typically use BMI as an easily calculated surrogate marker for body composition. It is calculated from height and weight, and it relates to risks of morbidity and mortality as well energy requirements. It is not a perfect substitution; some populations (e.g., football players, bodybuilders) may have a high BMI primarily due to their increased muscle mass. However, it is adequate to detect and quantify overweight/obesity in the majority of Americans because most Americans who have BMIs in the overweight and obese ranges have an excess of body fat.

BMI = wt (in kg)/height (in m²)

Classification of underweight, normal weight, overweight, and obesity in adults is based on BMI-related mortality data (Table 19.1).[2,4,5]

19.3   ENERGY BALANCE

Energy is stored in the body as triglyceride or glycogen in a number of tissues including adipose tissue, skeletal muscle, and liver. Triglyceride is a more efficient means of energy storage because each gram liberated 9.3 kcal when oxidized in comparison to glycogen, which liberates 4.1 kcal when oxidized. Additionally, glycogen is stored as a gel requiring roughly three times its weight in water. In a 70 kg (154 lb) man, approximately 2,500 kcal of glycogen is stored in skeletal muscle and 400 kcal are stored in the liver. The energy stored in triglyceride far exceeds this with 3,000 kcal stored in skeletal muscle, 450 kcal in the liver, and 120,000 kcal in adipose tissue.

TABLE 19.1
BMI and Weight Classification

BMI	Classification
<18.5 kg/m²	Underweight
18.5–24.9 kg/m²	Normal weight
25–29.9 kg/m²	Overweight
30–34.9 kg/m²	Class I obesity
35–39.9 kg/m²	Class II obesity
>40 kg/m²	Class III obesity

The total energy expenditure or energy required by an individual can be determined by the equation below:

Total Energy Expenditure (TEE) = Basal Metabolic Rate (BMR) + Activity + Thermic Effect of Food

BMR is the amount of energy consumed at rest. The amount of energy needed to maintain 1 kg of lean body mass is remarkably constant for individuals with a similar height. BMR is also known as resting metabolic rate (RMR), basal energy expenditure (BEE), or basal energy requirement (BER). *The differences in BMR between individuals reflect differing body composition.* The total energy expenditure, however, can vary widely from person to person based on activity level. This includes all activity (exercising, fidgeting, housework, etc.). BMR can be determined experimentally with a calorimeter, but, for practical purposes, calculations can be used to estimate BMR. Many methods are available for calculating BMR. One of the classic calculations that approximates BMR is the Harris–Benedict equation:[6]

Men: BMR (in kcal/day) = 66.5 + (13.8 × wt in kg) + (5 × ht in cm)
            – (6.76 × age in years)
Women: BMR (in k/cal/day) = 655 + (9.56 × wt in kg) + (1.85 × ht in cm)
            – (4.68 × age in years)

Once BMR is determined, one can then determine the amount of calories expended in activity or physical activity level (PAL). PAL is the ratio of TEE to BMR. This varies far more from person to person than BMR and depends on BMI, age, and sex. The data for PALs has been derived from a doubly labeled water database for basal energy expenditure and metabolic equivalents (METS) for a number of activities.[7,8] PAL can be divided by average daily activity levels of individuals (Table 19.2). The BMR is then multiplied by the PAL to determine BMR + Activity.

The thermic effect of food is the heat that is produced by the metabolism and storage of nutrients. It is essentially the energy costs of digestion, transport, and storage of nutrients. The heat produced varies between macronutrients, but is 6 to 10% of TEE on average.

An adjusted body weight rather than actual body weight should be used in obese patients to avoid overfeeding.

TABLE 19.2
Physical Activity Levels (PAL)

Activity Level	PAL
Sedentary	1.0–1.4 (ex. no recreational exercise, minimal exertion during the day)
Low active	1.4–1.6 (ex. small amount of recreational exercise, job requiring some walking during the work day)
Active	1.6–1.9 (ex. fairly active during the day, plus some moderate to intense exercise)
Very active	1.9–2.5 (ex. endurance athletes)

Adjusted body weight = ideal body weight + ([actual body weight − ideal body weight] × [0.25])

When calories are consumed in excess of total energy expenditure, they are stored with the majority of energy, which is stored as triglyceride in adipose tissue. When more calories are expended than consumed, triglycerides are released from adipose tissue to be oxidized for energy and weight is lost. It is important to note, however, the calculations presented above are only estimations and can be affected by a variety of factors.

19.3.1 THERAPEUTIC LIFESTYLE CHANGES

The medical treatment of obesity involves not only identifying patients that need to lose weight, but also providing a structured, goal-oriented approach that can be modified depending on the clinical response. The components of this approach include diet, physical activity, and behavior modification. In discussing weight loss, it must be stressed to patients that changes they make are lifestyle changes and will be lifelong. If patients return to prior habits, they will regain their weight. It is important for the physician to provide long-term surveillance to ensure continued success of the patient, and, if needed, recruit additional support, such as dieticians, physical therapists, family members, or referral for behavior therapy.

19.3.2 DIET

Decreasing calorie intake should be considered the basis of any weight loss program. The National Institute of Health (NIH) currently recommends 300 to 500 kcal decrease in calories per day in persons with a BMI of 27 to 35 for a goal of 10% weight loss over six months (1/2 to 1 pound weight loss per week). For the same percent weight loss in persons with BMI >35, the NIH recommends decreasing calories by 500 to 1000 kcal/day (1 to 2 pound weight loss per week). While these recommendations are evidence based, practically speaking, determining a patient's total energy expenditure can be cumbersome as seen above and may be inaccurate primarily due to variations in energy expenditure. Therefore, a simple calorie guideline based on weight has been proposed as an easy way for clinicians to identify calorie goals for patients initiating therapeutic lifestyle changes (Table 19.3).[9] Very low calorie diets (VLCD), which vary in calories but are typically 800 kcal or less, have been used for weight loss. However, a meta-analysis has recently shown that although VLCDs are associated with significantly more weight loss in the short term, at one year there is no difference between low calorie diets and VLCD.[10] In addition, VLCDs need to be medically monitored due to their increased association with weight loss complications, thus, they are rarely recommended.

There are many "diets" currently in fashion. These vary the macronutrient content of the diet. Diets that restrict dietary fat have been extensively studied and do cause weight loss.[11] However, in a randomized control trial comparing a low-fat *ad libitum* diet and a low-calorie diet providing 1,200 to 1,500 kcal/day, the low-calorie diet was associated with almost double the weight loss of the low-fat diet. Additionally, a

TABLE 19.3

Suggested Energy Composition of Initial Reduced-Calorie Diet

Weight in Pounds	Suggested Energy Intake kcal/day
150–199	1000
200–249	1200
250–299	1500
300–349	1800
>300	2000

Source: Klein, S. AGA technical review on obesity. *Gastroenterology* 2002;123(3):882–932. With permission.

recent meta-analysis of 13 studies has shown that over six months, low carbohydrate diets may produce more weight loss than conventional low-fat diets.[12] This difference is lost by 12 months in most studies. The long-term effects of a low carbohydrate diet have not been extensively studied. Although in studies up to one year, there is a favorable outcome on cardiovascular risk factors; it is unclear if this effect is long lasting. Furthermore, a recent study of participants in the National Weight Control Registry, which is a registry of people who have lost at least 30 pounds and have maintained their weight loss for at least one year, found that although more participants were on a low carbohydrate diet as of 2003 compared with 1995 (17.1% and 5.9%, respectively), success in maintaining weight loss was still associated with consumption of a low-calorie moderate fat diet.[13] Currently, the NIH recommends 30% or less total calories from fat (8 to 10% saturated fat), 15% of total calories from protein, and 55% or more calories from carbohydrates. Again, any dietary change that causes a calorie deficit will cause weight loss and regardless of the method of weight loss, patients need a long-term commitment to the dietary change in order to be successful at losing and maintaining their weight loss.

Other than macronutrient composition, the diet plan should stress other components of healthy eating. Physicians should emphasize the importance of regular meals, as skipping meals can lead to overeating later in the day. Patients should also focus on portion control. Lastly, physicians should encourage food choices that are low calorie, but nutrient dense.

19.3.3 Exercise

Exercise is not a critical component of weight loss. Exercise performed by itself and not in conjunction with calorie reduction typically does not produce clinically significant weight loss;[14] however, exercise has many other beneficial metabolic effects. Exercise performed in conjunction with reducing weight has been shown to decrease loss of lean tissue seen during weight loss in both adults and elderly adults.[14–17] Exercise can also decrease baseline serum free fatty acids[18,19] and improve skeletal muscle insulin sensitivity to glucose metabolism.[20,21]

Although exercise is not crucial for weight loss, it is likely a key component of weight maintenance. The exercise required for weight maintenance is substantial, though, as one study found that 80 minutes/day of moderate activity (e.g., brisk walk) or 35 minutes of vigorous activity (e.g., running) was needed.[22] Another study found that an energy expenditure of 2,500 kcal/week (approximately 25 miles of walking) was associated with better weight maintenance than lower levels of energy expenditure.[23] Furthermore, 94% of the participants in the National Weight Control Registry regularly exercise, with an average of 2,700kcal/week in energy expenditure (approximately 27 miles walking).[13] In this population, decreases in physical activity have been associated with weight regain.

The current recommendations by the U.S. Department of Agriculture (USDA) for exercise are based on an individual's goals. To reduce the risk of chronic diseases in adulthood, the USDA recommends 30 minutes of moderate intensity (e.g., brisk walking) per day on most days of the week. To manage weight into adulthood, the USDA recommends 60 minutes of moderate to vigorous intensity exercise per day on most days of the week. To prevent weight regain in persons who have lost weight, the USDA recommends 60 to 90 minutes of moderate intensity exercise per day on most days of the week.

19.3.4 BEHAVIOR MODIFICATION

Behavior modification in the treatment of obesity is the process of identifying and then modifying lifestyle habits that contribute to a person's obesity. Behavior modification has three general principles: (1) it is goal oriented, (2) it is process oriented, and (3) it advocates small rather than large changes. Goals should be well defined and easy to quantify, e.g., performing moderate intensity exercise for 30 minutes 5 days a week. Process oriented means that the goals that are set are reasonable for patients to achieve, and it stresses prior planning to ensure that these goals are met. Small changes are recommended over large changes because making small stepwise changes are typically easier to maintain than large changes.

The components of behavior modification that support the general principles include: self-monitoring (recording food intake, physical activities, and behaviors daily), stimulus control (identifying triggers for eating and avoiding them), social support (recruiting friends and family to help achieve weight loss goals), cognitive restructuring (thinking positively about self and weight loss), problem solving (identifying barriers to success and finding ways to deal with them), and relapse prevention (managing episodes of overeating or weight regain).[24] Self-monitoring is one of the key components of behavior modification and should be stressed to patients.[25,26] A variety of tools are available to aid patients in self-monitoring. For example, the USDA's Web site (www.mypyramid.gov) contains a Web-based dietary plan as well as a dietary and physical activity tracker.

Although behavior modification has been shown to have an average of 9% weight loss,[25] group behavior modification therapy may be difficult to find, and, moreover, in many cases is too expensive for patients. Commercial weight loss centers also can be an option, but these may be too expensive as well for many patients. However, there are some simple steps that a physician can do in the office to promote behavior modification. First, identify a small change that the patient can make (e.g., switching from regular soda to diet soda). Second, make a plan for how that change will be carried out. Next, have the patient keep a record of that behavior change. At the next office visit, review the patient's record. Congratulate successes, but avoid criticism. Instead, if patients do not meet their goals, identify barriers to meeting their goals and discuss ways to deal with those barriers.

19.4 PHARMACOTHERAPY

Weight loss medications can enhance weight loss; however, they should only be used in conjunction with therapeutic lifestyle changes. It should be stressed to the patient that these medications are not a replacement for therapeutic lifestyle changes. In addition, weight loss medications should be considered a long-term medication, if not life-long. Patients will regain weight if the medications are stopped and should be counseled about this prior to starting the medications. Conversely, if the medication has not caused weight loss within one to two months, it will likely not cause further weight loss and should be stopped. Indications for use of weight loss medications include:

- BMI >30 kg/m^2 or BMI >27 kg/m^2 with concomitant obesity-related risk factors or diseases
- Unable to achieve weight loss goal despite therapeutic lifestyle changes
- No contraindications to use

There are multiple weight loss medications that are currently approved for use in the United States; however, only sibutramine and orlistat are approved for long-term use. Because these medications need to be used long-term, only the drugs that are approved for long-term use will be discussed further.

19.4.1 Sibutramine

Sibutramine is a central reuptake inhibitor of norepinephrine and serotonin thought to act by suppressing appetite. Meta-analyses of long-term randomized control trials have shown that subjects taking sibutramine lose ~4.5% more weight than control subjects.[27,28] Furthermore, sibutramine has been shown to be effective in diabetic subjects[29] and intermittent use of the medication is as efficacious as continuous use at one year.[30] Again, all of these studies included therapeutic lifestyle changes in both the control and drug arms of the study. Sibutramine has been shown to be less effective without these lifestyle changes.[31]

Sibutramine can increase heart rate and blood pressure, and carries a risk of serotonin syndrome when combined with MAOIs (monoamine oxidase inhibitors), triptans, and opioids. Contraindications to its use include poorly controlled hypertension, coronary artery disease, angina, arrhythmias, congestive heart failure, stroke, transient ischemic attacks, seizure disorder, severe liver or kidney disease, and concomitant use of MAOIs. The most common side effects are dry mouth, headache, constipation, and insomnia. Most insurance carriers do not cover sibutramine, and the cost for a month's supply varies from $100 to $140.

19.4.2 ORLISTAT

Orlistat binds to intestinal lipases and prevents the digestion and absorption of fat in the intestine. Patients taking orlistat are instructed to consume 30% or less of their daily calories as fat. Under this condition, prescription strength orlistat will block roughly 30% of ingested fat from being digested and absorbed, although the actual percentage may vary from person to person.[32] Meta-analyses of long-term orlistat use demonstrate approximately 3% more weight loss at one year than with therapeutic lifestyle changes alone,[33,34] and twice as many subjects lost >5% and >10% of their total body weight on orlistat compared with placebo.

The most common side effects of orlistat include: abdominal pain, fatty/oily stool, increased defecation, liquid stools, fecal urgency, flatulence, flatus with discharge, fecal incontinence, and oily evacuation. Most side effects do improve over time while still on the medication.[35] Approximately 5% of patients taking orlistat will develop deficiencies in fat soluble vitamins; therefore, a multivitamin should be prescribed with orlistat and taken separately.[35] Orlistat also may interfere with the absorption of lipophilic medications. Orlistat should not be given simultaneously with these medications and serum drug levels of the lipophilic drug should be monitored frequently. Prescription orlistat costs $250 to $300 for a one-month supply. A nonprescription form is also available, which is essentially half of the prescription dose. The nonprescription form costs approximately $60 for a one-month supply, but is not as effective as the prescription dose.

19.5 BARIATRIC SURGERY

Bariatric surgery can be an effective method of weight loss for some obese patients. These surgeries do come with risk; however, the weight loss achieved with bariatric surgery improves diseases that are associated with obesity and, in some cases, completely reverses them.[36] Moreover, data from long-term studies have shown that, although some weight regain does occur, significant weight loss is maintained and obesity-related disease mortality is decreased after bariatric surgery.[37,38]

Bariatric surgery also should be performed only as an adjunct to therapeutic lifestyle changes. Indications for surgery include:

- BMI > 40 kg/m^2 or BMI 35 to 40 kg/m^2 with life-threatening cardiopulmonary disease, severe diabetes, or lifestyle impairment.
- Failure to achieve weight loss with other treatment modalities.

Contraindications to bariatric surgery include a history of medical noncompliance, psychiatric illness, and high risk of death during the procedure. Success of the surgery requires involvement of a team of medical, surgical, psychiatric, and nutrition experts. The most common current techniques include laparoscopic adjustable gastric banding and roux-en-y gastric bypass and will be discussed further below; less common techniques include biliopancreatic diversion and biliopancreatic diversion with duodenal switch. Patients should be aware of multiple complications, risks associated with the procedure, and that complication rates are lower at centers with more experience.[39]

19.5.1 Roux-en-Y Gastric Bypass (RYGB)

RYGB was first reported in 1967 by Mason and Ito. It is the most commonly performed bariatric surgery.[40] The procedure is both restrictive and malabsorptive, and it may have effects on the neuroendocrine system regulating appetite and satiety.[41] First, a small (10 to 30 ml) pouch is made out of the stomach either by stapling across or complete transection. Then, the small intestine is divided 30 to 60 cm distal to the ligament of Treitz. The segment of bowel proximal to the division is the biliopancreatic limb, and the portion distal to the division is the roux limb. The roux limb is anastomosed to the gastric pouch. The biliopancreatic limb is anastomosed 75 cm from the gastrojejunostomy in a standard RYGB procedure. For the super obese patient, the distance between the gastrojejunostomy and the jejunostomy may be as much as 150 cm.

The procedure can be done open or laparoscopically. Patients undergoing RYGB, regardless of open or laparoscopic technique, typically loose ~60% of their excess body weight.[36,42] The complications of open RYGB include: hemorrhage, wound infection, arrhythmias, pulmonary emboli, hernias, staple line disruption, dumping syndrome, anastomotic strictures, and anastomotic leaks. These can occur in 5 to 10% of patients.[43] The laparoscopic approach does have several advantages including less wound complications, less blood loss, faster recovery, but also may be associated with increased risk of anastomotic strictures. Patients will need nutritional counseling before and after the procedure with nutrient supplementation starting at the time of surgery with regular follow-up as nutritional deficiencies are common in RYGB patients.

19.5.2 Laparoscopic Adjustable Gastric Banding (LAGB)

The LAGB procedure involves the surgical placement of a silicone band around the upper stomach, just distal to the gastroesophageal junction. The band is connected to a port that is implanted subcutaneously. The port can be accessed to infuse or withdraw saline to adjust the circumference of the band.

Weight loss for LAGB is ~50% of excess weight at two years on average.[36,42] With additional adjustments of the band after the initial weight loss, additional weight loss may be achieved and in some cases may reach levels similar to RYGB. However, the efficacies of these two treatments have never been studied in a randomized trial. The risks of the procedure are less than those of RYGB and include: local infection, erosion of the band into the mucosa, band prolapse, and esophageal dilatation. The 30-day mortality rate is 0.1% in the hands of experienced surgeons.[36,42]

19.6 CONCLUSIONS

Obesity treatment is important for the health of our obese patients. Weight loss and weight maintenance are challenging, but even a 5% reduction in weight is associated with significant health improvements. It is important for the clinician to emphasize therapeutic lifestyle changes when discussing weight loss. Moreover, clinicians should be open to using adjunctive treatments, such as pharmacotherapy or bariatric surgery to enhance weight loss and weight maintenance in their patients.

REFERENCES

1. Ogden CC, McDowell M, and Flegal, K. Obesity among adults in the United States— No statistically significant change since 2003–2004. U.S. Department of Health and Human Services, Centers for Disease Control and Prevention, National Center for Health Statistics, Washington, D.C., 2007.

2. Calle EE, Thun MJ, Petrelli JM, Rodriguez C, Heath CW, Jr. Body-mass index and mortality in a prospective cohort of U.S. adults. *N Engl J Med* 1999;341(15):1097–105.

3. Goldstein DJ. Beneficial health effects of modest weight loss. *Int J Obes Relat Metab Disord* 1992;16(6):397–415.

4. Troiano RP, Frongillo EA, Jr., Sobal J, Levitsky DA. The relationship between body weight and mortality: a quantitative analysis of combined information from existing studies. *Int J Obes Relat Metab Disord* 1996;20(1):63–75.

5. Manson JE, Willett WC, Stampfer MJ, et al. Body weight and mortality among women. *N Engl J Med* 1995;333(11):677–85.

6. Roza AM, Shizgal HM. The Harris Benedict equation reevaluated: resting energy requirements and the body cell mass. *Am J Clin Nutr* 1984;40(1):168–82.

7. Shetty P. Energy requirements of adults. *Pub Health Nutr* 2005;8(7a):994–1009.

8. Black AE, Coward WA, Cole TJ, Prentice AM. Human energy expenditure in affluent societies: an analysis of 574 doubly-labelled water measurements. *Eur J Clin Nutr* 1996;50(2):72–92.

9. Klein S, Wadden T, Sugerman HJ. AGA technical review on obesity. *Gastroenterology* 2002;123(3):882–932.

10. Gilden Tsai A, Wadden TA. The evolution of very-low-calorie diets: an update and meta-analysis [ast]. *Obesity* 2006;14(8):1283–93.

11. Yu-Poth S, Zhao G, Etherton T, Naglak M, Jonnalagadda S, Kris-Etherton PM. Effects of the National Cholesterol Education Program's Step I and Step II dietary intervention programs on cardiovascular disease risk factors: a meta-analysis. *Am J Clin Nutr* 1999;69(4):632–46.

12. Hession M, Rolland C, Kulkarni U, Wise A, Broom J. Systematic review of randomized controlled trials of low-carbohydrate vs. low-fat/low-calorie diets in the management of obesity and its comorbidities. *Obes Rev* 2009;10(1):36–50.

13. Phelan S, Wyatt HR, Hill JO, Wing RR. Are the eating and exercise habits of successful weight losers changing? [ast]. *Obesity* 2006;14(4):710–6.

14. Garrow JS, Summerbell CD. Meta-analysis: effect of exercise, with or without dieting, on the body composition of overweight subjects. *Eur J Clin Nutr* 1995;49(1):1–10.

15. Ballor DL, Poehlman ET. Exercise-training enhances fat-free mass preservation during diet-induced weight loss: a meta-analytical finding. *Int J Obes Relat Metab Disord* 1994;18(1):35–40.

16. Frimel TN, Sinacore DR, Villareal DT. Exercise attenuates the weight-loss-induced reduction in muscle mass in frail obese older adults. *Med Sci Sports Exerc* 2008;40(7):1213–9.

17. Villareal DT, Banks M, Sinacore DR, Siener C, Klein S. Effect of weight loss and exercise on frailty in obese older adults. *Arch Intern Med* 2006;166(8):860–6.

18. de Glisezinski I, Moro C, Pillard F, et al. Aerobic training improves exercise-induced lipolysis in SCAT and lipid utilization in overweight men. *Am J Physiol Endocrinol Metab* 2003;285(5):E984–90.

19. Oscai LB, Patterson JA, Bogard DL, Beck RJ, Rothermel BL. Normalization of serum triglycerides and lipoprotein electrophoretic patterns by exercise. *Am J Cardiol* 1972;30(7):775–80.

20. Dengel DR, Pratley RE, Hagberg JM, Rogus EM, Goldberg AP. Distinct effects of aerobic exercise training and weight loss on glucose homeostasis in obese sedentary men. *J Appl Physiol* 1996;81(1):318–25.
21. Houmard JA, Tanner CJ, Slentz CA, Duscha BD, McCartney JS, Kraus WE. Effect of the volume and intensity of exercise training on insulin sensitivity. *J Appl Physiol* 2004;96(1):101–6.
22. Schoeller DA, Shay K, Kushner RF. How much physical activity is needed to minimize weight gain in previously obese women? *Am J Clin Nutr* 1997;66(3):551–6.
23. Jeffery RW, Wing RR, Sherwood NE, Tate DF. Physical activity and weight loss: does prescribing higher physical activity goals improve outcome? *Am J Clin Nutr* 2003;78(4):684–9.
24. Brownell KD, Wadden TA, LEARN Education Center. The LEARN program for weight control: lifestyle, exercise, attitudes, relationships, nutrition. Special medication ed. Dallas: American Health Pub. Co.: LEARN Education Center [distributor], 1998.
25. Wadden TA, Sarwer DB, Berkowitz RI. Behavioural treatment of the overweight patient. *Baillieres Best Pract Res Clin Endocrinol Metab* 1999;13(1):93–107.
26. Hollis JF, Gullion CM, Stevens VJ, et al. Weight loss during the intensive intervention phase of the weight-loss maintenance trial. *Am J Prevent Med* 2008;35(2):118–26.
27. Apfelbaum M, Vague P, Ziegler O, Hanotin C, Thomas F, Leutenegger E. Long-term maintenance of weight loss after a very-low-calorie diet: a randomized blinded trial of the efficacy and tolerability of sibutramine. *Am J Med* 1999;106(2):179–84.
28. Bray GA, Blackburn GL, Ferguson JM, et al. Sibutramine produces dose-related weight loss. *Obes Res* 1999;7(2):189–98.
29. Kaukua JK, Pekkarinen TA, Rissanen AM. Health-related quality of life in a randomised placebo-controlled trial of sibutramine in obese patients with type II diabetes. *Int J Obes Relat Metab Disord* 2004;28(4):600–5.
30. Wirth A, Krause J. Long-term weight loss with sibutramine: a randomized controlled trial. *JAMA* 2001;286(11):1331–9.
31. Wadden TA, Berkowitz RI, Womble LG, et al. Randomized trial of lifestyle modification and pharmacotherapy for obesity. *N Engl J Med* 2005;353(20):2111–20.
32. Zhi J, Melia AT, Guerciolini R, et al. Retrospective population-based analysis of the dose-response (fecal fat excretion) relationship of orlistat in normal and obese volunteers. *Clin Pharmacol Ther* 1994;56(1):82–5.
33. Li Z, Maglione M, Tu W, et al. Meta-analysis: pharmacologic treatment of obesity. *Ann Intern Med* 2005;142(7):532–46.
34. Padwal R, Li SK, Lau DCW. Long-term pharmacotherapy for overweight and obesity: a systematic review and meta-analysis of randomized controlled trials. *Int J Obes Relat Metab Disord* 2003;27(12):1437–46.
35. Davidson MH, Hauptman J, DiGirolamo M, et al. Weight control and risk factor reduction in obese subjects treated for 2 years with orlistat: a randomized controlled trial. *JAMA* 1999;281(3):235–42.
36. Buchwald H, Avidor Y, Braunwald E, et al. Bariatric surgery: a systematic review and meta-analysis. *JAMA* 2004;292(14):1724–37.
37. Adams TD, Gress RE, Smith SC, et al. Long-term mortality after gastric bypass surgery. *N Engl J Med* 2007;357(8):753–61.
38. Sjostrom L, Narbro K, Sjostrom CD, et al. Effects of bariatric surgery on mortality in Swedish obese subjects. *N Engl J Med* 2007;357(8):741–52.
39. Flum DR, Dellinger EP. Impact of gastric bypass operation on survival: a population-based analysis. *J Am Coll Surg* 2004;199(4):543–51.
40. Buchwald H, Williams SE. Bariatric surgery worldwide 2003. *Obes Surg* 2004;14(9):1157–64.

41. Cummings DE, Weigle DS, Frayo RS, et al. Plasma ghrelin levels after diet-induced weight loss or gastric bypass surgery. *N Engl J Med* 2002;346(21):1623–30.
42. Maggard MA, Shugarman LR, Suttorp M, et al. Meta-analysis: surgical treatment of obesity. *Ann Intern Med* 2005;142(7):547–59.
43. Pories WJ. Bariatric surgery: risks and rewards. *J Clin Endocrinol Metab* 2008;93(11_Supplement_1):s89–96.

20 Bariatric Surgery

Alessandrina Freitas and John F. Sweeney

CONTENTS

20.1 INTRODUCTION

Over the past 30 years, there has been a virtual explosion in the epidemic of obesity here in the United States. There are several causes for this dramatic increase of obesity: labor-saving devices, the decrease in physical activity, the increase in sedentary occupations and lifestyles, and the ready availability of high caloric food. This is problematic because obesity is associated with an increase in chronic debilitative diseases like diabetes, hypertension, hyperlipidemia, amongst others. The increase in these diseases is driving up healthcare costs dramatically. This chapter will review the history of bariatric surgery, indications for bariatric surgery, surgical procedures currently available, identification and management of postoperative complications, and the short- and long-term outcomes for the various operations discussed.

20.2 HISTORY OF BARIATRIC SURGERY

The birth of bariatric surgery can be traced to the 1950s at the University of Minnesota. Researchers there were evaluating the nutritional importance of the proximal and distal small intestine in a series of animal experiments. They discovered that bypassing most of the intestines while keeping the stomach intact induced a state of malabsorption that was associated with significant weight loss in a canine model. This so-called jejunoileal (JI) bypass was applied shortly thereafter and was initially deemed a huge success; patients could eat whatever they wanted and still lose weight. Unfortunately, too many patients developed complications, such as diarrhea, night blindness (from vitamin A deficiency), osteoporosis (from vitamin D deficiency), protein-calorie malnutrition, and kidney stones. The more worrisome complications included progressive hepatic fibrosis, cirrhosis, and eventual liver failure in a significant number of patients. These latter complications were felt to be secondary to toxic overgrowth of bacteria in the bypassed intestine. Because of these problems, the JI bypass is no longer a recommended surgical procedure for weight loss. An important lesson learned from this experience was that long-term follow-up by an experienced bariatric surgeon is required for all patients who undergo a bariatric procedure for weight loss.

20.3 INDICATIONS FOR SURGERY

Appropriate patient selection is essential for successful outcomes of bariatric surgery. Prior to consideration for a weight reduction procedure, the patient should have documented attempts at weight loss by nonoperative means. The National Institute of Health (NIH) guidelines for consideration for bariatric surgery are a body mass index (BMI) >40 or >35 with significant medical comorbidities attributed to obesity.

These comorbidites include, but are not limited to, hypertension, diabetes, hyperlipidemia, osteoarthritis, obstructive sleep apnea, and gastroesophageal reflux disease. Once these rather straightforward guidelines have been met, a more detailed evaluation of the patient is undertaken to ensure that the patient will be able to comply with the resultant lifestyle alterations. Psychiatric stability and the cognitive ability to generally understand the procedure and it's expected outcomes is paramount. The patient must be motivated and willing to participate in long-term follow-up. Finally, existing medical comorbidities must be evaluated to ensure that the patient can physically withstand the proposed operation and could be reasonably expected to benefit from long-term weight reduction.

Specific contraindications to bariatric surgery are few as long as the previous discussed criteria are met. Patients who cannot provide informed consent due to debilitating psychiatric disease or cognitive impairment and those who have an unacceptably high perioperative mortality risk should be excluded. Endocrine disorders that are associated with weight gain (e.g., hypothyroidism, Cushing's Syndrome) must be under control before surgery is considered.

Bariatric surgery is usually considered for patients in the 18- to 60-year-old range. Weight reduction surgery can be performed in patients older than 60 years of age as long as the patients have a satisfactory performance status. Weight reduction surgery in the adolescent population is becoming more common, despite some residual controversy as to its appropriate application and still limited, long-term outcome data. It is clear that adolescents who have undergone bariatric procedures achieve weight loss and resolution of comorbidities at a rate equal to, and perhaps superior than, adult populations. The earlier intervention in comorbid conditions before they have time to develop irreversible sequelae has been cited on numerous occasions as rationale for adolescent weight reduction surgery. Currently, procedures that have been applied to the adolescent population are the adjustable gastric band, Roux-en-Y gastric bypass, and sleeve gastrectomy. Until further information regarding outcomes is available, bariatric surgery in adolescents should only be performed as part of an institutional review board (IRB)-approved protocol.

20.4 SURGICAL PROCEDURES

Surgery is the only proven method to achieve long-term weight reduction in the morbidly obese. The evolving field of bariatric surgery is now comprised of operations that are based on restriction, malabsorption, or a combination of these two methods. Although all of these procedures are commonly performed through a laparoscopic approach, there are some patients that, due to extreme obesity, multiple previous abdominal surgeries, or comorbid physiology that makes CO_2 insufflation dangerous, in whom open surgery may be a more suitable option. Only the laparoscopic approach to these operations will be discussed here.

20.4.1 Restrictive Procedures

The concept of restrictive weight loss surgery is simple: reduce the amount of oral intake by limiting the gastric volume. Retention of food in the limited upper gastric pouch (vertical banded gastroplasty, adjustable gastric banding) and limited total reservoir size and increased intraluminal pressure (sleeve gastrectomy) produce early satiety. Purely restrictive procedures have the advantage of leaving the alimentary tract in continuity minimizing the risks of metabolic complications.

20.4.1.1   Vertical Banded Gastroplasty (VBG)

Thirty years ago, VBG was the most commonly performed weight loss surgery. Historically, patients undergoing a VBG had excellent early weight loss, but demonstrated a tendency to regain weight over the long term. Over the years, it has fallen out of favor due to the increased effectiveness of gastric bypass and the increased ease of adjustable gastric banding.

VBG can be done as an open, laparoscopic, or hand assisted procedure. An area 5 to 9 cm below the gastroesophageal junction is identified and the circular stapler is used to create a circular defect through the anterior and posterior gastric walls. The second stapler application is a linear staple line directed toward the angle of His (angle of entry of the esophagus into the stomach) from the superior aspect of the newly created circle. The restricting pouch is completed by the placement of a band to create a controlled outflow stoma.

20.4.1.2   Adjustable Gastric Banding

Currently there are two U.S. Food and Drug Administration (FDA)-approved adjustable gastric banding devices in the United States. It is the safest bariatric procedure performed today, with a 0.05% mortality.[1] The primary advantage of the adjustable gastric banding is the availability to modify stoma size over time in order to provide early satiety with minimal symptoms, such as vomiting or dysphagia. The addition or removal of saline is generally titrated to a weight loss of 1 or 2 lbs per week. Disadvantages include the ability to circumvent weight loss by ingestion of high calorie liquids and the need for frequent follow-up in the first two years for band adjustments. Conversion rate to an open procedure is roughly 1%.[1]

There are three basic steps for placement of an adjustable gastric band. These include dissection of the proximal stomach with creation of a retrogastric tunnel, band placement and fixation, and subcutaneous access port placement. Dissection of the proximal stomach is now commonly done via the pars flaccida technique to create a retrogastric tunnel. This results in a lower rate of gastric prolapse and gastric pouch dilation when compared to the older perigastric technique.[2,3]

Port placement varies based on surgeon preference, but generally follows a similar configuration. A 5 mm optical access trocar is placed at the left anterioaxillary line just off the costal margin.

Following CO_2 insufflation, a 15-mm port is placed in the left midclavicular line 15 cm inferior to the xiphoid process. A 12-mm port is placed in the right midclavicular line 15 cm below the xiphoid. A final 5-mm port is placed in the right anterior axillary line at the costal margin. The liver is elevated, allowing better visualization of the gastroesophageal junction. The band is inserted into the abdomen via the 15-mm port, where it is ready for later use. The gastric fundus is then caudally retracted and attachments between the fundus and diaphragm are divided (Figure 20.1). This allows for visualization of the angle of His, essential for the later passing

FIGURE 20.1 (See color insert following Page 112) Dissection of angle of His. (From Jones DB. *Atlas of Minimally Invasive Surgery.* Cine-Med Inc, 2006. With permission.)

of the band. Excision of perigastric fat pads, especially those around the gastroesophageal junction, is performed. The pars flaccida technique to create a retrogastric tunnel is carried out and the grasper is visualized at the previously dissected angle of His (Figure 20.2). The band is brought through this tunnel to encircle the upper stomach and is locked in place (Figure 20.3). A 5-mm instrument should be able to be passed between the stomach and band. The band is secured in placed with a tension-free anterior fundoplication, using permanent suture (Figure 20.4). The final portion of the procedure is placement of the access port that allows band adjustment over time. The tubing is delivered out through the 15-mm trocar site and is attached to the access port, leaving any excess tubing to lie freely within the peritoneal cavity. All intraperitoneal instruments can be removed and insufflation ceased.

FIGURE 20.2 (See color insert following Page 112) Pars flaccida approach for creation of retrogastric tunnel. (From Jones DB. *Atlas of Minimally Invasive Surgery.* Cine-Med Inc, 2006. With permission.)

FIGURE 20.3 (See color insert following Page 112) Lap band placement. (From Jones DB. *Atlas of Minimally Invasive Surgery.* Cine-Med Inc, 2006. With permission.)

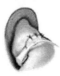

FIGURE 20.4 (See color insert following Page 112) Completed anterior fundoplication to prevent gastric prolapse. (From Jones DB. *Atlas of Minimally Invasive Surgery.* Cine-Med Inc, 2006. With permission.)

The access port is secured at four corners with permanent suture to the anterior rectus sheath. The band is left empty initially and all incisions are closed in the usual fashion.

An over-penetrated abdominal x-ray should be obtained in the recovery room to document band orientation. Contrast esophagraphy should be performed post-operatively if there is any question about pouch anatomy, or if there is concern for obstruction or perforation. Band adjustments are made in the office every six to eight weeks.

20.4.1.4   Vertical (Sleeve) Gastrectomy

Sleeve gastrectomy (Figure 20.5) initially was proposed as the first step of a two-stage surgery for the super obese patient. Following sleeve gastrectomy and weight loss, the patient would then undergo a bypass procedure. However, the sleeve gastrectomy is now being used as a stand alone operation for weight reduction. This restrictive procedure resects approximately 80 to 90% of the stomach, leaving behind only a narrow tube to function as an alimentary conduit. There is some concern over the lack of long-term postoperative data and some ambiguity on the most efficacious surgical technique. However, studies have demonstrated good results without any serious complications.[4]

There are several key steps to performing the sleeve gastrectomy, whether approached open or laparoscopically. Starting 3 to 6 cm from the pylorus and proceeding to the angle of His, a linear stapler is used to transect the vascular supply of the greater curvature. A Harmonic scalpel is applied to divide the gastroepiploic vessels and the short gastric vessels are individually ligated. A 32 to 48 French bougie is placed via the esophagus along the lesser gastric curvature. This allows a continuous, consistent guide for the sleeve caliber. As would be expected, use of a

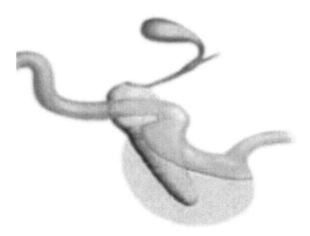

FIGURE 20.5 (See color insert following Page 112)   Completed appearance of a sleeve gastrectomy. (Tucker ON. Indications for sleeve gastrectomy. *J Gastrointest. Surg.* Springer. 4:664, 2008. With permission.)

larger caliber bougie results in a lower incidence of stricture.[5] Several firings of a linear stapler cutter are applied to transect the antrum, corpus, and fundus. The entire staple line is then inverted with a continuous seroserosal suture. The bougie is then removed and the gastric sleeve is examined endoscopically for any areas of stricture or leak. A gastrograffin swallow is performed on the first postoperative day to rule out any leaks or strictures and, if negative, the patient is begun on a clear liquid diet per protocol.

20.4.2 Malabsorptive Procedures

Modern malabsorptive procedures share a common design of an enteric limb in continuity with the stomach and a chemical limb carrying bile and pancreatic secretions. These limbs join together to form the common channel in which nutrients can be absorbed. The major improvement over early malabsorptive surgeries is the avoidance of bacterial proliferation in a portion of bowel without flow.

The degree of malabsorption is proportional to the length of bypass. All of these procedures bypass at least a portion of the stomach, duodenum, and early jejunum.

20.4.2.1 Biliopancreatic Diversion +/– Duodenal Switch

Biliopancreatic diversion is the most technically challenging bariatric procedure performed today. It results in a high percentage of weight loss, but also carries the most significant morbidity and mortality of any of the weight loss surgeries. Thirty day mortality following biliopancreatic diversion or duodenal switch is 1.1%.[6]

20.4.3 Restrictive/Malabsorptive Combinations

20.4.3.1 Roux-en-Y Gastric Bypass

The RYGB accounts for up to 80% of bariatric procedures performed in the United States today. Thirty day operative mortality is 0.5%.[6,7] The restrictive portion of the procedure is the creation of a 15 to 30 ml gastric pouch. Malabsorption is employed via a variable-length Roux limb that is anastomosed to the gastric pouch.

The operation begins by identifying the ligament of Treitz. The proximal jejunum is divided approximately 40 cm distal to the ligament of Treitz with a linear stapling device. A Roux limb is created by measuring approximately 75 to 150 cm from the tip of the divided distal small bowel. There is no evidence supporting a specific Roux limb length as long as it is greater than 75 cm in length. A side-to-side jejunojejunostomy is established at this point between the proximal biliopancreatic limb and the Roux limb to reestablish gastrointestinal (GI) continuity. With this accomplished, a 15 to 30 ml gastric pouch is created by dividing the stomach with an endoscopic stapling device. A gastrojejunostomy is then fashioned between the gastric pouch and the tip of the Roux limb. This can be accomplished using a circular stapler, a linear stapler, or by hand sewing the anastomosis. Intraoperative endoscopy is undertaken to evaluate the anastomosis, check for bleeding, and perform an intraoperative leak test (Figure 20.6).

FIGURE 20.6 (See color insert following Page 112)   Completed appearance of a Roux-en-Y gastric bypass. (From Jones DB. *Atlas of Minimally Invasive Surgery*. Cine-Med Inc, 2006. With permission.)

20.5   COMPLICATIONS: IDENTIFICATION AND MANAGEMENT

Regardless of the weight reduction surgery performed, the obese patient is at an increased risk for multiple perioperative complications. Some complications are universal in the bariatric population while others are specific to the type of procedure performed.

20.5.1   COMPLICATIONS COMMON TO ALL BARIATRIC PROCEDURES

20.5.1.1   Deep Venous Thrombosis/Pulmonary Embolism

Prevention of deep venous thrombosis (DVT) begins prior to anesthesia induction, with the application of sequential compression devices. Pharmacologic prophylaxis with heparin or low molecular weight heparin should be employed in all bariatric surgery patients. There is little evidence supporting the preferential use of one of these drugs or the duration of prophylaxis in the bariatric population. In the case of a known hypercoagulable disorder or history of previous DVT or thrombophlebitis, a preoperatively placed inferior vena cava filter should be considered. Some have also advocated preoperative evaluation of mean pulmonary artery pressure in those patients at very high risk and IVC filter placement if the pressure is found to be ≥40.[8]

The incidence of DVT following bariatric surgery is 2%. Body habitus preventing early ambulation, prevalence of venous stasis disease, and relative polycythemia from chronic hypoventilation all contribute to this number. The diagnosis of DVT in the obese patient can be challenging. The classic sign of unilateral swollen limb may be difficult to recognize. Therefore, a high clinical suspicion must be kept and the use of duplex venous ultrasound applied if there is any suspicion.

Pulmonary embolism (PE) can be suddenly fatal. Cardinal symptoms of tachycardia, pleuritic chest pain, respiratory distress, and desaturation not appropriately responsive to oxygen therapy should immediately raise suspicion for PE. Diagnosis can be made by computerized tomography (CT) scan or lung/ventilation (V/Q) scan.

20.5.1.2   Bleeding

Hemorrhage can present early in the postoperative course or be delayed (after 48 hours). An early postoperative bleed presents with hematemesis, bloody bowel movements, and, if severe, hypotension, tachycardia, and a precipitous fall in hematocrit. Bleeding more than 48 hours postoperative present with dark blood in the stool and may represent clot evacuation from the operative sites. Bleeding usually occurs from staple lines and may be intraluminal or intraabdominal. Estimates of hemorrhage following laparoscopic RYGB are 1.1 to 4%.[9]

Techniques to decrease the risk of postoperative hemorrhage are well known. These include the usual careful attention to hemostasis intraoperatively, over sewing of staple lines, and the use of staple line reinforcing products. Additionally, use of shorter staple height may result in better hemostasis by an increased compression of tissues.[9]

Like all surgically significant bleeding, the first priority of management is IV fluid resuscitation and transfusion of blood products as needed. Reoperation to localize and contain the source of bleeding may be necessary if the patient becomes unstable or the bleeding is brisk and ongoing. GI bleeding that presents late is less likely to require operative management.

20.5.1.3 Anastomotic Leak

Due to the greater number of involved staple lines, anastomotic leak is more common after malabsorptive surgery. However, this complication can be seen following restrictive procedures involving resection of gastric segments. Anastomotic leaks occur in 2 to 4% of surgeries involving a staple line or anastomosis.[10] Leak rates after RYGB are 1 to 5%[5] and most often involve the gastrojejunostomy or gastric transection site. Older age, male gender, diabetes, and sleep apnea have been cited as independent risk factors for anastomotic leak. Conversion from a previous restrictive procedure to a RYGB holds a greater risk for leak than primary RYGB.[7]

Anastomotic leaks can occur early or late in the postoperative course. Leaks within the first 48 hours are more likely to be related to technical problems at the anastomosis site and are more likely to warrant emergent reexploration. Leaks occurring 5 to 10 days postoperatively result from poor healing of the anastomosis or ischemia. These late leaks have a more indolent presentation.

Tachycardia is the first sign of an anastomotic leak. Other signs and symptoms include fever, tachypnea, hypoxia, hiccups, and anxiety.[8,10] By the time a patient complains of increased abdominal or back pain, he or she may be systemically ill. If a leak goes unrecognized, progression to overt peritonitis, sepsis, and death may be rapid. A gastrograffin upper GI study should be routinely performed prior to initiating clear liquids and repeated if there is concern for a leak and the patient's condition allows.

Reoperation may be necessary to repair a failed anastomotic site, especially if the leak is large and/or the patient's condition deteriorates. If the leak is small and the patient is clinically stable, percutaneously placed drains, restriction of PO intake with parenteral nutritional support as needed, and antibiotics may be sufficient intervention.

20.5.1.4 Wound Infection

Wound infections are one of the most common postoperative complications seen in the bariatric population. Prophylactic antibiotics strictly administered prior to incision is the best preventive measure. One of the major benefits of the laparoscopic approach to these procedures is the much lower rates of wound infection using the laparoscopic approached as opposed to open surgery.

Several factors contribute to the relatively high rate of wound infections following bariatric surgery. Morbidly obese body habitus and the often coexisting diabetes, complicate normal wound healing. Additionally, the diminished immune defense capacity associated with morbid obesity is well documented.[11–13]

Cellulitis without underlying infection may require only antibiotics. However, the thick layer of poorly vascularized subcutaneous fat disrupted during the surgery provides the ideal environment for liquefaction and subsequent infected fluid collections. Treatment of these infections is antibiotics, reopening and drainage of the wound, and allowing the open wound to heal by secondary intention.

20.5.1.5 Failure to Lose Weight or Regaining of Weight

Regardless of procedure performed, 15% of patients do not achieve the goal of 50% of excess body weight lost after bariatric surgery.[14] Reasons include diet noncompliance, such as the intake of high calorie liquids or forced overeating after restrictive procedures and intestinal adaptation following malabsorptive surgery. Physical disruption of the staple line in a nontransected RYGB results in an unrestricted gastric volume and decreased weight loss. Nutritional counseling, before and after surgery, is helpful in reducing the patient choice factors that contribute to weight loss failure.

20.5.2 COMPLICATIONS OF RESTRICTIVE PROCEDURES

20.5.2.1 Gastric Prolapse

Gastric prolapse ("band slipping") is herniation of the stomach cephalad through the band, which enlarges the pouch and causes band malposition. The incidence of herniation after adjustable gastric banding is now 1 to 2%,[1,3] a great reduction since adoption of the pars flaccida technique. In comparison with the older perigastric technique, the pars flaccida technique provides better posterior fixation of the band. Anterior fundoplication secures the anterior aspect of the band. Leaving the band empty initially decreases postoperative vomiting and also decreases herniation.

20.5.2.2 Pouch Dilation

In patients who have had restrictive procedures, forced eating of a greater volume than can be accommodated by the gastric reservoir can result in discomfort, vomiting, and nutritional deficiency.

Over time, the ingestion of a larger volume than can be comfortably accommodated may lead to pouch dilation and resultant decreased weight loss. Gastric pouch dilation also may result from outflow obstruction by the band. Patients complain of dysphagia and gastroesophageal reflux. Simply removing some of the fluid via the port can resolve this complication.[1,14]

20.5.2.3 Band Erosion

This is a rare complication (0 to 7%).[1,14] When it does occur, it is usually a slow process and may be asymptomatic. A loss of restrictive function and recurrent port site infections should prompt investigation of band erosion. Faults in surgical technique, such as gastric microperforation or fundoplication over the buckling device contribute to its occurrence.[9] Band erosion can be evaluated by esophagogastroduodenoscopy (EGD).

20.5.2.4 Port/Tube Dysfunction

Mechanical disruptions of the port and tubing system of adjustable gastric bands, such as tube kinking/disconnection or port malfunction, render the band ineffective and prevent it from being adjusted. Therefore, these problems necessitate operative correction in order to maintain weight loss.

Tube kinking can be avoided by leaving the tubing long and freely floating within the peritoneal cavity and by port placement a distance away from the fascial defect to allow for a gradual curve in the tubing.

Port site infections are very rare and should immediately raise concern for band erosion.

20.5.2.5 Need for Band Removal

Factors, such as failure to lose weight, band erosion, and patient intolerance of symptoms, may all necessitate removal of the band. Removal, which occurs in 0.6 to 6%,[1,2] can usually be accomplished laparoscopically. Depending on the patient wishes and need for additional weight loss, these patients may be converted to a malabsorptive procedure.

20.5.3 COMPLICATIONS OF MALABSORPTIVE PROCEDURES

20.5.3.1 Small Bowel Obstruction

Bowel kinking or mechanical stricture at an anastomotic site can result in perioperative bowel obstruction. Identification may be made by upper gastrointestinal studies with small bowel follow through showing an isolated narrowing or acute angle. If suspicion remains after a nondiagnostic obstructive series, a CT scan should be performed. Reoperation may be necessary in the early postoperative period to relieve the obstruction. Small bowel obstruction may also present much later in the postoperative course. In these late obstructions, the culprit is either adhesive bands or the development of an internal hernia. Even if the mesenteric spaces were meticulously closed intraoperatively, the sutures may become loosened and the spaces reemerge after significant weight loss.

A bowel obstruction in a patient following an RYGB should always prompt immediate surgical evaluation and intervention to prevent bowel strangulation.

20.5.3.2 Marginal Ulceration

Ulcer formation at the anastomotic site occurs in up to 15% of patients following RYGB.[12] Factors that contribute to ulceration are large gastric pouch with many productive parietal cells, use of nonabsorbable sutures, decreased perfusion of anastomotic sites, and nonsteroidal antiinflammatory drug (NSAID) use. Peak incidence of marginal ulceration is in the second postoperative year.[14] Symptoms include retrosternal burning, nausea and vomiting, and dyspepsia. Medical management with acid suppressive medications (proton pump inhibitors), and sulcrafate is usually successful. If resolution of symptoms is not achieved after a six-week course, upper endoscopy is done for definitive diagnosis. Biopsies for *Heliobacter pylori* should be taken during endoscopy. An upper GI contrast study is also performed to rule out gastro-gastric fistula. For severe refractory symptoms, operative revision may be necessary.

If ulceration at the gastrojejunal stoma of RYGB is not controlled, stomal stenosis resulting in intractable vomiting and severe malnutrition occurs. Stenosis at stoma sites can be treated by endoscopy and successive balloon dilatation.

20.5.3.3 Malnutrition

Many obese patients suffer from some degree of preoperative malnutrition that can be exacerbated by the operation performed. There are also several well-documented nutrition complications common in the postoperative bariatric population.

20.5.2.4 Micronutrient Deficiencies

Micronutrient deficiencies are the most common complication following malabsorptive bariatric procedures. These deficiencies are often asymptomatic and routine yearly lifetime screening is prudent.

Iron deficiency eventually occurs in up to 75% of patients who have undergone a malabsorptive procedure.[10] This results from the duodenum being bypassed and, thus, losing the site of predominant iron absorption. Women of childbearing age are especially prone to iron deficiency anemia given the increased losses of menstruation. Daily supplements of 650 mg ferrous sulfate orally is prescribed for all patients.

Likewise, the loss of vitamin D-dependent calcium absorption in the bypassed duodenum often leads to calcium deficiency. The resultant bone mineral loss and propensity toward osteoporosis rarely is severe enough to cause pathologic fracture. At this time, routine bone density examinations are not recommended. Daily calcium supplementation of 1,200 mg is recommended.

An intrinsic factor is produced by the gastric parietal cells and is essential for absorption of vitamin B_{12} in the terminal ileum. Therefore, B_{12} deficiency can be problematic for RYGB and biliopancreatic diversion patients. Symptomatic peripheral neuropathy or overt megaloblastic anemia is rare, seen in less than 5% of patients.[10]

Fat soluble vitamin (A, D, E, K) deficiencies can all result from the decreased ileal absorptive time. However, this is rarely symptomatic. Other rare micronutrient deficiencies include zinc, thiamine, folate, and selenium. Unexplained fatigue, neurologic symptoms, or persistent vomiting should prompt a thorough evaluation for micronutrient deficiency.

20.5.2.5 Protein Malnutrition

Although less commonly encountered, protein malnutrition is a debilitating complication of malabsorptive surgery. This is seen most profoundly following biliopancreatic diversion, occurring in up to 11.9% of patients.[8] Protein malnutrition is also a problem following RYGB with a very short common channel. The average time to diagnosis of protein malnutrition is 18 months postoperatively.[14] Protein malnutrition presents with fatigue, edema, recurrent vomiting, high bowel frequency and steatorrhea, hypercoagulability, immune suppression, and hypoalbuminemia. Diagnoses is confirmed by low serum albumin and depressed total iron binding capacity. Mortality associated with severe protein malnutrition has been reported up to 1%.[14] All patients should receive nutritional counseling to intake 40 to 60 g of protein per day. In patients exhibiting signs of protein malnutrition, a high nitrogen diet should immediately be started and other routes of enteral or parental feeding explored as necessary. In patients with refractory protein malnutrition, operative revision or reversal may become necessary. However, repeat surgery in a patient with an extremely depressed capacity for wound healing must be carefully considered before reoperation.

20.5.2.6 Excessive Weight Loss

Excessive weight loss to a BMI less than 20 is a very rare complication of bariatric surgery. All of these patients should undergo contrast radiography and upper endoscopy to rule out mechanical causes, such as stricture or bowel obstruction. Psychiatric evaluation also should be performed and any underlying illness aggressively treated. High protein oral supplements and even parental nutrition may be necessary in some patients. In extreme cases, revision or reversal of the surgery is unavoidable.

20.6 OUTCOMES

Weight loss following bariatric surgery is commonly reported as the mean percentage of excess weight loss by the formula: (weight loss/excess weight) × 100. Excess weight is the discrepancy between preoperative weight and ideal weight. A large meta-analysis of 134 studies found the mean weight loss across all types of bariatric surgery to be 61.2%. This percentage varies by the type of surgery performed, with gastric banding procedures resulting in 47.5%, gastric bypass resulting in 61.6%, and biliopancreatic diversion resulting in 70.1% of excess weight lost.[6] Although the observed weight loss is numerically impressive, it should be noted that most patients following bariatric surgery are still obese. Resolution of preoperative comorbidities is perhaps a more meaningful way to measure outcomes following bariatric surgery.

20.6.1 DIABETES

All types of bariatric surgery have been observed to improve type 2 diabetes. Many patients are eventually able to discontinue use of hypoglycemic agents and maintain normal blood glucose and HbA1C levels. Complete resolution of diabetes has been quoted in a meta-analysis as 76.8% across all bariatric procedures.[6] Diabetes resolution is more likely following malabsorptive or combined malabsorptive/restrictive procedures. Interestingly, improvement and even resolution of diabetes often occurs within days of surgery, long before any significant weight loss has occurred. There are numerous theories attempting to explain this observation. Current research into the effect of bariatric procedures on gastrointestinal hormones including leptin, ghrelin, resistin, enteroglucagon, and cholecystokinin are likely to provide the reasoning to this well-documented phenomenon.

20.6.2 Hypertension

Blood pressure shows a predictable decrease following weight loss, with a reduction of 1% of body weight correlating with a 1 mm Hg decrease in systolic pressure and a 2 mm Hg decrease in diastolic pressure.[6] A greater than 40% reduction in the rate of systolic and diastolic hypertension has been observed in male bariatric surgery patients.[18] Improvement in blood pressure after bariatric surgery is independent of the type of surgery performed.

20.6.3 Obstructive Sleep Apnea

Obstructive sleep apnea (OSA) is an extremely common comorbidity of obesity. Obese patients are prone to airway collapse during nocturnal respiration due to fat deposition in the parapharyngeal region. OSA leads to complaints of chronic fatigue, daytime sleepiness, and excessive snoring or gasping for breath while asleep. OSA as an independent risk factor for hypertension, cardiac arrhythmias, myocardial infarction, pulmonary hypertension, and cor pulmonale. The incidence of sleep apnea in patients who present for bariatric surgery is 45% to greater than 70%.[15-17] This number increases to more than 94% for those with a BMI >60.[15] The association is so high that some practitioners advocate routine screening for OSA and referral for preoperative polysomnography as part of a routine preoperative evaluation. Multiple studies have shown significant improvement or resolution of OSA following bariatric surgery.[16,17]

20.6.4 Hyperlipidemia

Cholesterol is improved by weight loss after bariatric surgery. Improvements in low density lipoproteins (LDLs), high density lipoproteins (HDLs), and triglycerides have all been observed postoperatively.[18]

20.6.5 Osteoarthritis

Obese patients who present for bariatric surgery almost uniformly have some degree of musculoskeletal complaints. Excellent pain improvement has been observed after bariatric surgery, including one study that reported an 89% complete resolution of osteoarthritis pain in at least one joint.[19] The greatest decrease in musculoskeletal complaints is in the cervical and lumbar spine and in the feet.[20]

20.7 SUMMARY

Obesity is a major health problem in the United States and throughout much of the industrialized world. Nonsurgical treatments for obesity thus far have been unsuccessful in providing long-term weight loss. Bariatric surgery is the only effective, well-established weight loss treatment for the severely obese. However, bariatric surgery is invasive and obese patients are high risk surgical candidates. Bariatric surgery is an option for well-screened patients who are committed to long-term lifestyle changes and physician follow-up. Resolution or improvement in comorbidities, such as diabetes, hypertension, hyperlipidemia, obstructive sleep apnea, and osteoarthritis following bariatric surgery is well documented in the literature. Additionally, multiple studies have shown improved survival for severely obese patients who underwent bariatric surgery compared to patients who did not have operative intervention. The type of surgery most appropriate for a specific patient, the preoperative evaluation needed, and the long-term postoperative care depends on a multidisciplinary team led by an experienced bariatric surgeon.

REFERENCES

1. Fielding GA, Ren CJ. Laparoscopic adjustable gastric band. *Surg Clin N Am.* 85:129–140, 2005.
2. Ren CJ, Fielding GA: Laparoscopic gastric banding: surgical technique. *J Laparoendoscop Adv Surg Techni.* 13(4): 257–263, 2003.
3. Fielding GA, Allen JW: A step by step guide to placement of the LAP BAND adjustable gastric banding system. *Am J Surgery* 184:26S–30S, 2002.
4. Rubin M, Yehoshua RT, Stein M et al. Laparoscopic sleeve gastrectomy with minimal orbidity early results in 120 morbidly obese patients. *Obes Surg* 18:1567–1570, 2008.
5. Rubin M, Yehoshua RT, Stein M, Lederfein D, Fichman S, Bernstine H, Eidelman LA. Laparoscopic sleeve gastrectomy with minimal morbidity: early results in 120 morbidly obese patients. *Obes Surg.* 18:1567–1570, 2008.
6. Buchwald H et al. Bariatric surgery: a systematic review and meta analysis. *JAMA.* 292(14), Oct 2004.
7. Fernandez AZ, DeMaria EJ, Tichansky DS, Kellum JM, Wolfe LG, Meador J et al. Multivariate analysis of risk factors for death following gastric bypass for treatment of morbid obesity. *Ann Surg* 239, 698–702, 2004.
8. Byrne TK. Complications of surgery for obesity. *Surg Clin N Am.* 81:1181, 2001.
9. Nguyen NT et al. Gastrointestinal hemorrhage after laparoscopic gastric bypass. *Obes Surg.* 14:1308–1312, 2004.
10. Tessier, DJ, Eagan, JC. Surgical management of morbid obesity. *Cur Prob Surg.* 45:68–137, 2008.
11. Tanaka S, Inoue S, Isoda F et al. Impaired immunity in obesity: suppressed but reversible lymphocyte responsivenss. *Int J Obes.* 17:631–636, 1993.
12. Lamas O, Marti A, Martinez JA. Obesity and immunocompetence. *Eur J Clin Nutrit.* 56:42S–45S, 2002.
13. Christou NV, Jarand J, Sylvestre JL, McLean AP. Analysis of the incidence and risk factors for wound infections in open bariatric surgery. *Obes Surg.* 14:16–22, 2004.
14. McNatt SS, Longhi JJ, Goldman CD, McFadden DW. Surgery for obesity: a review of the current state of the art and future directions. *J Gastrointest Surg.* 11:382–402, 2007.
15. Lopez PP, Stefan B, Schulman CL, Byers PM. Prevalence of sleep apnea in morbidly obese patients who presented for weight loss surgery evaluation: more evidence for routine screening for obstructive sleep apnea before weight loss surgery. *Am Surg.* 74:834–838, Sept 2008.
16. Haines KL, et al. Objective evidence that bariatric surgery improves obesity-related obstructive sleep apnea. *Surgery.* 141(3):354–358, Mar 2007.

17. Rasheid S, Banasiak M, Gallagher SF, et al. Gastric bypass is an effective treatment for obstructive sleep apnea in patients with clinically significant obesity. *Obes Surg*.13:58–61, 2003.

18. Vogel JA, Franklin BA, Zalesin KC, et al. Reduction in predicted coronary heart disease risk after substantial weight reduction after bariatric surgery. *Am J Cardiol.* 99(2):222–226, Jan 2007.

19. Lementowski PW, Zelicof SB. Obesity and osteoarthritis. *Am J Orthoped.* 37(3):148–51, Mar 2008.

20. Hooper MM, Stellato TA, Hallowell PT, et al. Musculoskeletal findings in obese subjects before and after weight loss following bariatric surgery. *Int J Obes.* 31:114–120, 2007.

21 Obesity and Gastrointestinal Cancers

Yume Nguyen and Bhaskar Banerjee

CONTENTS

21.1 INTRODUCTION

Obesity is linked to many chronic health conditions including stroke, coronary heart disease, diabetes mellitus, gallbladder disease, dyslipidemia, respiratory dysfunction, and certain forms of cancer. Obesity has become a growing epidemic in many regions of the world and in the United States over one-third of adults are overweight or obese. Overweight or obesity results from a chronic state of positive energy balance due to an excess of nutritional intake relative to energy expenditure. Excess weight has been associated with increased mortality from all cancers combined and for cancers of several specific sites. The exact figures are uncertain, but some studies estimate overweight and obesity account for 20% of all deaths from cancer in women and 14% in males.[1] Obesity is associated with a number of malignancies including leukemia, non-Hodgkin lymphoma, multiple myeloma, breast, cervical, colorectal, esophageal, gallbladder, kidney, liver, ovarian, pancreatic, prostate, stomach, and uterine cancers. In addition to increasing the risk of developing cancer, some studies show that obese or overweight patients have a poorer outcome once diagnosed with cancer. In addition to having more advanced disease at the time of diagnosis, obese patients have a higher rate of recurrence of prostate/breast cancer, have a worse response rate to chemotherapy, and have more complications perioperatively.

Compounding the problem, obese persons are less likely to undergo cancer screening exams, such as colonoscopy or mammography. This may be due to the patient factors, such as embarrassment or a perception that the exam would be too difficult to undergo. Physician or other healthcare provider factors also may contribute to this relatively low rate of screening. Referral for routine screening may not be offered to obese patients due to other health problems that may overshadow routine health maintenance or a perception that these procedures may be technically difficult. For some morbidly obese patients, many tests are simply not available to them due to the inability to support the excess weight or large size.[2,3]

This chapter will focus on obesity as a risk factor in the development of gastrointestinal cancers; however, it is worth mentioning that some cancer treatments often cause weight gain. The Childhood Cancer Survivor Study showed that acute lymphoblastic leukemia (ALL) survivors who received cranial radiation therapy at a young age are at higher risk for obesity compared to a sibling control group.[4] It has been speculated that this finding may be associated with a leptin receptor polymorphism in patients with ALL.[5] Other cancer treatments, such as steroid medications or hormones, may promote weight gain as well.

21.2   POTENTIAL MECHANISMS

Much interest and intense research has focused on the underlying mechanism responsible for the link between obesity and cancer. It is now known that adipose tissue is an actively secreting endocrine organ. There are several biologically active adipocytokines, or adipokines, associated with obesity, such as adiponectin, leptin, vascular endothelial growth factor (VEGF), TNF-alpha, insulin, insulin-like growth factor-1 (IGF-1), as well as several factors associated with inflammation and oxidative stress. Much attention has been paid to these adipokines to search for a causal or associated link between obesity and cancer. These adipokines regulate several physiologic processes, such as appetite, insulin sensitivity and regulation, immunity, inflammation, and angiogenesis.

Leptin is a hormone secreted by adipocytes and is involved in appetite regulation and energy homeostasis via its influence at the hypothalamus level. Leptin levels, which correlate with the amount of fat stores, affect the inflammatory and immune response and enhance cellular proliferation and antiapoptotic activity in colonic tissue.[6] The inappropriate response and altered immune response may contribute to the dysregulated growth of tumorigenesis. Adiponectin is produced exclusively by adipocytes and, unlike other adipokines, its levels are decreased in obesity states. It has been shown in vitro to inhibit angiogenesis and tumor proliferation. It is postulated that adiponectin affects the obesity–cancer association by acting as a negative regulator of endothelial cell proliferation.[7] The role of insulin in regulating glucose homeostasis and supplying energy to cells and tissues for cellular growth and differentiation may be a key link in the promotion of uncontrolled cell growth associated with tumor formation. Insulin exerts its effect via transmembrane receptor activation and downstream intracellular signaling. Ultimately, transcription of certain genes and translation of proteins may impact cellular proliferation and growth, which can have an influence on tumor development. Insulin also has affects on the synthesis and biological availability of the male and female sex steroids, including androgens, progesterone, and estrogens. Insulin is likely linked to carcinogenesis by acting directly on cells or indirectly via its interaction with insulin-like growth factor-1 (IGF-1) or other endocrine hormones, such as estrogens. Insulin increases levels of IGF-1 that has been implicated in several types of cancers and its receptor is overexpressed in many different tumors. Its effect on tumorigenesis may be through its indirect action on various oncogenes, such as p53 tumor suppressor gene.[8] Both insulin and IGF-1 *in vitro* inhibits apoptosis and promotes cellular proliferation.[9]

21.3   INFLAMMATION AND CANCER

It is widely accepted that chronic inflammation is associated with an increased risk of developing cancer, and a state of chronic low-grade systemic inflammation accompanies obesity. Several studies have been conducted that show that exercise and/or calorie restriction can reduce certain inflammatory markers.[10,11] Physical activity and calorie consumption are both modifiable factors and are targets for directed intervention in the carcinogenesis process. As such, substances that mediate the effects of calorie restriction or physical activity are being sought out as they possess substantial chemotherapeutic potential. However, the mechanism that underlies the antitumor effect of calorie restriction and physical activity is poorly understood.

21.4   CALORIE RESTRICTION

Calorie restriction (CR) has long been known to decrease inflammation and improve longevity through unclear mechanisms. Restriction of calories by 10 to 60% in animal studies has been shown to decrease cell proliferation, increasing apoptosis through antiangiogenic processes. The potent anticancer effect of caloric restriction is clear, but caloric restriction alone is not generally considered to be a feasible strategy for cancer prevention in humans. Identification and development of preventive strategies that "mimic" the anticancer effects of low energy intake are currently underway because it is not feasible to calorie restrict to such an extreme degree in humans. The independent effect of energy intake on cancer risk has been difficult to estimate because body size and physical activity are strong determinants of total energy expenditure.

The exact mechanism responsible for the CR-mediated antitumor effects is unknown. The benefits derived from calorie restriction may be mediated by IGF-1, which stimulates the cell cycle, leptin, and insulin production. During times of calorie restriction, IGF-1 levels are reduced and IGF-1 receptors are increased, which creates a net negative circulating level of IGF-1. Others have focused on the NF-E2–related factor 2 (Nrf2) pathway, which activates antioxidant enzymes when triggered by caloric restriction. Some investigators have focused on the mitochondria for answers relating to the question of CR and antitumor effects. It appears that mitochondria, the site of free-radical production, in the calorie-restricted mice have fewer free radicals and may be regulated by PGC1-α.[12] Resveratrol, a naturally occurring antioxidant chemical found in red wine, acts on the gene SIRT1, which produces enzymes that stimulate mitochondrial growth. This appears to suppress tumor formation and growth in animal studies of cancer.[13,14]

21.5 PHYSICAL ACTIVITY

The mechanisms that account for the inhibitory effects of physical activity on the carcinogenic process are reduction in fat stores, activity-related changes in sex hormone levels, altered immune function, effects in insulin and insulin-like growth factors, reduced free radical generation, and direct effect on the tumor. Epidemiologic evidence posits that the cascade of actions linking overweight and obesity to carcinogenesis are triggered by the endocrine and metabolic systems. Perturbations to these systems result in the alterations in the levels of bioavailable growth factors, steroid hormones, and inflammatory markers.

21.6 COLON CANCER

Cancer of the colon and rectum is the second most common malignancy in the United States and the third deadliest cancer. It is well known that obesity increases the risk of developing colon cancer in men, but data on colon cancer risk in women has been conflicting. Some estimates suggest an overall increased 30 to 60% risk of developing colon cancer, but a recent meta-analysis suggests the risk is less than previously reported at 20% or a relative risk (RR) of 1.21.[15] The majority of studies have focused on body mass index (BMI) or weight as an indicator of obesity, but later studies have also highlighted the importance of central adiposity by utilizing anthropometric measurements, such as waist circumference or waist-to-hip ratios. Individuals within the highest percentile of waist circumference have a greater than 50% increased risk of colorectal cancer (CRC) compared to the lowest waist circumference. This risk increases incrementally by 4% with every 2-in increase in waist circumference[15] These studies highlight that colon cancer is possibly related more to the metabolic syndrome with emphasis on abdominal or visceral adiposity rather than simply increased size or weight.

Not only do the obese have a higher risk for developing colon cancer, they are more likely to have a poor or inadequate prep for colonoscopy. A BMI of ≥ 25 is an independent risk factor for an inadequate bowel prep for colonoscopy and the likelihood of a poor prep increases further with higher BMI values.[16] Retained stool in a poorly prepped colon increases the chance of neoplastic polyps being missed at the colonoscopy exam. A more aggressive prep, e.g., over two days may be needed for obese patients.

Although many studies group cancers of the colon and rectum together, as they do share some environmental risks, rectal cancer has been shown to differ in their etiology and behavior. Unfortunately, few studies have been done focusing on rectal cancer alone and the link between obesity and rectal cancer has been weak. Whether an association exists remains a source of controversy.

21.6.1 Gender Difference

The association of colon cancer and obesity is stronger in men than women with a RR of 1.44 (95% CI, 1.32 to 1.58) and 1.09 (95% CI, 1.01 to 1.17), respectively. The reason for this gender disparity is unclear, but may be related to the difference in fat distribution between men and women and estrogen status. Some recent studies maintain that CRC risk and obesity are maintained in subgroups of women, namely premenopausal females <50 years of age. The period following menopause is a state of low endogenous estrogen. Adipose tissue becomes the primary site of estrogen production, which is not highly regulated by the hypothalamic-pituitary-ovarian axis. HRT (hormone replacement therapy) has been shown to decrease the risk of colon cancer in postmenopausal women in observational as well as intervention studies.[17,18] It has been theorized that estrogen modifies colon cancer development and may be beneficial, whether from endogenous or exogenous sources, in post-menopausal females by counteracting the tumor promoting effects of insulin. This benefit is not seen in premenopausal females because the availability of estrogen is tightly regulated.

The European Prospective Investigation into Cancer and Nutrition (EPIC) trial, which included >350,000 European subjects with >6 years of follow-up, found that elevated body weight and BMI were associated with increased risk of colon cancer in men, but not women. However, when utilizing waist circumference, WHR, and height as measures of obesity, there was an increased risk in both sexes. After strati-fying for postmenopausal women on HRT, there was no association found utiliz-ing anthropometric measurements in this population. Furthermore, postmenopausal women not on HRT had a statistically significant association between waist circum-ference and colon cancer.[19] Slattery and colleagues presented conflicting data to that of the EPIC trial. They note a positive association in premenopausal women and those on HRT, but no association in the postmenopausal population regardless of HRT status.[20] Furthermore, in the NIH–AARP U.S. cohort, they found that colon cancer risk was associated with obesity in younger and older females and HRT had no effect on this finding.[21]

Other studies also have evaluated the relationship between obesity and colon adenomas, a precursor to colon cancer. These studies have been largely consistent with previous data, which reveal that the risk of colorectal adenoma is increased with obesity in premenopausal females, but decreased in postmenopausal females, especially those on HRT.[22]

21.6.2 Physical Activity

Migration and epidemiologic studies reveal a higher prevalence of colorectal can-cer in Western industrialized countries. Several environmental and lifestyle fac-tors have been implicated as causing this trend including diets high in fat, low in fiber, sedentary lifestyle, and alcohol consumption. Several investigators have looked into these individual confounders of obesity as independent risk factors for CRC development. Many studies have consistently shown an inverse relation-ship between physical activity and colon cancer. About a 40 to 50% reduction in incidence was noted in these studies amongst individuals at the highest level of activity.[23] These findings have been seen in studies specifically for women in the Nurses' Health Study Research Group.[24] In the EPIC trial, they found similar risk reduction with physical activity with evidence of a dose-response effect, specifically in the right colon.[25] These findings have not been seen in rectal cancer. Interestingly, Meyerhardt and colleagues found that increased physical activity after the diagnosis of stage I to III CRC is associated with improved cancer-specific and overall mortality.[26]

21.6.3 DIET

Dietary factors that potentially increase the risk of CRC include low fruit, vegetable, or fiber intake, high red meat or saturated fat consumption, and exposure to caffeine or alcohol. The significance of low fruit, vegetable, and fiber intake has been called into question because of contradictory results from large observational studies and negative results from randomized trials.

21.6.4 UNDERLYING MOLECULAR BASIS

The underlying mechanism responsible for the association of excess weight and CRC is an area of intense research. Factors that are associated with colon cancer, such as a sedentary lifestyle, high fat/low fiber diet, and obesity are also associated with diabetes and insulin resistance. As such, the link between colon cancer and hyperinsulinemia has been studied extensively. Obesity, and specifically visceral adiposity, is associated with elevated levels of insulin and IGF-1. Some investigators have proposed that the elevated level of insulin promotes colonic tumor growth. In the Cardiovascular Health Study Cohort, an observational study of 5,849 participants over 65 years of age, found that individuals in the highest quartile of fasting glucose were at 80% higher risk of developing incident colorectal cancer compared with those in the lowest quartile (RR 1.8; 95% CI 1.0 to 3.1).[27]

21.7 ESOPHAGEAL AND GASTRIC CARDIA ADENOCARCINOMA

Barrett's esophagus (BE) is the precursor lesion of most adenocarcinomas of the esophagus and gastric cardia. The true prevalence of BE is unknown as most are asymptomatic. Predicting those patients with BE who are at high risk of progressing to esophageal adenocarcinoma (EAC) is also difficult. With the increasing incidence of EAC and the poor prognosis associated with this diagnosis, there is great interest in furthering our interest in this disease. One- and five-year survival remains dismal at 44% and 13%, respectively. Several risk factors for development of Barrett's have been identified including gastro-esophageal reflux disease (GERD), central obesity, and male gender.

The rise in EAC correlates with the increasing obesity epidemic in Western countries. Obesity, especially central adiposity, has long been associated with the development of BE. However, recent meta-analysis finds obesity to be an indirect risk factor due to its underlying association with GERD, and, once GERD occurs, increasing BMI has no effect on progression to BE.[28] It is postulated that obesity promotes GERD possibly via increased intraabdominal pressure, relaxed lower esophageal sphincter (LES), and higher rates of hiatal hernias.

A few studies have focused specifically on BMI and EAC controlling for GERD symptoms and found that BMI is an independent risk factor suggesting that the risk is not mediated by GERD alone.[29,30] Abdominal obesity, which is more common in males, is associated with EAC and may account for the gender difference seen in EAC and gastric cardia adenocarcinomas.[31] The reasons underlying why obesity is not directly related to BE but is directly associated with EAC and gastric cardia adenocarcinomas are still unknown. It does appear that increasing BMI is associated with increasing risk of these cancers even within normal weight subjects.[32] Of note, esophageal squamous cell carcinoma and gastric noncardia adenocarcinoma are not associated with BMI.

21.8 PANCREATIC CANCER

Pancreatic cancer (PC) is the fourth leading cause of cancer mortality in Western countries. The five-year overall survival rate remains dismal at less than 5% and mortality rates are nearly equal to incidence rates. Despite advances in treatment, the mortality from pancreatic cancer has not improved over the past few decades. The best chance of survival is when the disease is localized at diagnosis; however, less than 10% of cases are found at an early stage. Prevention by identifying risk factors for pancreatic cancer may be the key to improving mortality from this deadly cancer. Approximately 80% of pancreatic cancers are adenocarcinomas, and the peak incidence occurs in the sixth to seventh decade of life. Cigarette smoking is the strongest known risk factor. Others factors having a weaker link to pancreatic cancer include diabetes, chronic pancreatitis, certain hereditary and familial cancer syndromes, and obesity, especially in men.

Although obesity as a risk factor was found less consistently in women, the Women's Health Initiative examined central obesity specifically in postmenopausal women, as determined by waist-to-hip ratio as opposed to general obesity as determined by elevated BMI, in relation to pancreatic cancer and found women in the highest waist-to-hip quintile had 70% [95% CI 10 to 160%] excess risk compared to the lowest quintile.[33] In the largest prospective cohort study, The American Cancer Society Cohort, mortality from pancreatic cancer was increased in these subjects with a BMI >30 kg/m^2 with relative risks between 1.26 to 2.76 for categories of increasing BMI.[1]

The link between obesity and pancreatic cancer may arise as a result of several mechanisms and is likely to be multifactorial. Observational studies have found associations between insulin resistance or diabetes and pancreatic cancer, but it is unclear if it is involved in the etiology or is a result of the malignant process. A case-control study revealed higher levels of adiponectin, but lower levels of leptin in tissue specimens of confirmed pancreatic cancer adjusting for risk factors of PC.[34] The relationship to these adipokines in the pathogenesis of PC is unclear. In addition, a few studies suggest that high consumption of fruits, vegetables, and increased physical activity may reduce pancreatic cancer risk.[35,36]

21.9 HEPATOCELLULAR CARCINOMA

Hepatocellular carcinoma (HCC) is the most common primary malignancy of the liver. Incidence of HCC is increasing worldwide, but rates remain highest in Asian countries and sub-Saharan Africa. The major risk factor for HCC is cirrhosis of the liver due to viruses (Hepatitis B and C virus), toxins (including alcohol), metabolic (diabetes, nonalcoholic fatty liver disease or NAFLD, hemochromotosis), and autoimmune (primary biliary cirrhosis, autoimmune hepatitis).

Nonalcoholic fatty liver disease (NAFLD) or nonalcoholic steatohepatitis (NASH) likely mediates the association between obesity and HCC. Obesity, particularly abdominal obesity, is one element of the metabolic syndrome that is a risk factor for developing NASH or NAFLD. A small percentage of NAFLD subjects progresses to cirrhosis and a proportion of these may develop HCC. Amongst liver transplant recipients with so-called cryptogenic cirrhosis, obesity was an independent risk factor for developing HCC (Odds ratio 11.1, p = 0.02).[37] It is hypothesized that burned out NASH represented a large proportion of these previously termed cryptogenic cirrhosis cases. Also, in patients with chronic hepatitis C, overweight and obesity were shown to be independent risk factors of HCC, with a hazard ratio of 1.86 (95% confidence interval, 1.09 to 3.16; P = .022) and 3.10 (95% confidence interval, 1.41 to 6.81; P = .005), respectively, as compared with the underweight patients.[38] Obesity and insulin resistance often occur concomitantly and population studies have demonstrated that diabetes is also an independent risk factor for HCC even in the absence of known chronic liver disease.[39] It is unclear whether treatment for NAFLD or NASH will prevent progression to cirrhosis or alter the risk of HCC.

REFERENCES

1. Calle, E.E., et al., Overweight, obesity, and mortality from cancer in a prospectively studied cohort of U.S. adults. *N Engl J Med*, 2003. **348**(17): 1625–38.
2. Ferrante, J.M., et al., Colorectal cancer screening among obese versus non-obese patients in primary care practices. *Canc Detect Prev*, 2006. **30**(5): 459–65.
3. Rosen, A.B. and E.C. Schneider, Colorectal cancer screening disparities related to obesity and gender. *J Gen Intern Med*, 2004. **19**(4): 332–8.
4. Garmey, E.G., et al., Longitudinal changes in obesity and body mass index among adult survivors of childhood acute lymphoblastic leukemia: a report from the Childhood Cancer Survivor Study. *J Clin Oncol*, 2008. **26**(28): 4639–45.
5. Ross, J.A., et al., Genetic variation in the leptin receptor gene and obesity in survivors of childhood acute lymphoblastic leukemia: a report from the Childhood Cancer Survivor Study. *J Clin Oncol*, 2004. **22**(17): 3558–62.
6. Liu, Z., et al., High fat diet enhances colonic cell proliferation and carcinogenesis in rats by elevating serum leptin. *Int J Oncol*, 2001. **19**(5): 1009–14.
7. Brakenhielm, E., et al., Adiponectin-induced antiangiogenesis and antitumor activity involve caspase-mediated endothelial cell apoptosis. *Proc Natl Acad Sci USA*, 2004. **101**(8): 2476–81.

8. Takahashi, K. and K. Suzuki, Association of insulin-like growth-factor-I-induced DNA synthesis with phosphorylation and nuclear exclusion of p53 in human breast cancer MCF-7 cells. *Int J Canc*, 1993. **55**(3): 453–8.

9. Yakar, S., D. Leroith, and P. Brodt, The role of the growth hormone/insulin-like growth factor axis in tumor growth and progression: lessons from animal models. *Cytokine Growth Fact Rev*, 2005. **16**(4–5): 407–20.

10. Hursting, S.D., et al., Calorie restriction, aging, and cancer prevention: mechanisms of action and applicability to humans. *Annu Rev Med*, 2003. **54**: 131–52.

11. Sohal, R.S. and R. Weindruch, Oxidative stress, caloric restriction, and aging. *Science*, 1996. **273**(5271): 59–63.

12. Anderson, R.M., et al., Dynamic regulation of PGC-1α localization and turnover implicates mitochondrial adaptation in calorie restriction and the stress response. *Aging Cell*, 2008. **7**(1): 101–11.

13. Fulda, S. and K.M. Debatin, Resveratrol modulation of signal transduction in apoptosis and cell survival: a mini-review. *Canc Detect Prev*, 2006. **30**(3): 217–23.

14. Lavu, S., et al., Sirtuins—novel therapeutic targets to treat age-associated diseases. *Nat Rev Drug Discov*, 2008. **7**(10): 841–53.

15. Moghaddam, A.A., M. Woodward, and R. Huxley, Obesity and risk of colorectal cancer: a meta-analysis of 31 studies with 70,000 events. *Canc Epidemiol Biomark Prev*, 2007. **16**(12): 2533–47.

16. Borg B.B., Gupta, N.K., Zuckerman, G.R., Banerjee, B., and Gywali, C.P., Obesity and other predictors of poor bowel preparation for colonoscopy. *Clin Gastro and Hepatol*, 2009. **7**: 270–275.

17. Rossouw, J.E., et al., Risks and benefits of estrogen plus progestin in healthy postmenopausal women: principal results from the Women's Health Initiative randomized controlled trial. *JAMA*, 2002. **288**(3): 321–33.

18. Chlebowski, R.T., et al., Estrogen plus progestin and colorectal cancer in postmenopausal women. *N Engl J Med*, 2004. **350**(10): 991–1004.

19. Pischon, T., et al., Body size and risk of colon and rectal cancer in the European Prospective Investigation into Cancer and Nutrition (EPIC). *J Natl Canc Inst*, 2006. **98**(13): 920–31.

20. Slattery, M.L., et al., Body mass index and colon cancer: an evaluation of the modifying effects of estrogen (United States). *Canc Causes Contr*, 2003. **14**(1): 75–84.

21. Adams, K.F., et al., Body mass and colorectal cancer risk in the NIH-AARP cohort. *Am J Epidemiol*, 2007. **166**(1): 36–45.

22. Wolf, L.A., et al., Do factors related to endogenous and exogenous estrogens modify the relationship between obesity and risk of colorectal adenomas in women? *Canc Epidemiol Biomark Prev*, 2007. **16**(4): 676–83.

23. Colditz, G.A., C.C. Cannuscio, and A.L. Frazier, Physical activity and reduced risk of colon cancer: implications for prevention. *Canc Causes Contr*, 1997. **8**(4): 649–67.

24. Martinez, M.E., et al., Leisure-time physical activity, body size, and colon cancer in women. Nurses' Health Study Research Group. *J Natl Cancer Inst*, 1997. **89**(13): 948–55.

25. Friedenreich, C., et al., Physical activity and risk of colon and rectal cancers: the European prospective investigation into cancer and nutrition. *Canc Epidemiol Biomark Prev*, 2006. **15**(12): 2398–407.

26. Meyerhardt, J.A., et al., Physical activity and survival after colorectal cancer diagnosis. *J Clin Oncol*, 2006. **24**(22): 3527–34.

27. Schoen, R.E., et al., Increased blood glucose and insulin, body size, and incident colorectal cancer. *J Natl Canc Inst*, 1999. **91**(13): 1147–54.

28. Cook, M.B., et al., A systematic review and meta-analysis of the risk of increasing adiposity on Barrett's esophagus. *Am J Gastroenterol*, 2008. **103**(2): 292–300.

29. Chow, W.H., et al., Body mass index and risk of adenocarcinomas of the esophagus and gastric cardia. *J Natl Canc Inst*, 1998. **90**(2): 150–5.

30. Lagergren, J., R. Bergstrom, and O. Nyren, Association between body mass and adenocarcinoma of the esophagus and gastric cardia. *Ann Intern Med*, 1999. **130**(11): 883–90.

31. Corley, D.A., A. Kubo, and W. Zhao, Abdominal obesity and the risk of esophageal and gastric cardia carcinomas. *Canc Epidemiol Biomark Prev*, 2008. **17**(2): 352–8.

32. Abnet, C.C., et al., A prospective study of BMI and risk of oesophageal and gastric adenocarcinoma. *Eur J Canc*, 2008. **44**(3): 465–71.

33. Luo, J., et al., Obesity and risk of pancreatic cancer among postmenopausal women: the Women's Health Initiative (United States). *Br J Cancer*, 2008. **99**(3): 527–31.

34. Dalamaga, M., et al., Pancreatic cancer expresses adiponectin receptors and is associated with hypoleptinemia and hyperadiponectinemia: a case-control study. *Canc Causes Contr*, 2009. **20**(5): 625–33.

35. Freelove, R. and A.D. Walling, Pancreatic cancer: diagnosis and management. *Am Fam Physic*, 2006. **73**(3): 485–92.

36. Hanley, A.J., et al., Physical activity, anthropometric factors and risk of pancreatic cancer: results from the Canadian enhanced cancer surveillance system. *Int J Canc*, 2001. **94**(1): 140–7.

37. Nair, S., et al., Is obesity an independent risk factor for hepatocellular carcinoma in cirrhosis? *Hepatology*, 2002. **36**(1): 150–5.

38. Ohki, T., et al., Obesity is an independent risk factor for hepatocellular carcinoma development in chronic hepatitis C patients. *Clin Gastroenterol Hepatol*, 2008. **6**(4): 459–64.

39. Davila, J.A., et al., Diabetes increases the risk of hepatocellular carcinoma in the United States: a population based case control study. *Gut*, 2005. **54**(4): 533–9.

22 Nutrition and Colon Cancer Prevention

Petr Protiva

CONTENTS

22.1   INTRODUCTION

Colorectal cancer is a common malignancy in the United States. There are approximately 149,000 new cases diagnosed annually, and about 50,000 people die of this disease each year. Colorectal cancer accounts for about 9% of cancer-related deaths, making it the second most common cancer-related death in the United States. Several factors contribute to an increased risk of developing colorectal cancer, including genetic and environmental factors. Although genetic factors will result in a significant risk increase, most cases of colorectal cancer are sporadic with no family history of the disease. Numerous other factors have also been associated with an increased risk of developing colorectal cancer including inflammatory bowel disease, diabetes mellitus or insulin resistance, cholecystectomy, excessive alcohol intake, a history of smoking, a history of pelvic radiation, ureterocolic anastomosis, acromegaly, and prior treatment for Hodgkin's lymphoma. Additionally, there are positive associations between colorectal cancer and human immunodeficiency virus as well as coronary artery disease; less clear associations exist between colorectal cancer and Barrett's esophagus or breast cancer 1 gene (BRCA1) status.

Nutrition and nutritional status also are important modulators of colorectal cancer development. Studies suggest that obesity, defined as a body mass index (BMI) greater than 30, may contribute a 1.5- to 2-fold increased relative risk of colorectal cancer and also raises the risk of dying of this disease. Numerous epidemiological studies have demonstrated that nutrition is an important risk factor for colorectal cancer; nevertheless, its effect is difficult to quantify and is modest at best. Best estimates suggest that a balanced, prudent diet rich in fruits and vegetables and low in animal protein and saturated fats is associated with only about a 25 to 50% relative risk reduction compared to a Western-style diet. However, colorectal cancer is a prevalent disease and even a modest risk reduction without side effects may translate into major personal and societal benefits. Therefore, significant research efforts have been devoted to studying the impact of individual dietary components on colorectal cancer risk. Yet, considerable controversy exists, as nutritional habits are chronically difficult to quantify even in a controlled interventional trial, let alone in population-based studies. This chapter will discuss the evidence of dietary intervention and habits on colorectal cancer risk.

22.2   CALORIES AND OBESITY

High caloric food intake that is not balanced by increased energy expenditure leads to obesity. The extent to which food with high caloric content contributes to cancer, independent of obesity or BMI, is not known, but increased BMI and obesity are associated with an increased risk of colon cancer and adenomas. Two large prospective cohort studies have demonstrated an increased risk for colorectal carcinoma associated with high BMI. Additionally, it was shown that patients who are obese also appear to have a higher risk of dying from colorectal cancer. It appears that this holds true especially for abdominal adiposity, and patients with increased abdominal fat tend to have more insulin resistance and higher circulating insulin levels. Both insulin resistance and high insulin-like growth factor 1 (IGF-1) levels are known to be associated with a colorectal neoplasm risk in humans and in animal models.[1,2] A recent systematic review and meta-analysis of prospective observational studies involving analyses of 221 datasets and 141 articles, including 282,137 incident cases from the past four decades, concluded that a 5 kg/m^2 increase in BMI was associated with a relative risk (RR) of 1.24 (1.20 to 1.28, 95% CI, P <0.001) for colon cancer in men and a RR of 1.09 (1.05 to 1.13, 95% CI, P <0.001) in women. There was also a significantly increased risk (RR of 1.09: 1.06 to 1.12, 95% CI, P <0.001) observed for rectal cancer in men, but not in women.[3]

22.3   ANIMAL PROTEINS AND FATS

Diets high in red animal meat appear to promote colon carcinogenesis. There is probably not a single mechanism by which red meat consumption promotes colon carcinogenesis, but current theories suggest that (1) cooking meat at a high temperature forms carcinogenic heterocyclic amines and polycyclic aromatic hydrocarbons, (2) carcinogenic N-nitroso compounds are formed in meat endogenously, and (3) heme iron in red meat can promote carcinogenesis because it increases cell proliferation in the mucosa through lipoperoxidation and/or cytotoxicity of fecal water. Nitrosation may also increase the toxicity of heme in cured products.[4] Additionally, high protein/high calorie diets may increase IGF-1 signaling, which is also associated with an increased risk of colorectal neoplasm.[2] Indeed, several large epidemiological studies showed an increased risk for individuals with the highest intake of red or processed meat consumed over long periods. A study involving more than 148,000 individuals concluded that consumption of a high ratio of red meat to poultry and fish also represents a risk.[5] A recent meta-analysis of 23 publications that reported results from prospective studies on red meat and/or processed meat consumption in relation to the risk of colon or colorectal cancer, was conducted. This meta-analysis reported a RR for colorectal cancer of 1.2 (1.11 to 1.31, 95% CI) for processed meats and 1.28 (1.15 to 1.42, 95% CI) for red meats, comparing the highest with the lowest category of intake.[6] The excess risk seems to affect only the distal colon, and a high intake of red meats is also associated with an increased risk of rectal cancers.

The data on fat intake and colon cancer is controversial, but it seems that total fat does not appear to modulate colon cancer risk. However, it is possible that excess intake of particular types of fat may affect the risk differently. There is a theory that high fat diets promote carcinogenesis in the colon via promotion of IGF signaling and insulin resistance or via fecal bile acids. Another interesting theory suggests that diets high in cholesterol and/or n-6 polyunsaturated fats may promote carcinogenesis by inducing an inflammatory reaction in the stromal compartment.[7] Nevertheless, it is difficult to disentangle the effects of high calorie diets from the effects of fats, as most diets rich in fats are also high in energy content. Even in a controlled clinical trial setting, it is difficult for subjects to maintain low fat diets over long periods of time (years). It appears that excess calories from any source lead to weight gain and an increase in the risk of multiple cancers, including colon cancer.[8]

22.4   FRUITS, VEGETABLES, AND FIBER

A high intake of fresh fruits and vegetables is encouraged because of their general health benefits that extend beyond cancer prevention. Several factors are thought to be responsible for this preventive effect. Fruits and vegetables provide nondigestible fiber bulk, may prevent constipation, and reduce the exposure to intraluminal carcinogens. They also contain small bioactive molecules and vitamins that may prevent cancer by targeting various molecular pathways known to promote carcinogenesis. Colonic bacteria ferment fibrous residues in plants' nondigestible material that leads to high intraluminal levels of short-chain fatty acids, such as butyrate, that may affect differentiation, apoptosis, and epigenetic regulation of gene expression in the colorectum.

In general, prospective studies provide weaker evidence than case-control studies on the association of fruit and vegetable consumption with reduced cancer risk.[9] The discrepancies may be related to recall and selection biases in case-control studies. In contrast, the association may have been underestimated in prospective studies because of the combined effects of imprecise dietary measurements and limited variability of dietary intakes within each cohort. A pooled analysis of 14 cohort studies concluded that fruit and vegetable intakes were not strongly associated with colon cancer risk overall, but may be associated with a lower risk of distal colon cancer.[10] Diets rich in fruit and deep-yellow vegetables, dark-green vegetables, onions, and garlic are also modestly associated with a reduced risk of colorectal adenoma, a precursor of colorectal cancer.[11] The evidence comes from the Prostate, Lung, Colorectal, and Ovarian Cancer Screening Trial (PLCO) (1993–2001), where 3,057 cases with at least one prevalent histologically verified adenoma of the distal large bowel were compared with 29,413 control subjects. Ongoing debate exists on whether certain fruits and vegetables or organically farmed crops are more likely to reduce the risk, especially when compared to industrially produced crops that are generally perceived to contain less bioactive phytochemicals. Indeed, some plants rich in polyphenolic compounds exhibit strong anticancer or chemopreventive activity in preclinical models,[12,13] and human studies are under way. However, in general, those studies are performed with plant extracts or pure isolated compounds and, thus, cannot serve as an argument for preventive activity of the original edible plant.

Some epidemiology studies suggested that the preventive effect of plant food on colon cancer also may be mediated by its fiber content. A large European study (n = 519,978) showed that dietary fiber was inversely related to colon cancer incidence (adjusted RR of 0.58, 95% CI 0.41 to 0.85), comparing the highest to lowest quintiles of fiber intake.[14] However, the data were not controlled for folate intake. The large U.S. cohort study did not show an association between cancer risk and fiber intake, including fiber in cereals.[15,16] Randomized, controlled polyp prevention trials found that fiber supplementation did not have a significant impact on recurrence of colorectal adenomas.[17,18] A meta-analysis of five studies also concluded that fiber did not affect the incidence or recurrence of adenomatous polyps.[19] Similarly, when other dietary risk factors were taken into account, a pooled analysis of 13 prospective cohort studies (725,628 men and women followed up to 20 years) showed no association of fiber with the risk of colorectal cancer.[20] Overall there is compelling evidence that inadequate folate intake enhances the risk of colorectal cancer; however, artificial folate oversupplementation may lead to accelerated carcinogenesis most likely in individuals with existing cancerous or precancerous lesion.

22.5 CALCIUM AND VITAMIN D

Numerous epidemiologic studies have suggested that calcium or dairy products may lower the risk of colorectal neoplasia. Data from a prospective epidemiologic study in over 45,000 Swedish men, age 45 to 79 years, with a mean follow-up of between 6 and 7 years, showed a reduction in colorectal cancer incidence when analyzed for the highest versus the lowest quartile for calcium intake (mean odds ratio of 0.68: 95% CI: 0.51, 0.91; P for trend =0.01). Using multivariate analysis, the data from this study suggested that there might be a threshold effect at about 1,200 to 1,400 mg of calcium per day.[21] Because high calcium intake is also linked to prostate cancer, there may be a minimum safe level of calcium intake, around 700 mg/day, that confers protection against colorectal cancer without significantly increasing prostate cancer risk. Two other epidemiologic studies, with 8- and 19-year follow-ups, showed an inverse relationship between calcium intake and incidence of colorectal cancer.[22,23] In the Health Professionals Follow-up Study and the Nurse's Health Study, the risk of distal colon cancer was reduced in subjects who took up to 1,250 mg/day elemental calcium versus <500 mg/day (RR 0.58, 95% CI 0.32 to 1.05).[24]

Calcium supplementation appears to prevent the recurrence of colorectal adenomas and is recommended as the primary or secondary prevention by the American College of Gastroenterology.[25] In a randomized, controlled, double-blind, multicenter trial of 930 subjects with a history of colorectal adenoma, calcium supplementation was associated with a significant, though moderate, reduction in the risk of recurrent colorectal adenomas, with an adjusted risk ratio of 0.81 (95% CI, 0.67 to 0.99; P = 0.04, placebo vs. 1,200 mg elemental calcium supplementation).[26] An analysis of three trials including 1,485 subjects with previously removed adenomas who were randomized to calcium versus placebo supplementation also showed that the recurrence of adenomas was significantly lower in subjects randomized to calcium supplementation (RR: 0.80, CI: 0.68, 0.93; P-value = 0.004).[27] However, the Women's Health Initiative (n = 36,282) did not find a significant decrease in incidence or stage of colorectal cancer in the group, which had been randomly assigned to receive 500 mg calcium and vitamin D 200 IU twice daily, compared to the placebo.[28] The average age of women at the start of randomization was 62 years, and follow-up was 7 years. This interval may have been too short to find an effect on cancer incidence. Long-term follow-up for subjects from the women's health initiative (WHI) trial is under way.

It is not clear how calcium protects from the development of colon cancer. It may offer protection by reducing epithelial cell proliferation in the colon, either directly by acting via the calcium sensing receptor,[29] through the cardiac L-type calcium channel present in the colon[30] or indirectly by binding secondary bile acids and ionized fatty acids.[31–34] Moreover, there is a functional interaction between calcium and vitamin D with an implication for colon cancer prevention.[29]

Vitamin D is a fat-soluble molecule that acts principally through interaction with a high-affinity binding protein vitamin D receptor (VDR), which is a member of the steroid receptor, super family ligand-dependent, transcription factor. Binding of calcitriol to VDR induces a configurational change and the receptor then heterodimerizes with the retinoid X receptor and the complex binds to vitamin D responsive elements in the nucleus. This interaction induces gene transcription, which results primarily in cell cycle arrest, differentiation, and apoptosis. Furthermore, there are nonreceptor-dependent actions of vitamin D upon the cell, which include activation of calcium channels, at least in the small intestine and colon.[35] There are several known polymorphisms in the VDR that are functionally associated with differences in bone density and in serum calcitriol levels, but the effect on the action of vitamin D on the colon is unclear.[36] In fact, one study showed that VDR polymorphism genotypes and haplotypes did not directly alter colorectal adenoma recurrence risk, but the reduction in risk associated with a high intake of dairy products was confined to individuals with ApaI aA/AA genotype.[37]

Epidemiologic data show that exposure to sunlight results in a reduction in the incidence of many cancers, but most clearly of colorectal cancer. There is a distinct north to south latitude difference in colorectal cancer development.[38] Six of seven studies on colorectal cancer showed a significant reduction of cancer and one was borderline significant.[39] A prospective study of serum levels of vitamin D revealed a 55% reduction in cancer development in the highest compared to the lowest quartile.[40] Perhaps one of the most important observations is that of interplay between vitamin D levels, calcium intake, and colon cancer risk, originating from subsequent analyses of a polyp prevention trial.[26] The data showed that most of the effect of calcium in lowering the incidence of recurrent adenomas occurred in individuals who had baseline levels of serum 25 hydroxyvitamin D above the median (about 29 ng per ml) with little effect in individuals with lower levels.[41] Therefore, it is the combination of calcium and vitamin D that is important in altering adenoma recurrence. An additional 10-year follow-up study on subjects from the calcium and polyp prevention trial[26] showed that, in calcium-supplemented subjects, the beneficial effect upon adenoma recurrence extended for another five years after subjects stopped taking supplemental calcium (40% less adenoma recurrence when compared to placebo control subjects).[42] Interestingly, colon cancer chemopreventive activity of hormonal replacement therapy may be, at least partially, mediated through vitamin D action in the colorectum.[43]

22.6   FOLATE, VITAMIN B$_6$, AND VITAMIN B$_{12}$

The area of nutritional supplements and vitamins involved in one carbon metabolism is a focus of intense research, as methylation of DNA and proteins is involved in nucleic acid synthesis, epigenetic regulation of gene expression, and modulation of intracellular signaling pathways. Folic acid, vitamins B$_6$ and B$_{12}$ as well as dietary choline, methionine, and betaine participate in single carbon metabolism and increase the complexity of data analysis in human chemoprevention studies. Translational studies examining the effect of both folate supplementation and depletion–repletion regimens on the colon and circulating biomarkers were conducted, and the gene expression and DNA methylation data is being carefully analyzed in hopes of shedding more light on this complex topic.[44]

Folate is present in green, leafy vegetables, fruits, cereals, grains, nuts, avocados, lentils, beans, and meats. Folic acid, the form of the vitamin included in food supplements, has the same biologic effects as folate, but is more bioavailable. The role of folate in cancer prevention is uncertain. Alcohol consumption and the presence of genetic polymorphisms in the folate metabolizing pathway makes interpreting the data from studies difficult. Folate intake has been associated with a decreased risk for colon and other cancers, especially in individuals who consume alcohol, in observational studies. Subjects with the methylenetetrahydrofolate reductase (MTHFR) genotype, which leads to lower enzymatic activity, have a reduced risk of colon cancer[45] as well as cancers of the esophagus, stomach, and pancreas.[46] Combined results from the Nurses Health Study and the Health Professionals Follow-Up Study showed an inverse relationship between folate intake and the risk of developing adenomatous polyps.[47] The Nurses Health Study demonstrated a decreased risk of colon cancer in women who took multivitamins containing folic acid for at least 15 years (RR 0.25, CI 0.13 to 0.51).[48] However, the results from the Women's Health Initiative showed that, although an increased intake of dietary folate and vitamin B$_6$ lowered colorectal cancer risk, supplementation with folic acid and vitamin B$_6$ did not.[49] A recent nested case-control study within the Alpha-Tocopherol, Beta-Carotene Cancer Prevention Study showed that serum vitamin B$_6$ was inversely associated with colon cancer (odds ratio: 0.30 (95% CI, 0.11 to 0.82)) in the highest versus lowest quintile, but folate and other one-carbon-related biomarkers were not associated with colon or rectal cancer.[50] Alcohol consumption interferes with folate availability and raises the risk of colon cancer. One study showed that the increased risk of colon cancer associated with alcohol is not seen in men with the highest folate intake.[51]

In contrast to biologic and observational evidence supporting a role in cancer prevention, results from randomized trials are controversial. The largest controlled trial to evaluate folic acid supplementation in patients with colorectal adenomas, the Aspirin/Folate Polyp Trial found no decrease in new adenomas at three- and six-year follow-ups. In this trial, 1021 subjects with prior adenomas were randomized in 4 arms and 2/4 arms received 1 mg folic acid for three to six years. The incidence of at least one advanced lesion was 11.6% for folic acid and 6.9% for placebo (RR = 1.67; 95% CI 1.00 to 2.80; p =. 05). The RR of having >3 polyps = 2.3 (CI = 1.2 to 4.3, p = 0.02). Prostate cancer developed in 7.3% of those receiving folic acid versus 2.8% among placebo group (p <0.01).[52] In HOPE-2 trial involving 5m522 subjects, active arm received 2.5 mg folic acid, 1 mg B_{12}, 50 mg B_6 × 5 years. The RR of colon cancer was 1.4 (95% CI, 0.9 to 2.8). Only one trial that used a high dose (5 mg) of daily folate supplementation concluded that, at a high dose, folic acid supplementation is associated with a significant reduction in the recurrence of colonic adenomas, but only 49 in the folic acid group and 45 in the placebo group completed this study.[53]

22.7 SELENIUM AND ANTIOXIDANTS

Preclinical animal studies suggest that selenium intake reduces the risk of a variety of tumors. An inverse association between selenium and cancer also was shown in several epidemiological studies.[54,55] However, while selenium levels up to 130 ng/ml correlate with low cancer mortality, this data from 14,000 patients also suggests that levels above 130 ng/ml correlate with an increase in mortality.[56] Data from a randomized trial examining the link between selenium and skin cancer also reported a significant reduction of mortality for cancers of the lung, colon (nearly 50% decreased risk), and prostate; nevertheless, one should note that the primary outcome in this study was skin cancer and selenium treatment did not protect against development of basal or squamous cell carcinomas of the skin.[57] Extended follow-up analyses of the data revealed that selenium supplementation was also associated with a decreased risk for developing adenomatous polyps.[58]

Findings from randomized trials on the association between antioxidant use and cancer risk have been mostly negative. The Women's Antioxidant Cardiovascular Study (n = 7,627), a double-blind, placebo-controlled 2 × 2 × 2 factorial trial of vitamin C, natural-source vitamin E, and beta carotene concluded that these supplementations offer no overall benefits in the primary prevention of total cancer incidence or cancer mortality.[59]

REFERENCES

1. Ealey, K.N., Xuan, W., Lu, S., and Archer, M.C. 2008. Colon carcinogenesis in liver-specific IGF-I-deficient (LID) mice. *Int. J. Cancer* **122**:472–476.
2. Schoen, R.E., Weissfeld, J.L., Kuller, L.H., Thaete, F.L., Evans, R.W., Hayes, R.B., and Rosen, C.J. 2005. Insulin-like growth factor-I and insulin are associated with the presence and advancement of adenomatous polyps. *Gastroenterology* **129**:464–475.

3. Renehan, A.G., Tyson, M., Egger, M., Heller, R.F., and Zwahlen, M. 2008. Body-mass index and incidence of cancer: a systematic review and meta-analysis of prospective observational studies. *Lancet* **371**:569–578.

4. Santarelli, R.L., Pierre, F., and Corpet, D.E. 2008. Processed meat and colorectal cancer: a review of epidemiologic and experimental evidence. *Nutr. Cancer* **60**:131–144.

5. Chao, A., Thun, M.J., Connell, C.J., McCullough, M.L., Jacobs, E.J., Flanders, W.D., Rodriguez, C., Sinha, R., and Calle, E.E. 2005. Meat consumption and risk of colorectal cancer. *JAMA* **293**:172–182.

6. Larsson, S.C., and Wolk, A. 2006. Meat consumption and risk of colorectal cancer: a meta-analysis of prospective studies. *Int. J. Cancer* **119**:2657–2664.

7. Biasi, F., Mascia, C., and Poli, G. 2008. The contribution of animal fat oxidation products to colon carcinogenesis, through modulation of TGF-beta1 signaling. *Carcinogenesis* **29**:890–894.

8. Willett, W.C. 2001. Diet and cancer: one view at the start of the millennium. *Cancer Epidemiol. Biomarkers Prev.* **10**:3–8.

9. Riboli, E., and Norat, T. 2003. Epidemiologic evidence of the protective effect of fruit and vegetables on cancer risk. *Am. J. Clin. Nutr.* **78**:559S–569S.

10. Koushik, A., Hunter, D.J., Spiegelman, D., Beeson, W.L., van den Brandt, P.A., Buring, J.E., Calle, E.E., Cho, E., Fraser, G.E., Freudenheim, J.L. et al. 2007. Fruits, vegetables, and colon cancer risk in a pooled analysis of 14 cohort studies. *J. Natl. Cancer Inst.* **99**:1471–1483.

11. Millen, A.E., Subar, A.F., Graubard, B.I., Peters, U., Hayes, R.B., Weissfeld, J.L., Yokochi, L.A., and Ziegler, R.G. 2007. Fruit and vegetable intake and prevalence of colorectal adenoma in a cancer screening trial. *Am. J. Clin. Nutr.* **86**:1754–1764.

12. Protiva, P., Hopkins, M.E., Baggett, S., Yang, H., Lipkin, M., Holt, P.R., Kennelly, E.J., and Bernard, W.I. 2008. Growth inhibition of colon cancer cells by polyisoprenylated benzophenones is associated with induction of the endoplasmic reticulum response. *Int. J. Cancer* **123**:687–694.

13. Wang, L.S., Hecht, S.S., Carmella, S.G., Yu, N., Larue, B., Henry, C., McIntyre, C., Rocha, C., Lechner, J.F., and Stoner, G.D. 2009. Anthocyanins in black raspberries prevent esophageal tumors in rats. *Cancer Prev. Res. (Phila. PA)* **2**:84–93.

14. Bingham, S.A., Day, N.E., Luben, R., Ferrari, P., Slimani, N., Norat, T., Clavel-Chapelon, F., Kesse, E., Nieters, A., Boeing, H. et al 2003. Dietary fibre in food and protection against colorectal cancer in the European Prospective Investigation into Cancer and Nutrition (EPIC): an observational study. *Lancet* **361**:1496–1501.

15. Fuchs, C.S., Giovannucci, E.L., Colditz, G.A., Hunter, D.J., Stampfer, M.J., Rosner, B., Speizer, F.E., and Willett, W.C. 1999. Dietary fiber and the risk of colorectal cancer and adenoma in women. *N. Engl. J. Med.* **340**:169–176.

16. Giovannucci, E., Rimm, E.B., Stampfer, M.J., Colditz, G.A., Ascherio, A., and Willett, W.C. 1994. Intake of fat, meat, and fiber in relation to risk of colon cancer in men. *Cancer Res.* **54**:2390–2397.

17. Alberts, D.S., Martinez, M.E., Roe, D.J., Guillen-Rodriguez, J.M., Marshall, J.R., van Leeuwen, J.B., Reid, M.E., Ritenbaugh, C., Vargas, P.A., Bhattacharyya, A.B. et al. 2000. Lack of effect of a high-fiber cereal supplement on the recurrence of colorectal adenomas. Phoenix Colon Cancer Prevention Physicians' Network. *N. Engl. J. Med.* **342**:1156–1162.

18. Schatzkin, A., Lanza, E., Corle, D., Lance, P., Iber, F., Caan, B., Shike, M., Weissfeld, J., Burt, R., Cooper, M.R. et al. 2000. Lack of effect of a low-fat, high-fiber diet on the recurrence of colorectal adenomas. Polyp Prevention Trial Study Group. *N. Engl. J. Med.* **342**:1149–1155.

19. Asano, T., and McLeod, R.S. 2002. Dietary fibre for the prevention of colorectal adenomas and carcinomas. *Cochrane. Database. Syst. Rev.* CD003430.

20. Park, Y., Hunter, D.J., Spiegelman, D., Bergkvist, L., Berrino, F., van den Brandt, P.A., Buring, J.E., Colditz, G.A., Freudenheim, J.L., Fuchs, C.S. et al. 2005. Dietary fiber intake and risk of colorectal cancer: a pooled analysis of prospective cohort studies. *JAMA* **294**:2849–2857.

21. Larsson, S.C., Bergkvist, L., Rutegard, J., Giovannucci, E., and Wolk, A. 2006. Calcium and dairy food intakes are inversely associated with colorectal cancer risk in the Cohort of Swedish Men. *Am. J. Clin. Nutr.* **83**:667–673.

22. Garland, C., Shekelle, R.B., Barrett-Connor, E., Criqui, M.H., Rossof, A.H., and Paul, O. 1985. Dietary vitamin D and calcium and risk of colorectal cancer: a 19-year prospective study in men. *Lancet* **1**:307–309.

23. Pietinen, P., Malila, N., Virtanen, M., Hartman, T.J., Tangrea, J.A., Albanes, D., and Virtamo, J. 1999. Diet and risk of colorectal cancer in a cohort of Finnish men. *Cancer Causes Control* **10**:387–396.

24. Wu,K., Willett,W.C., Fuchs,C.S., Colditz,G.A., and Giovannucci,E.L. 2002. Calcium intake and risk of colon cancer in women and men. *J. Natl. Cancer Inst.* **94**:437–446.

25. Bond,J.H. 2000. Polyp guideline: diagnosis, treatment, and surveillance for patients with colorectal polyps. Practice Parameters Committee of the American College of Gastroenterology. *Am. J. Gastroenterol.* **95**:3053–3063.

26. Baron, J.A., Beach, M., Mandel, J.S., van Stolk, R.U., Haile, R.W., Sandler, R.S., Rothstein, R., Summers, R.W., Snover, D.C., Beck, G.J. et al. 1999. Calcium supplements for the prevention of colorectal adenomas. Calcium Polyp Prevention Study Group. *N. Engl. J. Med.* **340**:101–107.

27. Shaukat, A., Scouras, N., and Schunemann, H.J. 2005. Role of supplemental calcium in the recurrence of colorectal adenomas: a meta-analysis of randomized controlled trials. *Am. J. Gastroenterol.* **100**:390–394.

28. Wactawski-Wende, J., Kotchen, J.M., Anderson, G.L., Assaf, A.R., Brunner, R.L., O'Sullivan, M.J., Margolis, K.L., Ockene, J.K., Phillips, L., Pottern, L. et al. 2006. Calcium plus vitamin D supplementation and the risk of colorectal cancer. *N. Engl. J. Med.* **354**:684–696.

29. Chakrabarty, S., Wang, H., Canaff, L., Hendy, G.N., Appelman, H., and Varani, J. 2005. Calcium sensing receptor in human colon carcinoma: interaction with Ca(2+) and 1,25-dihydroxyvitamin D(3). *Cancer Res.* **65**:493–498.

30. Wang, X.T., Nagaba, Y., Cross, H.S., Wrba, F., Zhang, L., and Guggino, S.E. 2000. The mRNA of L-type calcium channel elevated in colon cancer: protein distribution in normal and cancerous colon. *Am. J. Pathol.* **157**:1549–1562.

31. Buset, M., Lipkin, M., Winawer, S., Swaroop, S., and Friedman, E. 1986. Inhibition of human colonic epithelial cell proliferation *in vivo* and *in vitro* by calcium. *Cancer Res.* **46**:5426–5430.

32. Newmark, H.L., Wargovich, M.J., and Bruce, W.R. 1984. Colon cancer and dietary fat, phosphate, and calcium: a hypothesis. *J. Natl. Cancer Inst.* **72**:1323–1325.

33. Van der, M.R., Kleibeuker, J.H., and Lapre, J.A. 1991. Calcium phosphate, bile acids and colorectal cancer. *Eur. J. Cancer Prev.* **1** (Suppl 2):55–62.

34. Wargovich, M.J., Eng, V.W., and Newmark, H.L. 1984. Calcium inhibits the damaging and compensatory proliferative effects of fatty acids on mouse colon epithelium. *Cancer Lett.* **23**:253–258.

35. Lamprecht, S.A., and Lipkin, M. 2003. Chemoprevention of colon cancer by calcium, vitamin D and folate: molecular mechanisms. *Nat. Rev. Cancer* **3**:601–614.

36. Slatter, M.L., Yakumo, K., Hoffman, M., and Neuhausen, S. 2001. Variants of the VDR gene and risk of colon cancer (United States). *Cancer Causes Control* **12**:359–364.

37. Hubner, R.A., Muir, K.R., Liu, J.F., Logan, R.F., Grainge, M.J., and Houlston, R.S. 2008. Dairy products, polymorphisms in the vitamin D receptor gene and colorectal adenoma recurrence. *Int. J. Cancer* **123**:586–593.

38. Garland, C.F., and Garland, F.C. 1980. Do sunlight and vitamin D reduce the likelihood of colon cancer? *Int. J. Epidemiol.* **9**:227–231.

39. Garland, C.F., Garland, F.C., Gorham, E.D., Lipkin, M., Newmark, H., Mohr, S.B., and Holick, M.F. 2006. The role of vitamin D in cancer prevention. *Am. J. Public Health* **96**:252–261.

40. Pilz, S., Dobnig, H., Winklhofer-Roob, B., Riedmuller, G., Fischer, J.E., Seelhorst, U., Wellnitz, B., Boehm, B.O., and Marz, W. 2008. Low serum levels of 25-hydroxyvitamin D predict fatal cancer in patients referred to coronary angiography. *Cancer Epidemiol. Biomarkers Prev.* **17**:1228–1233.

41. Grau, M.V., Baron, J.A., Barry, E.L., Sandler, R.S., Haile, R.W., Mandel, J.S., and Cole, B.F. 2005. Interaction of calcium supplementation and nonsteroidal anti-inflammatory drugs and the risk of colorectal adenomas. *Cancer Epidemiol. Biomarkers Prev.* **14**:2353–2358.

42. Grau, M.V., Baron, J.A., Sandler, R.S., Wallace, K., Haile, R.W., Church, T.R., Beck, G.J., Summers, R.W., Barry, E.L., Cole, B.F. et al. 2007. Prolonged effect of calcium supplementation on risk of colorectal adenomas in a randomized trial. *J. Natl. Cancer Inst.* **99**:129–136.

43. Protiva, P., Cross, H.S., Hopkins, M.E., Kallay, E., Bises, G., Dreyhaupt, E., Augenlicht, L., Lipkin, M., Lesser, M., Livote, E. et al. 2009. Chemoprevention of colorectal neoplasia by estrogen: potential role of vitamin D activity. *Cancer Prev. Res. (Phila. PA)* **2**:43–51.

44. Protiva, P., Hopkins, M.E., Manson, J.B., Liu, Z.H., Nelson, C., Marshall, J.R., Lipkin, M., and Holt, P.R. 2007. Effect of folate supplementation on gene expression in human recto-sigmoid mucosa. *Gastroenterology* **132**:A440 (Abstr.).

45. Slattery, M.L., Potter, J.D., Samowitz, W., Schaffer, D., and Leppert, M. 1999. Methylenetetrahydrofolate reductase, diet, and risk of colon cancer. *Cancer Epidemiol. Biomarkers Prev.* **8**:513–518.

46. Larsson, S.C., Giovannucci, E., and Wolk, A. 2006. Folate intake, MTHFR polymorphisms, and risk of esophageal, gastric, and pancreatic cancer: a meta-analysis. *Gastroenterology* **131**:1271–1283.

47. Giovannucci, E., Stampfer, M.J., Colditz, G.A., Rimm, E.B., Trichopoulos, D., Rosner, B.A., Speizer, F.E., and Willett, W.C. 1993. Folate, methionine, and alcohol intake and risk of colorectal adenoma. *J. Natl. Cancer Inst.* **85**:875–884.

48. Giovannucci, E., Stampfer, M.J., Colditz, G.A., Hunter, D.J., Fuchs, C., Rosner, B.A., Speizer, F.E., and Willett, W.C. 1998. Multivitamin use, folate, and colon cancer in women in the Nurses' Health Study. *Ann. Intern. Med.* **129**:517–524.

49. Zhang, S.M., Moore, S.C., Lin, J., Cook, N.R., Manson, J.E., Lee, I.M., and Buring, J.E. 2006. Folate, vitamin B_6, multivitamin supplements, and colorectal cancer risk in women. *Am. J. Epidemiol.* **163**:108–115.

50. Weinstein, S.J., Albanes, D., Selhub, J., Graubard, B., Lim, U., Taylor, P.R., Virtamo, J., and Stolzenberg-Solomon, R. 2008. One-carbon metabolism biomarkers and risk of colon and rectal cancers. *Cancer Epidemiol. Biomarkers Prev.* **17**:3233–3240.

51. Giovannucci, E., Rimm, E.B., Ascherio, A., Stampfer, M.J., Colditz, G.A., and Willett, W.C. 1995. Alcohol, low-methionine—low-folate diets, and risk of colon cancer in men. *J. Natl. Cancer Inst.* **87**:265–273.

52. Cole, B.F., Baron, J.A., Sandler, R.S., Haile, R.W., Ahnen, D.J., Bresalier, R.S., Keown-Eyssen, G., Summers, R.W., Rothstein, R.I., Burke, C.A. et al. 2007. Folic acid for the prevention of colorectal adenomas: a randomized clinical trial. *JAMA* **297**:2351–2359.

53. Jaszewski, R., Misra, S., Tobi, M., Ullah, N., Naumoff, J.A., Kucuk, O., Levi, E., Axelrod, B.N., Patel, B.B., and Majumdar, A.P. 2008. Folic acid supplementation inhibits recurrence of colorectal adenomas: a randomized chemoprevention trial. *World J. Gastroenterol.* **14**:4492–4498.
54. Clark,L.C. 1985. The epidemiology of selenium and cancer. *Fed. Proc.* **44**:2584–2589.
55. Combs, G.F., Jr. 2005. Current evidence and research needs to support a health claim for selenium and cancer prevention. *J. Nutr.* **135**:343–347.
56. Bleys, J., Navas-Acien, A., and Guallar, E. 2008. Serum selenium levels and all-cause, cancer, and cardiovascular mortality among U.S. adults. *Arch. Intern. Med.* **168**:404–410.
57. Clark, L.C., Combs, G.F., Jr., Turnbull, B.W., Slate, E.H., Chalker, D.K., Chow, J., Davis, L.S., Glover, R.A., Graham, G.F., Gross, E.G. et al. 1996. Effects of selenium supplementation for cancer prevention in patients with carcinoma of the skin. A randomized controlled trial. Nutritional Prevention of Cancer Study Group. *JAMA* **276**:1957–1963.
58. Reid, M.E., Duffield-Lillico, A.J., Sunga, A ., Fakih, M., Alberts, D.S., and Marshall, J.R. 2006. Selenium supplementation and colorectal adenomas: an analysis of the nutritional prevention of cancer trial. *Int. J. Cancer* **118**:1777–1781.
59. Lin, J., Cook, N.R., Albert, C., Zaharris, E., Gaziano, J.M., Van, D.M., Buring, J.E., and Manson, J.E. 2009. Vitamins C and E and beta carotene supplementation and cancer risk: a randomized controlled trial. *J. Natl. Cancer Inst.* **101**:14–23.

Index

13C-labeled breath test, 84
14C-glycocholic acid breath test, 199
14C-xylose breath test, 199
24-hour recall, 22
5-HT$_3$ receptor antagonists, 77

A

Abdominal bloating
  in celiac disease, 99
  in delayed gastric emptying, 83
  response to probiotics in IBS, 117
Abdominal distension
  in malabsorption, 194
  response to probiotics in IBS, 117
Abdominal pain
  in Crohn's disease, 127
  in delayed gastric emptying, 83
Abetalipoproteinemia, 302
Absorption, physiology, 192–193
Achalasia, 43, 45
  therapy, 50
Acid neutralization, Sippy Diet for, 2
Acid suppression, for GERD, 49
Acute cellular rejection, 244
Acute hepatitis, nutrition therapy in, 280
Acute liver failure (ALF)
  carbohydrate metabolism in, 276
  effect on nutritional state, 274
  energy expenditure in, 275
  fat metabolism in, 277
  nutrition therapy in, 280–281
Acute nausea and vomiting, 74
Acute pancreatitis
  achieving nutrient recommendations with
    TPN, 260
  APACHE II criteria, 255
  artificial nutrition in, 256–260
  Atlanta classification for severity, 255
  Balthazar score, 255
  blood glucose control in, 256
  c-reactive protein (CRP) monitoring in, 255
  carbohydrate metabolism in, 256
  choice of optimal formula, 263–265
  choosing PN or EN in, 258–260
  clinical approach for nutritional support in,
    260–265
  clinical patterns, 253
  continuous jejunal feeding in, 260
  energy requirements in, 260
  enteral feeding for, 160

  exocrine macronutrient stimulation in,
    257–258
  fasting in, 256
  hyperlipidemia in, 257
  improved outcomes with enteral or TPN, 256
  indications for parenteral nutrition, 260
  lipid metabolism in, 257
  mild to moderate, 261
  negative nitrogen balance in, 257
  nutrition in, 253–254
  nutritional status in, 254–255
  oral refeeding in, 264–265
  outcome predictors, 254–256
  probiotics benefits in, 263
  protein metabolism in, 257
  route of feeding in, 262–263
  severe, 254, 262–265
  severity assessment, 255–256
  substrate metabolism during, 256–257
  systemic inflammatory response syndrome
    (SIRS) in, 254
  urinary trypsinogen activation peptide (TAP)
    monitoring in, 255
Acute phase proteins, 27
Adaptation. *See* Small intestine
Adaptive immune response, in celiac disease, 97
Adipokines
  links to cancer, 344
  role in NAFLD, 307
Adiponectin, 307, 344
  inhibition of angiogenesis by, 344
Adipose tissue
  action of insulin on, 305
  metabolic activity in, 307, 344
  TPN considerations, 209
Adjustable gastric banding, 330–332
Adjusted body weight, 317, 318
  TPN considerations, 208
Adolescents, bariatric surgery for, 329
Adrenal insufficiency, 80
Adverse effects
  of antiemetic/prokinetic agents, 77, 85
  of insulin sensitizing agents, 310
  of orlistat, 322
  of sibutramine, 321
  with protein hydrolysates, 9
Aeroallergen-specific IgE, 67
Albumin levels, 26, 27, 28
  in cirrhosis, 278
  TPN considerations, 206
Alcohol consumption, and folate availability, 358

365